Intensive
Care

Intensive Care

How Congress Shapes Health Policy

THOMAS E. MANN
NORMAN J. ORNSTEIN
Editors

American Enterprise Institute
and
The Brookings Institution
Washington, D.C.

Library of Congress Cataloging-in-Publication Data:
Intensive care : how Congress shapes health policy / Thomas E.
Mann and Norman J. Ornstein, editors.
 p. cm.
 Includes bibliographical references and index.
 ISBN 0-8157-5464-7. — ISBN 0-8157-5463-9 (pbk.)
 1. Medical policy—United States. 2. United States. Congress.
3. Health care reform—United States. I. Mann, Thomas E.
II. Ornstein, Norman J.
RA395.A3I494 1995
362.1'0973—dc20

95-4436
CIP

9 8 7 6 5 4 3 2 1

The paper used in this publication meets the minimum
requirements of the American National Standard for
Information Sciences—Permanence of Paper for Printed Library
Materials, ANSI Z39.48-1984

Typeset in Palatino

Composition by AlphaTechnologies/mps, Inc.
Charlotte Hall, Maryland

Printed by R. R. Donnelly and Sons Co.
Harrisonburg, Virginia

Preface

THIS BOOK is the final product of the Renewing Congress Project, a joint effort of the American Enterprise Institute and the Brookings Institution designed to give an independent assessment of Congress and to offer recommendations for improving its effectiveness and restoring its legitimacy within the American political system.

The Renewing Congress Project has over the past three years issued three reports and an edited volume to provide members of the House and Senate and outside observers with a perspective on congressional reform. The first report, issued shortly after the 1992 elections, focused on the House of Representatives and emphasized the need to strengthen the ability of its leaders to set an agenda and act on it, increase the quality of deliberation and debate, improve relations between the parties, reform the campaign finance system, and clean up the House's internal support system.

In June 1993 the second report addressed the full agenda of the Joint Committee on the Organization of Congress, including ethics, committees, the budget process, floor deliberation, and staffing in both chambers, as well as relationships between Congress and the other branches. This report laid out a model for how Congress should operate and provided detailed recommendations for institutional renewal. A number of the project's specific recommendations were incorporated into the Joint Committee's final report.

The Renewing Congress Project issued a third report in February 1994 in response to the Joint Committee's recommendations. This report identified strengths and weaknesses in the Joint Committee's work and suggested how it could be improved and promoted by party leaders.

Congress, the Press, and the Public, published in September 1994, explored the relationship between news media portrayal of Congress and public animosity toward it. The book was based on a conference held in May 1993 that brought together some fifty journalists, congressional specialists, and media and public opinion scholars to discuss attitudes toward Congress. The discussion explored the historical relationship between the press and Congress, the roots of current opinions and press coverage, and strategies for improving the image and public understanding of Congress.

This book expands on the project's earlier work by closely examining the policymaking process in Congress in an issue area that has been a central point of discussion and debate in recent years. The book explores how Congress has organized and equipped itself to make health policy and then examines in detail two recent episodes in health policymaking—the 1988–89 adoption and repeal of medicare catastrophic coverage and the 1993–94 failure to pass national health reform.

Many people have contributed to this book, and to the other activities and products of the Renewing Congress Project, by participating in roundtable discussions and conferences, conducting research, writing memoranda and commissioned papers, and providing critiques of draft documents. We are especially grateful to the many members of Congress and their staffs who spent hours with us discussing their concerns about the institution.

Carey Macdonald and Amy Schenkenberg provided valuable research assistance on this volume. Judy Chaney and Inge Lockwood helped prepare the manuscript for publication. Steph Selice edited the manuscript, Laurel Imig verified it, Karen McClure proofread the pages, and Julia Petrakis compiled the index. We are grateful to all of them.

Financial support for the Renewing Congress Project is provided by a number of private foundations, including the Robert Wood Johnson Foundation, which is the prime sponsor of this book; the Carnegie Corporation of New York; the John D. and Catherine T. MacArthur Foundation; the Ford Foundation; the Henry Luce Foundation, Inc.; and the John D. Olin Foundation, Inc.

Interpretations and conclusions presented here are solely ours and those of the authors and should not be ascribed to the persons whose assistance we have acknowledged, to any group that funded the research reported here, or to the trustees, officers, or other staff members of the American Enterprise Institute or the Brookings Institution.

Thomas E. Mann
Director of Governmental Studies
The Brookings Institution

Norman J. Ornstein
Resident Scholar
American Enterprise Institute

Washington, D.C.
July 1995

Contents

Chapter 1

Introduction

Thomas E. Mann and Norman J. Ornstein

THIS BOOK HAD its origin not in President Clinton's comprehensive health care reform proposal but rather in efforts
to reform Congress as an institution. The Renewing Congress Project, a
joint undertaking of the American Enterprise Institute and the Brookings Institution, was launched in 1992 to assist a fledgling initiative
within Congress to respond constructively to the broad public critique
of the institution and its members. The Project issued a series of reports
designed to shift the focus of reform from punishing Congress to
strengthening it. Proposals for changing organizational structures and
processes were evaluated in terms of a broader conception of the appropriate place of Congress in the American political system.[1] The reports
were devoted largely to a general diagnosis of the institutional mala-
dies of the contemporary Congress. We therefore decided it would be
instructive to supplement the analysis by looking more closely at one
important policy arena, to see what could be learned about how process
shapes policy and how that process might be improved in turn.

Health care policy was an obvious choice. The United States is
unique among modern industrial democracies in both the high percentage of its national product devoted to health care and the absence of
universal health insurance coverage. Analysts have long debated the
roots of this American exceptionalism, but most attach major importance to the political institutions through which policy is made. The fact
that the United States would take another run at national health insurance in the 103rd Congress encouraged us to make health policy the
focus of our case study, but other considerations also weighed in its
favor.

For the purposes of our project, health care had the advantage of
posing institutional problems for Congress in the course of routine
policymaking. Its jurisdiction is spread over numerous committees and

subcommittees in the House and Senate. Its fate in Congress, on policy changes large and small, is closely linked to the twists and turns of the complex budget process. Its highly technical nature raises questions of whether and how Congress can equip itself with the critical information needed to make sensible decisions. Finally, the dizzying array of intergovernmental and contractual arrangements for health care policy implementation confronts Congress with the major challenge of overseeing a vast administrative apparatus.

Understanding how Congress shapes health care policy—on matters ranging from ambitious plans to achieve universal health insurance coverage to annual appropriations for public health agencies—should shed light on the strengths and weaknesses of Congress and on how it might be improved. It might also make a modest contribution to the growing body of scholarship on how institutional arrangements affect governmental performance.

Congressional Structures and Processes

Part one of this book examines how Congress has organized and equipped itself to make health care policy.

Jurisdiction

In chapter 2 Lawrence Evans explores the nature and consequences of the congressional division of labor on health issues—how jurisdiction is distributed across committees in the House and Senate, and how that jurisdictional fragmentation affects policymaking. One of the most widespread criticisms of the contemporary Congress is that competition among committees sharing jurisdiction over major issue areas (such as energy, environment, and health) prevents the development of coherent policy, expands opportunities for delay, undermines legislative accountability, and promotes parochialism. Evans argues that jurisdictional ambiguity "is unavoidable in any system of committee boundaries because major issues are often complex and inseparable from other policy concerns, and because issues tend to change shape over time." The question is not whether members of Congress and affected interests will fight over turf; it is instead how those battles affect policy outcomes and the policymaking process.

In the case of health care, the scope of the underlying policy area virtually guarantees that almost every committee will have a legitimate claim to some piece of the action. The Ways and Means and Commerce Committees hold the lion's share of health jurisdiction (medicare, medicaid, the U.S. Public Health Service) in the House, but other committees have jurisdiction over the Employee Retirement Security Act (ERISA), medical malpractice, rural health and nutrition, and the major federally managed health care systems. Much health legislation (40 percent in a recent Congress) is referred to more than one committee. Health jurisdiction is somewhat less fragmented in the Senate, where two committees—Finance and Labor and Human Resources—dominate and multiple referrals are a rarity.

Evans argues that the impact of health committee jurisdiction is contingent on the nature of the specific issue under consideration. On highly visible and controversial matters, power tends to shift from committees upward to leaders and outward to the full chamber, thereby reducing the role of committees and the impact of jurisdiction on policymaking. On less salient, more constituency-oriented issues, the key decisions are likely to be made in committee, making jurisdiction critically important to policymaking.

There were jurisdictional disputes in the 1993–94 national health care reform battle—turf fights broke out in both the House and Senate among competing committees and their leaders—but they were more irritant than obstacle to comprehensive reform. As Evans points out, having five separate committees working simultaneously on health care reform in the two chambers may well have kept the reform process from coming to an end in the spring of 1994, when building majorities for any ambitious proposal posed severe problems. On the other hand, a temporary ad hoc panel might well have made the political infeasibility of comprehensive reform apparent and expedited the crafting of a compromise measure. In any case, it would be a mistake to argue that jurisdictional fragmentation was a major factor in the failure of national health care reform.

Evans found jurisdiction more consequential on policies governing veterans' health benefits. Giving jurisdiction to the Veterans' Affairs Committees (narrowly based panels that serve largely as advocates of the veterans community) produces parochial policies and insulates health policymaking for veterans from broader debates on national health issues. Folding this jurisdiction into one of the major health committees would make good sense on process and policy grounds, but the political costs of doing so are high.

Evans concludes by noting that changes instituted by the new Republican majority in the 104th Congress to limit committee autonomy—including abolishing joint referrals and using temporary panels and other ad hoc mechanisms to expedite the flow of legislation—may well further limit the impact of committee boundaries on health policymaking.

Budgeting

If the importance of committee jurisdiction for health policymaking is limited, contingent, and diminishing, congressional budget procedures appear to play a major and sometimes dominant role. In chapter 3 Joseph White assesses the impact of budgeting on health policymaking by examining three distinct episodes: medicare and medicaid policymaking through budget reconciliation, appropriations for AIDS treatment and research, and national health care reform.

In an era of large deficits and the fiscalization of policy debate, the institutions within Congress for exercising its power of the purse affect the way health care policy is made. Largely in response to pressure to do something about the deficit, those institutions have been expanded in recent years to include budget resolutions, reconciliation, scorekeeping, discretionary spending caps, and "paygo" rules in addition to the normal authorizing and appropriations processes. White considers whether these institutions, and the larger politics of deficit reduction, encourage or discourage sensible health care policy.

In the case of health entitlements, budget processes and politics led both to the creation of a powerful regulatory cost control regime for medicare (including hospital prospective payment and physician fee schedules) and to an expansion of medicaid coverage to children and pregnant women. Crafted in the context of reconciliation legislation, these policy changes were made largely as part of an inside game, with little public attention and floor debate. The pressure to reduce the deficit, the dynamic of budget scorekeeping, and the need for substantial support from liberal Democrats to pass every deficit-reduction package created opportunities for policy initiatives not ordinarily associated with Republican administrations.

The federal government's response to the AIDS epidemic is largely a story of the appropriations process and therefore illustrative of the impact budget institutions have on health programs that are subject to annual appropriations. White chronicles the evolution of AIDS policy from the syndrome's initial appearance as a new and threatening disease (when it elicited broad support in Congress for increased funding of epidemiological studies, medical research, and modest prevention efforts) to its current status as a more established problem (with controversy over AIDS testing and public education, and competition from other public health threats in determining budget priorities). The case of AIDS policymaking through appropriations is typical of the more general dynamics of the appropriations process. This is especially true of its relatively nonpartisan and agency-oriented character and the power of Congress and the agencies vis-à-vis the president in setting priorities within an overall spending target.

White is less sanguine about the impact of budget procedures on national health reform. Although many factors contributed to the demise of health care reform in 1994, the congressional budget process was a major contributor. The imperative of deficit neutrality and the technical requirements and demands of Congressional Budget Office (CBO) scoring affected the design of the plan proposed by the Clinton administration, the terms of debate, and the schedule of drafting and legislative consideration of alternative plans. In forcing attention to costs, budget processes are inherently biased against the creation of new government commitments. But the stringent procedures of the new congressional budget process set a hurdle higher than any previous social policy initiative has ever had to surmount. Of course, that hurdle is there for a reason—it serves other values that Americans consider important, including fear of budget deficits.

Information

The critical role in national health care reform played by CBO underscores the increasing demands for information on the likely effects of alternative policy options. Congress enacted the original medicare and medicaid programs with little internal capacity or external resources to evaluate their costs and benefits. Thirty years later, an extraordinary array of public and private entities provides technically sophisticated health policy information. In chapter 4 Mark Peterson explores what kinds of information are needed to design and assess health policy initiatives and whether Congress actually uses that information in a manner that resembles rational policy deliberation.

Peterson argues that to draft and enact legislation acceptable to the public that has a reasonable chance of fulfilling its objectives (thereby minimizing their own political and programmatic uncertainty), members of Congress need three distinct types of information. These are ordinary knowledge, formed through everyday observation and interaction, which represents subjective, commonsense understanding of how the world works and how events can be explained; distributional knowledge, based on information about the impact of policy options on particular interests, the likely winners and losers, and the intensity of response expected from affected constituencies; and policy-analytic knowledge, which flows from systematic, unbiased inquiry into the objectives and effects of government programs. The supply of ordinary and distributional knowledge about national health reform available to members was abundant, based on a flood of anecdotal information supplied by constituents and lobbyists as well as an extraordinary outpouring of polling and focus group readings of public opinion and reports from interest groups. Congress was not in the dark about what the American public thought or how organized interests and geographical constituencies would be affected.

In addition, following the dramatic expansion of its in-house analytic capabilities during the 1970s—through the increase in professional staffs and the upgrading and creation of new support agencies—Congress had ample policy-analytic information available to challenge executive branch officials and to test the empirical claims of interest groups. Yet in the case of national health care reform, the use of that policy-analytic information was constrained by disagreement among experts (which produced an aura of dueling policy analysis reports) and the overriding importance of strongly held, largely ideological views of representatives and senators and gut reactions of ordinary citizens.

Peterson concludes by arguing that although policy analysis is often overwhelmed by a politics informed by ordinary and distributional knowledge, its availability in Congress serves as an important counter to unsubstantiated claims of interested parties, a critical basis for distinguishing fact from fiction. Recent moves by the new Republican majority to reduce Congress's own analytic capabilities—by slashing committee staffs and support agencies while sparing personal office staffs—is likely to enhance the power of politics over information.

Oversight

Two of the new support agencies created by Congress—the Prospective Payment Assessment Commission (ProPAC) and the Physician Payment Review Commission (PPRC)—have come to play a crucial role in congressional oversight of federal health programs and in the design of cost control measures for such programs. As Mark Nadel argues in chapter 5, oversight can no longer be accurately described as Congress's neglected function. In an era of large budget deficits and continuous fiscal constraints, opportunities for legislating new programs have all but vanished. Policymaking increasingly consists of shaping the administration and revision of existing programs, which heightens the importance of oversight to members of Congress. This is particularly true in the health policy arena, where large federal programs with automatic cost escalators absorb an ever-larger share of the federal budget.

Nadel reviews the techniques of oversight—informal staff and member contact with agency officials, hearings, and evaluations by congressional support agencies—as well as the targets of those activities. Oversight might be triggered in various ways: by a scheduled reauthorization of legislation, press reports of scandal or malfeasance, a funding crisis, or completion of a formal program evaluation. Members of Congress respond to different incentives in pursuing oversight: from the protection of broad constituencies (such as recipients of medicare, or women's groups concerned about gender differences in biomedical research), to the representation of more parochial concerns (such as formulas for allocating medicaid funds among the states), to the advancement of their own policy preferences.

This naturally leads to concerns that oversight is too reactive and unsystematic, with little coordination among committees sharing health care jurisdiction and no central strategy for comprehensive review of federal health programs. Nadel concludes this is less of a problem in practice than in theory. The sheer level of oversight activity and the continuous monitoring of programs by support agencies produces broad, high-quality surveillance by Congress, which in turn leads to changes in the underlying legislation. The use of oversight as a policymaking tool is likely to increase with a Republican Congress bent on reducing the size of government. The question, as Mark Peterson first asked it, is whether the retrenchment in committee staffs and support agencies diminishes the analytical basis for that oversight.

Health Policymaking

Part two of the book examines in detail two recent episodes in health policymaking—the 1988–89 adoption and repeal of medicare catastrophic coverage and the 1993–94 failure to pass national health reform.

Catastrophic Coverage

In chapter 6 journalist Julie Rovner, who covered both of the health policy cases examined here, recounts how an initially bipartisan and consensual effort to extend benefits to medicare recipients led to a humiliating reversal barely a year after the legislation was signed into law. The ignominious fate of the Medicare Catastrophic Coverage Act of 1988 foreshadowed and (more importantly) contributed to Congress's inability to enact national health reform a half-decade later.

Rovner describes the substantive and political forces that put catastrophic coverage on the agenda and moved it to passage. Rising out-of-pocket expenses as well as the burdens of prescription drugs and long-term care (neither covered by medicare) were threatening a growing number of elderly citizens. Those citizens constituted a powerful political bloc that was well-organized and voted at higher rates than their younger counterparts. Both parties saw political gain in addressing the concerns of older people. The Reagan administration was looking to mend fences with elderly Americans after its proposed cuts in social security; the Democrats, having just regained the majority in the Senate and having installed an ambitious new Speaker in the House, were eager to move forward with a health care agenda.

These forces created a window of opportunity for legislative action, but they rested on a fragile foundation of public support. First of all, the benefits of new federal catastrophic coverage were not apparent to many recipients. More than half of all medicare beneficiaries had medigap policies of one sort or another that provided supplementary coverage. Some enjoyed subsidized coverage from their former employers. Another 10 percent qualified for medicaid, which protected them from virtually all out-of-pocket medical costs. The latter two groups might understandably consider the new federal benefit an unnecessary duplication of coverage. Second, the oppressive budget deficit meant that the cost of the program expansion had to be paid by the beneficiaries. Because the premiums ("user fees") were pegged to family income, some middle- and upper-income senior citizens saw themselves as the losers. Third, most medicare recipients were unaware of how a serious illness could affect their finances. This lack of basic information about the existing law made the public all the more susceptible to scare tactics used by groups opposed to the legislation. The seeds of its repeal were evident by the time the bill was signed into law.

Rovner argues that the contemporary Congress—with its fragmented power and hypersensitivity to public preferences—is not well structured to deal with such complex, redistributive issues. Indeed, given the catastrophic experience of Congress in attempting to fix medicare in 1988–89, it is a wonder that policymakers approached national health care reform in 1993 with such ambition and optimism.

National Health Care Reform

Two chapters are devoted to the failed attempt during 1993 and 1994 to enact comprehensive health care reform. Chapter 7, another case study by Julie Rovner, provides a chronological account of this debate. The chronology runs from Harris Wofford's upset victory in the November 1991 special Senate election in Pennsylvania (which catapulted health reform onto the agenda of both major political parties) to the September 26, 1994, announcement by Senate Majority Leader George Mitchell officially pulling the plug on the effort, many weeks after any realistic chance of comprehensive reform had evaporated.

Rovner describes the forces operating in 1992 that led many observers to believe health care reform was inevitable. The extraordinarily high and rapidly rising costs of health care in the United States, coupled with the increasing number of uninsured Americans, led many diverse interests to the negotiating table. Large companies were desperate to curb the spiraling cost of health insurance for their employees. Organized labor saw how escalating health care costs were leading to lower wages and higher cost-sharing for workers. Doctors found their autonomy increasingly threatened by managed care. Hospitals faced budgets strained by the growing costs of uncompensated care and the resistance paying customers felt toward the inevitable cost shifting. Insurance companies saw the need for more settled market conditions. State offi-cials were anxious to cope with runaway medicaid spending, while federal policymakers grudgingly concluded that budget deficits could not be shrunk without curbing the increase in health care spending. Wofford's election and the subsequent positioning by presidential can-didates leading up to the November 1992 election persuaded members of Congress that a broader public constituency for comprehensive health care reform did indeed exist.

Rovner then retraces the steps taken in the great health reform battle of 1993–94. She begins with the development of a comprehensive plan within the Clinton administration to its public unveiling in a presiden-tial address to a joint session of Congress. Rovner describes the delayed submission of the 1,342-page bill to Congress, the strategies and tactics of supporters and opponents of reform, the shifting pattern of public support for the Clinton plan, the struggles within five committees in the House and Senate and subsequently by majority leaders in both cham-bers to fashion a plan that could attract majority support on the floor, the first-ever floor debate in the Senate, and the ultimately futile search for an acceptable middle ground by a bipartisan group of senators. Finally, she concludes with the concession by congressional leaders that no action on health care reform was possible in the 103d Congress.

Why did reform that at the outset seemed inevitable fail so com-pletely? Rovner argues that the contemporary Congress is poorly posi-tioned to deal effectively with large divisive issues, ones that entail substantial costs as well as benefits and create both losers and winners. The absence of an informed and durable base of public support left Congress even more riven by partisanship and hypersensitive to the arguments of those interests opposing major elements of comprehen-sive reform. The imperatives of the budget process ultimately forced reform advocates to be so explicit about costs and mechanisms that there was no avoiding the redistributional character and complexity of their plans.

In the concluding chapter of this book, Allen Schick examines what the saga of health care reform can teach about Congress. His conclusion is crystal clear: President Clinton's failure confirms rather than upsets the conventional wisdom of how external forces (the president, public opinion, and interest groups) and internal conditions (committees, po-litical parties, leaders, and rules and procedures) shape what Congress does. Once those external forces and internal conditions are taken into account, the failure of health care reform could have been expected and is not surprising or anomalous.

President Clinton put health care reform on the agenda, focused the attention of the nation and Congress on the issue, and set the terms by which congressional action would be measured. But setting the agenda is a far cry from dictating the legislative outcome; presidents are much more successful at the former than the latter. In fact, by threatening to veto any package that fell short of providing universal coverage, the president limited the ability of congressional Democrats to devise passable legislation.

Congress's failure to formulate an acceptable alternative also resulted from its difficulty reading and satisfying public opinion. Most Americans nominally supported universal coverage but not any explicit means for achieving it. In the end what proved decisive was the overall satisfaction the 85 percent of Americans with insurance coverage felt regarding their health care and what they feared might be entailed (in higher costs, lower benefits, reduced quality, or intrusive government) in extending coverage to the rest of the citizenry. Opponents of comprehensive reform skillfully and often unfairly portrayed the Clinton plan in ways that reinforced anxieties that predated their efforts.

If contradictions in public opinion impeded reform, Schick argues, so too did divisions among and within interest groups with a major stake in the issue. Health care reform fell victim to hyperpluralism—the fracturing of interests into smaller and more specialized groups. The redistributive character of the legislation created winners and losers within each sector, and the ad hoc coalitions assembled to bridge these divides proved too fragile to cement a majority. Efforts to build broad-based coalitions in support of comprehensive reform were undermined by skillful reverse lobbying by congressional opponents of the president's plan. The Clinton administration's attempts to buy group support produced unstable or ineffective results. Negotiations to mollify the small business community through generous subsidies were a spectacular failure, as opponents worked to mobilize opposition at the grass-roots level.

These external forces (powerful groups mobilized in opposition, a confused and wary public, and a presidential demand for legislation that could not pass) may well have been sufficient to doom health care reform, but Congress also contributed to that failure. The ordinary legislative process was not up to the challenge of moving such an extraordinary legislative initiative. The routine referral of health care legislation to the committees of jurisdiction, the early formation and reinforcement of sharp party differences, and the presumption of regular order on the floor of the House and Senate posed obstacles that congressional leaders could not overcome through ad hoc efforts to build majorities at the end of the process.

Schick draws several lessons about Congress and the policy process from his analysis of how a bill failed to become a law. A weak president who makes strong demands on Congress will likely end up with nothing to show for it. Incremental demands are more likely to pass than are comprehensive demands. Assembling a majority behind ambitious, controversial legislation requires extraordinary measures by congressional leaders, including early intervention and strong central guidance. But once committees are entrusted with the arduous task of formulating legislation, their mandate should be to produce *passable* legislation, not simply to secure the minimum winning coalition to get the measure out of committee. The more unified party is the stronger party, and unity is more easily obtained in opposition. Finally, major policy change needs bipartisan support. Early on, the administration and the Democratic congressional leadership wrote off Republican support, either because it was unavailable or was deemed not worth the price. Yet the price of going it alone was the complete failure of reform.

Improving Congressional Performance

As the individual contributions to this book make clear, comprehensive health care reform faced daunting obstacles in 1993 and 1994. One need not have been a structural determinist to have put long odds on President Clinton's chances of succeeding. The nature of the issue makes health care finance an especially difficult policy challenge. Health care reaches deeply into the economy and society, touching every individual and enterprise. The American system is a mature one, characterized by extraordinary complexity and variability and not easily transformed by new policy choices. Health care reform is inherently redistributive, creating losers as well as winners in every sector of society with little relief possible from a deficit-starved public till. It also evokes primitive ideological responses from politicians, all the more so given the lack of agreement among the experts on the desirability and likely consequences of alternative policy actions. Moreover, the immediate political context was far from favorable. The president operated on a narrow and fragile electoral base during a political time when forces championing more limited government are in the ascendancy. In addition, the public had little confidence that government officials could deliver on their promises, Democratic majorities in both houses of Congress belied the absence of an ideological majority sympathetic to the president's initiative, and the health care "crisis" lost some urgency as the economic recovery proceeded apace.

And yet it is also clear from this book that governmental structure does matter, in a myriad of ways. At the most general level, our Madisonian system of separated institutions routinely frustrates major policy change in the absence of crisis or widespread agreement. From the narrower vantage point presented here, the way Congress organizes itself and conducts its business determines in part which areas of policy or potential policy it considers; when it considers them; what information it seeks and uses; what frameworks animate its analysis and shape its conclusions; what pressures are brought to bear on itself and other actors in the process; which means, from oversight to law-drafting to budget-making, it uses to work its will; and what constitutes the necessary majorities for legislation to find its way into public law.

Congressional structure, and the strategic and tactical choices made by the president and congressional leaders to deal with the constraints and opportunities of that structure, contributed to the failure of health reform, just as it had shaped other episodes of health policymaking in recent years. The question then arises: Are there lessons to be drawn from these interactions of congressional structure and health policymaking that suggest steps Congress can and should take to improve the quality of the health care policy process and its outcomes? We conclude with some reflections on the implications of this book's findings for congressional reformers.

Creating New Committee Jurisdictions

Jurisdiction over health care policy is fragmented in Congress; nearly every standing committee has some piece of the pie. Some congressional reformers have called for consolidating all health matters into one supercommittee. But to do so would inevitably mean doing violence to other jurisdictional matters, such as taxation, education, or labor. In reality, there is no practical way to pull all health jurisdictions together.

But that is not to say that such jurisdictions are all sacrosanct. Some jurisdictional reform makes great sense. For one, health care for veterans (now considered in both houses in their respective Veterans' Affairs Committees) should be considered primarily in the major health panels, Finance in the Senate and Commerce in the House. Veterans' health care is a major part of the national health care system, involving major health facilities and a large segment of the population. Over the next decade, the millions of World War II veterans, now individuals in their late 60s and older, will place large demands on the Veterans Administration (VA) system, altering in the process the demands placed on medicare, medicaid, and the rest of the health delivery process. Subsequently, the demand for such care will drop, probably precipitously. There are already questions about the continuation, expansion, and accessibility of VA hospitals, for example, that will become even more significant in the next several years. But to consider these questions only in the context of veterans, instead of in the broader context of health care programs and policy, is foolish.

Similarly, health research (which now is fragmented in several ways, including pieces in the Armed Services Committees, the House Science Committee, and the House and Senate Commerce Committees, along with the two Appropriations panels) should be consolidated as much as possible in House Commerce and Senate Labor and Human Resources. Some of the fragmentation has occurred for tactical reasons; for example, breast cancer research was put in the Department of Defense because that was where the money was.

But that tactical ploy only underscores the problem. Health research priorities should be set in the context of overall health needs and health policy priorities, not separately and independently because of group pressures or the priorities of individual members. To be sure, structural change alone will not solve a set of problems that are much more deep-seated and complex. Appropriations panel members with their own research priorities will always clash with members of substantive health panels, who have their own concerns. The demands and skills of interest groups—from the American Cancer Society to ACT-UP—will influence decisions regardless of where the jurisdictions lie. Floor decisions may overrule those of committees and subcommittees. But it would still make a difference if basic and applied research in health is considered together with other health issues as much as possible—not with broader R&D, defense, or other issues.

There may be other small pieces of jurisdiction that can also be consolidated in the major health committees. For example, the House some years ago moved medicaid from the Ways and Means Committee to the Energy and Commerce Committee, arguing that unlike medicare (which was in Ways and Means because of its tax base in the social security system), medicaid was not primarily a revenue-related issue. In the Senate, medicare and medicaid remain together under the Finance Committee's jurisdiction. Making the jurisdictions in the two bodies parallel, probably by moving medicaid to the Senate Labor and Human Resources Committee, would be wise.

But the larger issue of pulling health jurisdictions comprehensively into health supercommittees has another answer, one addressed by Lawrence Evans in chapter 2. The best way to deal with the problem of making comprehensive policy when jurisdictions are not themselves combined comprehensively is to create ad hoc committees when the need arises.

The power granted the Speaker of the House to create an ad hoc panel on a large issue that normally is centered in more than one committee was created in the House in the 1970s. This power was first used by Speaker Thomas P. (Tip) O'Neill, Jr., in 1977 to expedite consideration of a comprehensive energy bill, a top priority of President Jimmy Carter in his first year in office. O'Neill's alternative was to refer the energy issue to five or more committees, jointly (all at once) or sequentially (one after the other). Each committee would consider its own piece of the issue and then merge them before considering the issue on the House floor—by any standard, a clumsy, fragmented, and slow process.

Instead, O'Neill appointed Rep. Thomas "Lud" Ashley (D.-Ohio) to chair an ad hoc panel, drawing members from a range of committees with a piece of energy-related jurisdiction (including Interior and Insular Affairs, Ways and Means, Agriculture, Commerce, and others) to consider the whole issue together and mark up a bill. The ad hoc panel worked—expediting consideration of the bill; pulling its pieces together; and creating a package designed to appeal to the House as a whole, not just the various interests overrepresented on the individual committees.

When Speaker Tom Foley confronted the same basic choices with President Clinton's high-priority comprehensive health policy issue, he chose instead to use a joint referral process. In this case he gave the entire health bill to three committees simultaneously—Energy and Commerce, Education and Labor, and Ways and Means. As Julie Rovner's chapter on the 1994 health policy debate makes clear, that strategy did not work. Three committees with vastly different outlooks and problems were unable to produce a combined bill. With no deadlines, all the deliberations were delayed beyond the point where any momentum could be built up or legislative action completed in a timely way. One committee, Commerce, deadlocked internally; two bills did emerge, but neither the Ways and Means product nor that of Education and Labor had a chance of finding broader acceptance in the full House chamber. Leadership problems on Ways and Means and a lack of representativeness on Education and Labor exacerbated the overall problem.

In retrospect, an ad hoc committee would have enabled the Speaker of the House to craft a membership that was itself representative of the chamber as a whole, consider the broader context of comprehensive health policy, expedite the process to political advantage, and move a bill (albeit a less ambitious one) that might well have passed. As Allen Schick argues in chapter 8, this extraordinarily complex and controversial legislative initiative called for extraordinary procedures and direction from the congressional leadership. The new Republican leadership in the House, reflecting the freshness of their majority, appears much more inclined to use ad hoc procedures and other means of central steering on major party issues. An ad hoc committee approach might well make sense as Congress grapples with the federal component of health care policy under pressure to balance the federal budget. Pulling together a broader array of members of Congress to consider medicare, medicaid, and health issues for veterans, thus enabling them to consider the interrelationships among these three big policy areas and their relationship to the rest of the health delivery system, is an attractive alternative to working within the existing committee framework.

Examining the Budget Process

An overriding reality of policymaking in Washington today is that it is budget driven. Money, of course, has always mattered; but its impact was vastly different when budgeting was incremental as opposed to decremental, and before the massive array of budget rules permeated substantive policymaking. For the past decade and even longer, deficit pressures have crowded out much of the substantive agenda. Many health care policy issues end up on the agenda less because the policies per se need action or review than because the budget forces them to be put there. More and more, strategic decisions about how to frame policy or bring issues to the floor revolve around budget rules and exigencies.

When the Clinton health care initiative was first proposed, Senate Majority Leader George Mitchell openly floated the possibility of expediting action on it in 1993. He considered doing this by tying the plan together with the budget into one giant reconciliation bill late in the year, which would also preclude any filibuster on it. Throughout the process—from the formulation of legislative language in the White House to the development and consideration of every alternative—the CBO economic assumptions, cost projections, and scoring conventions became crucial both to the timing of the proposals and their chances of success. CBO Director Robert Reischauer inadvertently became one of the most significant players in health care policy, simply by virtue of his budget-related position.

In 1995 and 1996, the budget-driven nature of contemporary politics promises to be even more significant, despite (or perhaps because of) the low priority of comprehensive health care reform. The early focus in the 104th Congress shifted to the Contract with America, including the proposed constitutional amendment to balance the budget and the subsequent promise made by congressional Republicans to devise a spending and taxing plan that would reduce the deficit to zero over seven years.

That promise meant a necessary focus on medicare and medicaid as two of the largest areas of government spending (and two of the fastest growing over the coming decade). Budget resolutions approved by the House and Senate called for a major slowdown in the projected rate of increased spending in both programs. The substantive merits of medicare and medicaid policies were open to debate; but the key point is that the driving force behind the proposals was money, not substance.

Budget concerns are certainly legitimate—indeed necessary—reasons for changing policy. However, there are major dangers when budget policy drives substantive legislation. First, time pressures and timetables may end up out of synch (or worse) when considering substantive needs. The need to find money *now* for budget cuts; the need to conform with the timetables built into the 1974 Budget Act; the need to comply with the Byrd Amendment in the Senate and the temptation to consider health care policy under reconciliation to maximize political leverage—all may work against the kind of careful, deliberative process that would make for the best medicare or medicaid policy. In addition, these needs may force each policy area to be considered individually when sensible policymaking would suggest they be considered together.

At the same time, although budgeting is now done on a five- or even seven-year cycle, it is intrinsically short-term. The need is to meet an immediate target, in the next year, and worry about the long term later. Saving money in the short term—or finding ways to declare short-term savings—can create policies that are counterproductive and even disastrous over the long term.

There is another problem with policymaking via the budget process. The reconciliation part is such that sweeping policy decisions are made in a huge omnibus package. Orders are given to authorizing committees to alter laws—often without the kind of hearing and markup process that commonly accompanies major change, and often drafted by Budget Committee members and staffers, not the members and staff of the authorizing committees.

There is no way to divorce budget processes from substantive policies, and no desirable reason to do so. Health care policy decisions should not be considered outside a budget framework; whenever they have been, more long-term problems have been created than solved. Neither, however, should such decisions be driven largely (much less exclusively) by budget timetables and deficit concerns. Better ways need to be found to ensure that members and committees specializing in health care policy have a substantial say and work with reasonable timetables.

One reform strategy is to aim at altering the reconciliation process to give committees such as Ways and Means, Commerce, and Finance more leeway and more time to craft appropriate substantive policies to fit under prescribed budget limits. Leaving an opening for ad hoc committees to do the job, while still setting deadlines firm enough to prevent the authorizing panels from delaying change to protect the status quo, is another possible strategy.

Clarifying Oversight

As Mark Nadel makes clear in chapter 5, oversight is one of the major avenues for Congress to shape health policy. Oversight enables Congress to track the work of agencies such as the Health Care Financing Administration (HCFA) or the Department of Veterans Affairs, to nudge policy execution into matching congressional intent, to use the feedback from the oversight process to change existing law or policy. But oversight can be a haphazard process—generally done not by mandate or requirement but by the whim of committee or subcommittee chairs, or driven by the reauthorization of a program or because of allegations of wrongdoing.

Congress has tried before to use structural reform to spur more oversight, including proposals that would require all standing committees to have oversight subcommittees. Many committees do have such subcommittees; however, that alone does not mean that systematic oversight of substantive programs is guaranteed. Often, the oversight subcommittees (frequently named Oversight and Investigations) focus more on allegations of scandal than on the less politically appealing examination of program execution. Little in the experience of past reform efforts would give encouragement to the idea that reform can create an incentive for more regular and systematic oversight that otherwise does not exist.

In general, the best oversight is done by the subcommittees of the two appropriations committees, which must make appropriations decisions annually and thus see oversight as a vital part of their responsibility. Much additional oversight comes when programs are reauthorized— but not all programs, or even most of them, are subject to annual or even frequent reauthorization.

The problem in the health care arena is that much of the federal role in health policy is in programs not subject to annual appropriations or regular reauthorization. Medicare, of course, is the best example. Overseeing HCFA is an indirect and inadequate way of dealing systematically with programs like medicare or medicaid. One idea is to subject medicare to regular reauthorizations (perhaps every five years) to build in regular reflection on and examination of the program's implementation by the Ways and Means and Finance Committees.

In the current fiscal environment, the real danger is that systematic oversight of major health programs will be overwhelmed in the rush to meet deficit reduction targets. The challenge for Congress is to use the information gained from its regular oversight of medicare and medicaid (including the reports of its specialized health research units Pro-PAC and PPRC as well as GAO and other general support agencies) to fashion policy changes that have some reasonable chance of slowing the projected cost increases while maintaining adequate service for their beneficiaries. At the very least this means that Congress must retain an analytic capacity through its committee staffs and support agencies to assess how well current programs are being implemented and what the likely impact of various policy changes would be. If the new Republican majority is indeed determined to make additional cuts in the congressional bureaucracy, they would be well advised to train their sights on personal office staffs rather than committee staffs and support agencies.

Facilitating Deliberation

In our previous examinations of the intended role of Congress and the nature of congressional organization, we stressed the Framers' intention that the legislative process be a deliberative one. They believed it should be characterized by careful debate and discussion in the various forums of Congress, a process designed not to reflect immediate public passions or desires but to enlarge upon public views and preferences to achieve a public judgment. We have suggested that the deliberative function has atrophied in both houses of Congress.

That general discussion of deliberation and the need to enhance the deliberative process applies fully to congressional consideration of health care policy. Even where there was a heavy congressional focus and a lengthy, intense, and public process (as was true of the Medicare Catastrophic Coverage Act and the Clinton health policy plan), deliberation in the classic sense is not a central feature of the policymaking process, either in committees or on the House or Senate floors. Developments both outside Congress (the fractionating and mobilization of interests, the application of modern campaign tactics to the policy process, the growing ideological polarization among elites, and the rapidly changing mass media) and inside it (increasing permeability, hypersensitivity to public opinion, and partisanship) make it difficult for the institution to come to an informed, thoughtful, independent judgment on the pressing issues of the day.

The Republican capture of the House and Senate has ushered in a period of reform that offers some hope of improving the deliberative process. Moves in the House to consolidate committees, eliminate subcommittees, and reduce the number of committee and subcommittee assignments should help a bit in focusing the attention of representatives and avoiding scheduling conflicts. More can and should be done to further consolidate and realign committee jurisdictions and reduce committee assignments. With fewer assignments comes more ability to focus and more incentive to dig into programs and policies in detail—including more incentive for strong and substantive oversight.

The House also moved to rationalize scheduling to try to minimize conflicts between floor action and committee work. Early in the 104th Congress, the process did not work well, in part because of the grueling pace of the first hundred days. But far more rigor in adhering to the new rules is required if the process is to work. The House also barred proxy voting as a way to require representatives to show up to committee sessions—a salutary ban, but one that can work only if tighter restrictions on the numbers and sizes of panels (and especially of assignments) prevail.

Deliberation requires that committee work count and that committees do not simply go through the motions of producing legislative language that has been precooked by the party leadership or outside interests. Although the moves to centralize power in the House and the eagerness of the Republican leadership to set an agenda and act on it are laudable, committees must have the political space to fulfill their responsibility in the chamber's division of labor. A Congress that simply ratifies public preferences or group demands is abrogating its charge to "refine and enlarge the public view."

There is one other area where general reform in Congress would lead to a more deliberative process in health policymaking—floor debate. There has been little in both the House and Senate in recent years that merits the appellation "debate." Unconnected one-minute speeches intermixed with arcane discussion of parliamentary procedures and rules is far more common than the genuine, focused give-and-take the Framers assumed would be at the center of the deliberative environment.

In 1994, the House experimented with three Oxford-style debates in prime time, including one on health care. They were generally successful (albeit somewhat contentious and narrow) and, with four or five players on each side, somewhat confusing. But by the third debate—one on trade and human rights—the ground rules were stronger. Both the House and the Senate need to conduct regular, real debates on larger issues, not just specific bills, ideally with only one or two members on each side.

The dilemmas of health policy—providing adequate insurance coverage and care while restraining the growth of health care costs; balancing the responsibilities of individuals, companies, the states, and the federal government; providing adequate funding for research; and setting appropriate research priorities—will not be erased by changing how Congress does its business or looks at problems. But it is clear that the way Congress does its business does affect the way it looks at health care policy problems. Some changes can make a difference, and for the better.

Part One
Congressional Structures and Processes

Chapter 2

Committees and Health Jurisdictions in Congress

C. Lawrence Evans

THE STRUCTURE OF the committee system on Capitol Hill is a perennial target of criticism.[1] In 1993, for example, the House Republican members of the Joint Committee on the Organization of Congress sharply criticized Democrats on the committee for not supporting a substantial realignment of committee jurisdictions, particularly regarding health issues:

> The present structure of the committee system is the largest impediment to the effective functioning of the Congress. One need only consider the jurisdictional wrangling over referral of [President Clinton's] health care proposal to come to the conclusion that reform is required. . . . Our expectation is that, absent jurisdictional reform, the prospect for a coherent Federal policy in health care is problematic.[2]

Senator Barbara Mikulski (D.-Md.) provides more colorful observations about congressional committee structure: "If the Congress had invented the human body, we would not have a backbone. We would have this disk here and another one would be over there with the liver and somebody would get a waiver to have it with the kidney . . . we would be like one great big pseudopod amoeba just going through life."[3]

However, other participants and observers suggest that the impact of committee jurisdictions on congressional policymaking is often exaggerated—leadership and the degree of consensus on key issues are far more important in passing coherent federal policy. Rep. John Dingell, ranking Democrat on the House Commerce Committee, argues that "fights over jurisdiction . . . almost always reflect real policy differences. . . . Jurisdictional tension and competition between committees, if not carried to excess, can be healthy. . . . Most importantly, all the jurisdictional changes in the world will never substitute for strong leadership."[4]

Thus, although the system of committee jurisdictions on Capitol Hill is often criticized, the implications of jurisdictional boundaries for congressional policymaking are not clear-cut. My purpose in this chapter is to explore the nature and consequences of congressional committee jurisdictions as they relate to one major issue area—national health policy. How is jurisdiction over health issues distributed across the standing committees of the House and Senate? Does the substantial jurisdictional fragmentation seen in the health arena inevitably lead to fragmented, uncoordinated policymaking? How will jurisdictional politics change under the new Republican majority's aegis? And what steps might be taken to promote coherent policymaking in complex, overarching issue areas such as health policy?

My main argument is that the impact of jurisdiction on health policymaking in Congress varies by issue. On far-reaching, highly salient measures like comprehensive health care reform, jurisdiction is dispersed across five or more congressional committees. But when interest in a bill is broad-based and deep, congressional decisionmaking is also less committee-centered than on more routine measures, reducing the overall importance of committee boundaries in the legislative process. In contrast, on less visible, more consensual items, particularly when a single constituency is primarily affected, jurisdictional arrangements tend to have a more pervasive impact on congressional policymaking.

Importance of Jurisdiction

Although committees are still fundamental to policymaking in Congress, their importance and autonomy has declined somewhat in recent decades. No longer the insular legislative fiefdoms of the pre-1970s "textbook Congress," congressional committees now operate within a highly permeable environment in which legislators not on the panel of jurisdiction can participate in decisionmaking and potentially influence policy outcomes. Floor amendments to committee bills have increased over the past few decades. In the House, the multiple referral of legislation to more than one committee became common after a mid-1970s rule change, further undermining committee-based jurisdictional monopolies. In the Senate, the informal norms that once girded committee power have disintegrated, leading to rampant legislative individualism and a reluctance to systematically defer to committee recommendations. Party leaders in both chambers now also use a range of mechanisms, from ad hoc committees to informal party caucuses, to supplement or even bypass the various standing committees.[5]

In the House, the trend away from committee autonomy has been reinforced by the recent efforts of Republicans to further centralize power in the office of the Speaker of the House. Potentially the most powerful House leader in a generation, Newt Gingrich breached the seniority norm to place aggressive conservatives in key committee chairmanships.[6] The terms of committee chairs have been limited to six years, precluding the gradual accumulation of power by senior committee leaders.[7] In addition, the remarkable consensus about policy among House Republicans provides Gingrich with the political support necessary to exert strong partisan leadership. A key architect of the "Contract with America," Gingrich pledged to complete House action on the Contract within the first 100 days of 1995, which necessarily limited the duration and thoroughness of committee deliberation.[8] As of spring 1995, Senate Republicans were also considering proposals to strengthen their own leadership relative to the committee chairs, although the Senate has always been less committee-centered than the larger, more highly structured House of Representatives.

This long-term decline in committee autonomy, however, does not mean that congressional committees are no longer important arenas for policymaking, or that jurisdictional concerns no longer matter. Perhaps the best indicator of the continuing importance of turf is that members of the House and Senate care intensely about the jurisdictional prerogatives of the panels on which they serve. As former House Speaker Thomas Foley has observed, "Once one gets into the area of committee jurisdiction there is an enormous sense of proprietary concern on the part of those who are involved. . . . [Members] go to battle stations almost immediately."[9]

Consider the efforts by House Republicans to overhaul committee jurisdictions after winning control of the chamber. The morning after the 1994 election, Gingrich asked Rep. David Dreier to formulate options for realigning jurisdictions in the House. One of the proposals—

reportedly found in a wastebasket and leaked to the media—would have abolished five standing committees and fundamentally realigned the jurisdictions of most remaining panels.[10] Although supported by many Republican leaders, the proposal touched off a firestorm among incoming chairs of the affected panels. One Republican aide compared the jurisdictional squabbling to "a Middle Eastern bazaar."[11] Interest group lobbyists joined the fray, telephoning Gingrich in opposition to certain aspects of the jurisdictional shifts.[12] And in the end, Republican leaders backed away from comprehensive jurisdictional reform in favor of less sweeping changes.[13]

Members of Congress care about turf because the legislative role of a committee—and thus of its members—is rooted in the panel's jurisdiction and the issues it considers. In both chambers, committee jurisdictions derive from a combination of formal rules, unpublished precedent, and informal agreements between affected committees. The basic outlines of jurisdiction are described in chamber rules (Rule 10 in the House and Rule 25 in the Senate). First codified fifty years ago as part of the Legislative Reorganization Act of 1946, these formal committee jurisdictions are largely based on referral precedents from the late nineteenth and early twentieth centuries.[14] In the House, minor alterations in jurisdiction were made in 1974 and 1980, with more significant shifts occurring in January 1995. In the Senate, some significant jurisdictional changes were made in 1977. But the basic structure of formal committee boundaries still rests on the Legislative Reorganization Act of 1946, underscoring why current jurisdictional alignments draw so much criticism from legislators and congressional observers: The role of government and the nature of the issue agenda have changed dramatically since most of these jurisdictions were designed. Many key issues, such as national health policy, do not mesh cleanly with existing committee lines.

Although jurisdictional ambiguity is a source of concern, it probably is unavoidable in any system of committee boundaries because major issues are often complex and inseparable from other policy concerns, and because issues tend to change shape over time. Health policy, for example, is highly technical, touching on matters as diverse as child nutrition, medical malpractice, hazardous wastes, and alcoholism on Indian reservations. Even if it were possible to define precisely the outer boundaries of health issues, assigning all health-related items to a single committee would require that almost all domestic policy items be given to that panel, undermining the congressional division of labor. Jurisdictional ambiguity is also unavoidable because, over time, old issues change shape and new ones emerge. Space-based biomedical research, for example, does not fit cleanly into existing jurisdictions, in part because committee boundaries were set before these programs were developed. Unless jurisdictions are routinely updated—which would be difficult given the political stakes—many issues will not mesh well with existing formal boundaries. As a result, each chamber has developed a body of unpublished precedent to help determine jurisdiction over issues and bills when formal committee boundaries are vague or unclear.[15] Informal agreements about turf also have developed between committees leaders with overlapping jurisdictions.

In both the House and Senate, the majority party leadership is formally responsible for referring legislation to committee. However, in each chamber, the vast majority of referral decisions are made by the Parliamentarian's office, which generally employs technical criteria for assigning bills to committee. Still, on major issues important to the majority party's agenda, party leaders help settle jurisdictional questions. In 1993, for example, the House leadership played a key role in deciding which committees would receive portions of the Clinton health care reform package.

As with many procedural matters, bill referral practices differ by chamber. Most House bills are referred to a single panel, but legislation also can be multiply referred to two or more committees. When Democrats controlled the House, multiple referrals typically were joint referrals—that is, the affected panels would receive the entire bill (although usually agreeing informally to focus only on provisions within their jurisdictions). On certain bills, sequential referrals were employed, with a measure being sent first to a "primary" committee of jurisdiction for action, after which one or more additional panels would receive the legislation on a sequential basis.[16]

At the beginning of the 104th Congress, the majority Republicans abolished joint referrals, hoping to avoid the internecine turf fights that often erupted between competing chairmen during the years of Democratic control. Under the new rules, the Speaker of the House *must* designate a "primary" committee of jurisdiction when bills are multiply referred. Any additional panels receiving the bill operate subject to time constraints and can only consider items falling within their own jurisdictions. Thus, multiple referrals still occur because committee jurisdictions continue to overlap, but these multiple referrals are now more structured and less open-ended. During the Republican transition, Speaker Gingrich also suggested that, when jurisdiction over a bill is shared, the primary committee itself might be made responsible for delegating portions of the measure to other panels, but the likelihood of such cross-committee cooperation is unclear.[17]

In the Senate, the practice of multiple referral has been rare under both Republican and Democratic majorities. Instead, Senate referrals are almost always resolved in favor of the committee with "predominant jurisdiction." That is, when a bill touches on the jurisdiction of more than one panel, the committee with the more significant jurisdictional claim typically gets the entire measure. In 1992, for example, Senator Paul Wellstone introduced legislation that would have created a national health insurance program by amending the Public Health Service Act. The Wellstone program would have been financed by changes in the Internal Revenue Code, and would have abolished medicare, medicaid, the Armed Forces Health Care System (CHAMPUS), as well as certain veterans health care programs. Although the Senate Labor Committee has jurisdiction over the Public Health Service, the Armed Services Committee has jurisdiction over CHAMPUS, and veterans health care is within the domain of the Committee on Veterans' Affairs, the entire Wellstone bill was referred to the Finance Committee because Finance had the largest jurisdictional claim.[18]

House and Senate committees, of course, are not passive onlookers in the jurisdiction game, and they employ a range of tactics to protect or expand their turf. For instance, bill drafters can strategically frame legislative language to steer a bill toward a friendly panel.[19] When jurisdiction over a measure is unclear, the chairs of the affected panels often write letters to the majority leadership and/or parliamentarians arguing their case. Expansionist-oriented committees can request sequential referral of items in contested areas, hoping to build a pattern of referrals that might lead to more substantial jurisdictional prerogatives. Subject to certain constraints, expansionist panels can also attach provisions outside their jurisdictions to base bills within their domain. Former Commerce Chairman John Dingell—himself proficient at jurisdictional enhancement—has complained about other committee leaders using this tactic: "[W]hen a committee decides it wants to 'do' a particular issue, it starts designing bills to avoid the real committee of jurisdiction by drafting the subject matter into Acts in its own jurisdiction having no real relation to that subject matter. . . . Members should not be allowed to 'game' the system of jurisdiction and referrals by mere drafting."[20] In short, jurisdiction continues to matter on Capitol Hill because it helps determine who has the opportunity to legislate, thus influencing the strategic behavior of lawmakers, staff, lobbyists, and other participants in the legislative process.

Who Has Health?

Jurisdiction over health-related issues is dispersed across many different congressional committees because of the complexity and scope of the underlying policy area. Indeed, almost every committee has at least some jurisdiction that touches on health issues. Consider table 2-1, which summarizes the health jurisdiction of House authorizing committees. In the House, all authorizing jurisdictions except the Select Committee on Intelligence have a degree of jurisdiction over health issues. Most authorizing committees in the Senate also have some health-related jurisdiction. In addition to the various authorizing panels, the major nonauthorizing committees in both chambers deal with health matters. The appropriators, for example, allocate budget authority for a wide range of health care programs. The Budget Committees consider the broader, budgetary implications of federal health policy. And the House Rules Committee is responsible for structuring floor consideration of major health bills.

Still, certain committees clearly are more important than others in the health arena. The Clinton reform bill, for example, was primarily referred to three House panels by the Democratic leadership: Energy and Commerce (renamed in 1995 the Committee on Commerce) and Ways and Means, which both received the entire bill, and the Education and Labor Committee (renamed in 1995 the Committee on Economic and Educational Opportunities), which received most of the measure. Seven additional House panels were referred portions of the legislation, but their involvement was restricted and secondary. In the Senate, the Clinton proposal was not formally referred to a committee because of a jurisdictional dispute, but only the Finance Committee and Labor and Human Resources Committee had the jurisdiction necessary to mark up comprehensive reform bills.[21]

One way to evaluate the relative *importance* of committees in the health care arena is to look at the number of health-related measures

TABLE 2-1. *Health Care Components of House Authorizing Committee Jurisdictions*

Agriculture. Rural health care, food safety and nutrition.

Banking and Financial Services. Financial services as related to health care.

Commerce. Public health and quarantine, medicaid, medicare not financed by payroll deductions, applied biomedical research, insurance, and toxic substances.

Economic and Educational Opportunities. Medical training and professions, employee health and safety, health care for children and elderly people.

Government Reform and Oversight. Health care fraud and abuse, health care services and facilities in the District of Columbia, civil service health care programs, health statistics.

House Oversight. Health care for House members and employees.

International Relations. Foreign aid as relates to health care.

Judiciary. Pharmaceutical patents and trademarks, medical malpractice, antitrust as relates to health care industry, drug enforcement policy.

National Security. Health care for military personnel, military hospitals and health facilities.

Resources. American Indian and territorial health care.

Science. Basic research as relates to health care.

Transportation and Infrastructure. Construction of government health facilities, health standards in federal buildings, railroad employee health programs.

Small Business. Health care policy as relates to small businesses, health care firms as small businesses.

Veterans' Affairs. Veterans' health care, Veterans Administration hospitals and health facilities.

Ways and Means. Health care and facilities funded by earmarked revenues.

Sources: House Rules; *Congressional Yellow Book*; internal memoranda of the Joint Committee on the Organization of Congress (prepared by Paul Rundquist), 103rd Congress.

TABLE 2-2. *Health Bill Referrals to House Authorizing Committees*

Committee	Number	Percent
Agriculture	12	1.12
Banking and Financial Services	12	1.12
Commerce	429	39.94
Economic and Educational Opportunities	82	7.64
Government Reform and Oversight	45	4.19
House Oversight	9	0.84
International Relations	7	0.65
Judiciary	52	4.84
National Security	39	3.63
Resources	9	0.84
Rules	6	0.56
Science	4	0.37
Transportation and Infrastructure	6	0.56
Small Business	2	0.19
Veterans' Affairs	41	3.82
Ways and Means	319	29.70

Note: Although referral data are from the 102nd Congress (1991–92), committee names and jurisdictions reflect changes made in January 1995. Health referrals to since-abolished panels are included in totals for committees to which jurisdiction was transferred. Because of multiple referrals, total number of referrals exceeds total number of health bills.

Source: SCORPIO files, U.S. Library of Congress.

they receive. Tables 2-2 and 2-3 provide such information for all health-related legislation introduced in the House and Senate during the 102d Congress (1991–92), the two-year period immediately preceding the introduction and consideration of comprehensive health care reform. Drawing on bill abstracts and other information in the SCORPIO files compiled by the U.S. Library of Congress, I was able to identify all authorizing legislation with a substantial health care component introduced in the House and Senate during the 102d Congress, as well as where the legislation was referred.[22] In total, 648 health-related bills were referred to committee in the House; for the Senate, the number was 391.

Before examining the number of health measures going to individual committees, it is useful to consider the incidences of multiple referral in each chamber. In recent years, approximately 20 percent of all House bills have been multiply referred. For health legislation, however, the

TABLE 2-3. *Health Bill Referrals to Senate Authorizing Committees*

Committee	Number	Percent
Agriculture	9	2.28
Armed Services	14	3.55
Banking, Housing, and Urban Affairs	1	0.25
Budget	2	0.51
Commerce, Science, and Transportation	3	0.76
Energy and Natural Resources	1	0.25
Environment and Public Works	5	1.27
Finance	195	49.49
Foreign Relations	3	0.76
Governmental Affairs	10	2.54
Indian Affairs	6	1.52
Judiciary	5	1.27
Labor and Human Resources	107	27.16
Rules and Administration	2	0.51
Veterans' Affairs	31	7.87

Note: Referral data are from the 102nd Congress (1991–92). Because of multiple referrals, total number of referrals exceeds total number of health bills.
Source: SCORPIO files, U.S. Library of Congress.

proportion of multiple referrals is much higher—over 40 percent during the 102d Congress. The more comprehensive the health measure, the more likely it is to receive a multiple referral.[23] In the Senate, in contrast, the multiple referral of health bills is very rare—less than one percent during the 102d Congress. The relatively high proportion of multiple referrals for health bills in the House (and the low proportion in the Senate) matters because referring legislation to more than one panel expands the opportunities for legislative obstruction and makes the crafting of coherent policy more difficult.[24] However, the abolition of joint referrals by House Republicans should alleviate these problems somewhat.

Health Jurisdictions in the House

The number of health-related referrals received by individual House authorizing committees is summarized in table 2-2. Although the referral data used here precede the Republican takeover, committee names and jurisdictions have been updated to reflect the changes implemented in January 1995. The small number of health referrals to panels that were abolished at the beginning of the 104th Congress are included in the totals for the committees that received their jurisdictions.[25]

In both chambers, it is useful to distinguish between a first tier of lead health panels, with broad jurisdiction over health issues; a second tier of committees with significant but narrower jurisdiction; and other panels with more limited, tangential involvement in health care. From table 2-2, it is apparent that the Commerce Committee and Ways and Means Committee are the lead health panels in the House.[26] When Democrats organized the chamber, the Education and Labor Committee (now the Economic and Educational Opportunities Committee) also considered comprehensive health care initiatives, but (during the 102d Congress) it received less than 20 percent of the referrals going to Commerce and only about one-fourth of those going to Ways and Means. Of the remaining panels, Judiciary, Veterans' Affairs, National Security, and Government Reform and Oversight have the most health jurisdiction and together constitute the second tier of health committees. The involvement of remaining panels is circumscribed.

WAYS AND MEANS. The health domain of the Ways and Means Committee is rooted in its jurisdiction over the Social Security Act and the Internal Revenue Code. At one point, the Committee had jurisdiction over public health issues because of a since-repealed section of the Social Security Act, but the panel clearly emerged as a central arena for health care policy in the 1960s with the passage of medicare and medicaid. During the 1970s, the Ways and Means Committee drew the attention of House reformers (the Bolling Committee and its successor, the Hansen Committee) concerned about the panel's substantial institutional prerogatives and broad jurisdiction. As a result, in 1974 jurisdiction over the health care titles of the Social Security Act not directly financed by payroll deductions was shifted from Ways and Means to the Commerce Committee. Ways and Means remains a key actor in national health care policy, however, primarily because of its jurisdiction over the entire tax code and most of medicare.[27]

COMMERCE. The health care turf of the Commerce Committee originated during the nineteenth century from the panel's jurisdiction over inland water transportation and safety, and it has expanded through the years to include public health more generally.[28] This includes hundreds of programs within the Public Health Service dealing with issues such as mental health, disease control, family planning, hospital facilities, and applied biomedical research.

The health policy role of the Commerce Committee was significantly expanded by the 1970s Bolling/Hansen reforms, which transferred to the Committee jurisdiction over Title 5 (Maternal and Child Health) and Title 19 (medicaid) of the Social Security Act, as well as those aspects of Title 18 (part B of medicare) not funded by payroll deductions. The division of medicare jurisdiction between the Commerce Committee and Ways and Means Committee may seem arcane, but it illustrates well the subtleties of the bill referral process when committee jurisdictions overlap, as well as the problems inherent in piecemeal jurisdictional reform.[29]

Part A of the medicare program is an entitlement that provides premium-free insurance coverage to elderly and disabled persons for a range of hospital services. Part B of the medicare program covers certain physicians fees and is mostly financed by premiums. These distinctions have significant jurisdictional implications in the House. The Ways and Means Committee continues to have sole jurisdiction over part A of medicare. But the reforms of the 1970s formally shifted those aspects of part B of medicare not financed by special taxes to the jurisdiction of the Commerce Committee. Not surprisingly, it has turned out in practice to be highly difficult for legislators and staff to distinguish between these different areas of medicare jurisdiction. For example, legislative proposals affecting part B of medicare (physician services) often affect part A (hospital expenses), if only because doctors practice in hospitals and the two categories of medical services are highly related. Deciding which bills dealing with part B of medicare should go to Commerce versus Ways and Means has also been problematic.

As a result, following the Bolling/Hansen reforms, a pattern of referrals developed where legislation dealing with part B of medicare was referred jointly to both the Commerce Committee and Ways and Means. Most observers believe that the shared jurisdiction worked relatively well, with substantial communication between the two panels. Now that the Republican majority has abolished joint referrals, a new referral pattern for part B of medicare is emerging, with the Commerce Committee receiving the "primary committee" designation and Ways and Means playing a secondary role.

ECONOMIC AND EDUCATIONAL OPPORTUNITIES. During the years of Democratic control, health care bills were routinely referred to the former Committee on Education and Labor. Until the 103d Congress, however, the panel's jurisdictional claims over health care issues were much narrower than those of Commerce or Ways and Means. But as fundamental alterations in the Employee Retirement Security Act (ERISA) were considered, the Committee began demanding a larger role in health care policy. For instance, former Democratic Chairman William D. Ford sought referral of most key provisions of the Clinton health care package, citing his panel's jurisdiction over ERISA. The Committee eventually received six titles of the Clinton bill.

Under Democratic control, the jurisdictional assertions of Education and Labor were opposed by the Ways and Means Committee, then chaired by Rep. Dan Rostenkowski. The response from Commerce was muted by Ford's close relationship with Chairman John Dingell. However, these patterns of intercommittee comity and conflict will inevitably change now that party control has shifted and different members are wielding the gavel in all three committees. Although the new Republican majority has renamed Education and Labor the Committee on Economic and Educational Opportunities, the panel's jurisdiction is unchanged, and Republicans are unlikely to adopt an approach to health care reform that relies heavily on the programs considered by the panel. The Committee's involvement in the health area should decline.

SECOND TIER. Among the second tier of committees active in health care issues, the Judiciary Committee has jurisdiction over medical malpractice, fraud, and abuse, as well as privacy issues and antitrust policy as it relates to the provision of health care services. As a result, the panel was referred portions of Title V of the Clinton bill, which touched on these issues. More generally, in previous years certain House Republicans have adopted an approach to health care reform that relies on items within the jurisdiction of the Committee on Judiciary. Rather than proposing new benefits, these proposals often focus more on restructuring the industry, more effectively regulating medical fraud and abuse, and reducing the costs associated with medical malpractice. As a result, the role of the Judiciary Committee in health policy may increase with Republicans in the majority.

The jurisdictions of the other second-tier health panels include the major federally managed health care systems, and thus tend to be more constituency-specific than is the case with Judiciary. Included here are the Committees on National Security, Government Reform and Oversight, Resources, and Veterans' Affairs. National Security is responsible for military health care, as well as the health insurance program for military retirees and family members. The Government Reform and Oversight Committee has jurisdiction over health benefits for federal employees; the Indian Health Care Program is within the jurisdiction of the Committee on Resources; and Veterans' Affairs has jurisdiction over the massive veterans health care system.

Particularly on the health care items within their jurisdictions, the members of these panels traditionally have been motivated by goals of constituency service and reelection.[30] The environment of interested outsiders is mostly dominated by constituency groups such as veterans organizations and public employee unions. Committee members function as advocates for their clientele groups and have a relatively parochial perspective on health policy. Not surprisingly, the relevant interest groups view panel members as supportive of their interests.

With Republicans organizing the House, certain of these member-constituency linkages may decline. For example, under Democratic control, the Federal Employees Health Benefits Program was under the purview of the Committee on Post Office and Civil Services, which was highly responsive to the interests of public employees. But the panel was abolished at the beginning of the 104th Congress, and these issues were consolidated with other government operations issues in the new Committee on Government Reform and Oversight. With its broader jurisdiction and Republican majority, this panel is expected to be less responsive to the concerns of public employees. In contrast, the National Security and Veterans' Affairs Committees should continue to function as advocates for beneficiaries of the various health programs they oversee.

Still other House committees have a more limited degree of health-related jurisdiction. For example, legislation is referred to the House Agriculture Committee dealing with rural health care and nutrition issues. The Committee on Science considers basic biomedical research, and the Banking and Financial Services Committee has partial jurisdiction over health bills affecting the financial services industry. These jurisdictions are on the boundaries of health issues, and, for the most part, they have not played a substantial role in national health policy. When they do consider major health issues, such consideration is usually part of a multiple referral, with Commerce or Ways and Means playing the dominant role.

Health Jurisdictions in the Senate

Formal health jurisdiction is less diffuse in the Senate than it is in the House. Two committees form the first tier of Senate health committees. The Finance Committee is the primary committee on overall health policy, with the Labor and Human Resources Committee playing a significant, albeit secondary, role. Table 2-3 indicates that over three-fourths of health care referrals in the Senate in 1991–92 were to these two committees.

FINANCE. The Finance Committee has the largest health care jurisdiction in Congress, extending to all health programs under the Social Security Act or financed by dedicated revenues, including all of medicare and medicaid, as well as child and maternal health care. Thus, the Finance Committee's health jurisdiction is substantially broader than that of its House counterpart, the Ways and Means Committee. On medicare, for example, there is no need to coordinate action by two different panels in the Senate as there is in the House.

Reductions in the Finance Committee's huge jurisdiction have been considered over the years. In the early 1970s, the Senate Parliamentarian jointly referred a health care bill falling in the Finance jurisdiction to both the Finance Committee and the Labor and Human Resources Committee. According to one staffer, then Finance Committee chairman Russell Long went to Majority Leader Mike Mansfield and "virtually exploded," securing from Mansfield a commitment that such a joint referral would not be repeated.[31] The Stevenson Committee—created by the Senate in the mid-1970s to reform the Senate committee system—later considered and rejected a formal reduction in the Finance Committee's jurisdiction.[32]

LABOR AND HUMAN RESOURCES. As with House Commerce, the Senate Labor Committee's involvement in health policy is long-standing, rooted in the former Committee on Public Health and Quarantine, which it subsumed in 1921.[33] The Labor Committee's current jurisdiction combines certain health care items considered by the House Committee on Commerce (public health, biomedical research, alcoholism) with the health care jurisdiction of the House Committee on Economic and Educational Opportunities (employee health and safety, ERISA, children, and elderly persons). Thus, the Labor Committee's health jurisdiction is narrower than that of the Finance Committee but still substantial. Recent chairs of the Labor Committee include Republican Orrin Hatch (1981–86) and Democrat Edward Kennedy (1987–94), who share a strong interest in health issues, which were held at full committee. The current chair, Nancy Landon Kassebaum, has been less active on health policy. Whether controlled by Democrats or Republicans, the Labor Committee generally has been more liberal than the Finance Committee, as well as the Senate as a whole.

SECOND TIER. As with the House, certain Senate panels have health jurisdictions that focus on specific constituent groups. These include the Armed Services Committee, the Governmental Affairs Committee, the Veterans' Affairs Committee, and the Committee on Indian Affairs. The first three panels have jurisdictions identical to their House counterparts. The Senate Veterans' Affairs Committee considers veterans health care and traditionally has been highly responsive to the major veterans groups. Senate Armed Services has jurisdiction over health care for military personnel, dependents, and retirees, and the Senate Governmental Affairs Committee oversees public employee health programs.

However, unlike the House, there is a separate Senate committee focusing on American Indian affairs, including the Indian Health Care System. Created to consider the report of a federal commission about American Indians, the Select Committee on Indian Affairs was originally intended to exist for just one Congress but has been retained due to Member interest, pressure from interested groups, and inertia.[34] By design, the Committee focuses on linkages between the Indian Health Care System and other American Indian issues, rather than more broadly on national health care issues. According to Chairman John McCain, "[The Committee] exists to ensure that all levels of government possess the integrity, accountability, and capability to meet the needs of Indian citizens."[35] Remaining Senate panels, such as Agriculture, Environment and Public Works, and Judiciary, have a more limited, tangential involvement in national health policy.[36]

Implications

The distribution of health-related jurisdiction in both chambers is complicated, reflecting the structure and diversity of the nation's health care system. A core group of panels in each chamber has jurisdiction over the central health programs (medicare, medicaid, the Public Health Service), while other panels consider related issues (medical malpractice, privacy, rural health care), broadening the circle of committees with a degree of jurisdiction over health. Major segments of the health care system that serve specific constituencies (veterans, military personnel and retirees, public employees, American Indians) are overseen by committees focusing, to varying degrees, on the needs of these groups.

Most of the general criticisms made about committee jurisdictions in Congress are potentially relevant to the health area.[37] Health jurisdiction is fragmented, potentially complicating efforts to formulate and pass coherent, national legislation. Multiple referrals in the House expand the opportunities for committee-based obstructionism and delay. The dispersion of jurisdiction makes it harder to discern who is responsible for policy failures, undermining legislative accountability. The committees with relatively narrow, constituency-oriented jurisdictions may empower special interests and promote a parochial approach to policymaking.

However, health policy is a general term, encompassing many specific issues and initiatives, and the overall role of committees—including the impact of jurisdiction—depends on the nature of the specific issue under consideration. On issues that are controversial, nationally salient, and prominent on the agendas of the two main political parties, power within Congress tends to shift out of committee, upward to the leadership level and outward to the chamber as a whole.[38] Key decisions are less likely to be made in committee, and the impact of jurisdiction on decisionmaking is limited. However, on less salient or less controversial measures, or on technically complex bills where committee members have important informational advantages, the key legislative decisions are more likely to be made in committee. A full exploration of these issues is beyond the scope of this chapter, but two examples—comprehensive health care reform and veterans health policy—illustrate how the impact of jurisdiction can vary by issue.

Comprehensive Health Care Reform

The potential for jurisdictional infighting over President Clinton's proposal to overhaul the national health care system was apparent from the beginning of the reform process in 1993. However, the issue dominated the national political agenda during the 103d Congress; the electoral fates of the two congressional parties were at stake, and a wide range of legislators and outside groups were actively involved in the reform process. As a result, decisionmaking within Congress was less "committee-centered" than on less salient or less controversial measures, and committee boundaries did not shape the policymaking process or determine the outcome. Rather, health care reform failed during the 103d Congress for more fundamental reasons than the distribution of turf on Capitol Hill.

Key House and Senate committees began jockeying for jurisdiction over the Clinton health care proposal even before the ink was dry. For instance, in September 1993, Hillary Rodham Clinton, head of the Administration's task force on health care reform, had to testify before five different House and Senate committees in a single week. Each panel wanted to stake out the strongest possible jurisdictional claim to the forthcoming measure, and they refused to combine hearings.[39]

After a draft of the package was leaked a few weeks later, the House Education and Labor Committee produced a detailed jurisdictional analysis, using its control over ERISA to claim virtually all of the bill. As one committee member observed, "I'm sure a lot of committees are casting a wide net."[40] Energy and Commerce Chairman John Dingell warned Speaker Foley that an unrestricted joint referral of the Clinton bill would guarantee "a Tower of Babel approach in which conflicting claims and provisions yield a health care system even more irrational than today's."[41] Asked which portions of the bill he sought for Energy and Commerce, Dingell responded, "We have health."[42] But according to Ways and Means Chairman Dan Rostenkowski, "[t]here's no question Ways and Means probably has the largest of obligations in health reform."[43] Other panels sought substantial portions of the measure, including the Banking and Small Business Committees. As one Republican House member quipped, "I wouldn't be surprised if, by the time this is over, both the Merchant Marine Committee and the Ethics Committee have a hand in it."[44]

The jurisdictional dispute certainly had *potential* implications for policy. Of the three lead panels, the members of Energy and Commerce were the most ideologically representative of the full House. Ways and Means had a higher ratio of Democrats to Republicans than did Energy and Commerce, making it more receptive to the president's goals for health care reform, which tilted to the left. The Education and Labor Committee, with its firm liberal majority, was the panel most supportive of comprehensive reform—but also least representative of the parent chamber. Thus, where the different portions of Clinton's plan were referred had potential implications for the content of the legislation reported to the floor, as well as the overall direction of the reform debate. As it turned out, all three committees considered comprehensive health care reform, with varying degrees of frustration. As Dingell feared, Foley imposed no timetable on the three lead committees. The seven additional panels with limited referrals did not have to report until two weeks after the top three acted.

In the Senate, a similar power struggle—called "a giant spitting contest" by one staffer—broke out between the Finance Committee and the Labor and Human Resources Committee.[45] Daniel Patrick Moynihan, then chairman of the Finance panel, claimed sole jurisdiction over the Clinton bill, citing his committee's jurisdiction over revenue matters, medicare, and medicaid. But Labor Committee Chairman Edward Kennedy sought the bill for his panel, arguing that the measure's financing mechanism was not really a tax. Most important, Kennedy argued that his committee, with its firm liberal majority, would be more receptive to Clinton's approach to health care reform, while the more conservative Finance Committee might gut the measure. In contrast, Moynihan and others were concerned that the Labor panel would report a bill too liberal to pass the Senate. Said one Democrat, "It would be a colossal mistake for the 'new Democrat' President to have his one major piece of social legislation be Teddy Kennedy's legislation."[46]

As a result, three separate versions of the president's plan were introduced in the Senate in late November 1993: one by Majority Leader George Mitchell; a second, identical, version by Moynihan; and a third version by Kennedy, which deleted those sections clearly falling within the Finance Committee jurisdiction. Moynihan responded by objecting to the unanimous consent request to send Kennedy's version to the Labor Committee. Kennedy countered by threatening to block referral of the Clinton measure to the Finance panel. Under Senate rules, committees can originate bills and need not depend on the referral process to begin legislating. To break the jurisdictional impasse, the Labor and Finance Committees both chose to draft and then mark up their own measures.[47]

As the lead committees began work on health care reform in early 1994, there was a general expectation that these jurisdictional conflicts would continue—and that they might complicate efforts to produce a coherent reform package. As one perceptive observer warned: "The mission is all the more difficult procedurally because the increasingly balkanized House and Senate must contend with the jousting and jealousies that result from overlapping committee jurisdictions and competing chairmen. Those fights have already started and are likely to continue."[48] In fact, the importance of jurisdiction quickly receded because of the salience and controversy of the issue, and because the lead heath panels in both chambers were unable to devise reform proposals that could pass on the floor.

Health care reform activated a diverse range of organizations and interests, from the Health Insurance Association of America to the American Chiropractic Association. Members of Congress were buffeted with competing demands and an abundance of information. Legislators on and off the lead committees of jurisdiction sought to play a role in the reform debate. As House member Jim McDermott, a key Democrat on health issues, observed: "Usually a committee works on a bill, and then committee members say to the rest of us, 'Trust me, this is a good bill,' and we vote for it. But it's very dicey to accept a 'trust me' on this bill. . . . This isn't like voting to take some action in Bosnia; it affects every person in every member's district."[49]

According to a prominent health care lobbyist, "From Day One, we've approached this project as if we had to lobby the entire House."[50] Health care reform transcended the congressional committee system.

The committees of jurisdiction were also unable to serve as initial arenas for building consensus. The Senate Labor and Human Resources Committee was the first to report legislation, mostly modeled on the Clinton plan, but ranking Republican Nancy Landon Kassebaum warned, "This proposal has reached the end of its trail because it fails to offer a middle ground."[51] Similar comments were made about the two plans reported in June by House Education and Labor—one a more generous version of Clinton's plan, the other a single-payer proposal. After months of struggle, the Ways and Means Committee barely managed to report a reform measure, with former chairman Rostenkowski saying "I don't know that this bill will get 218 votes."[52] The Finance Committee reported bipartisan legislation in early July, but without the guarantee of universal coverage deemed critical by liberals. Most telling, on June 28, John Dingell notified the Speaker of the House that his panel was unable to agree on a bill.[53] The House and Senate majority leaders—Rep. Richard Gephardt and Senator George Mitchell—tried to stitch together health care reform packages that could pass in their respective chambers, but their efforts were unsuccessful.

In the House, jurisdictional disputes did resurface briefly in late July 1994, delaying Gephardt's attempt to develop a consensus package for House Democrats. The Gephardt bill was based on the measure reported by Ways and Means, which was structured to fall mostly within that panel's jurisdiction, rather than the jurisdictions of Energy and Commerce or Education and Labor. As a result, Democratic leaders made certain changes in the proposed legislation to guarantee a substantial health care role for all three committees in the future—assuming the proposal passed. According to a staff participant, "These discussions about jurisdiction struck many people as chewing up an inordinate amount of time given the calendar."[54] As another observer noted, "Some of these guys are acting as if they're going to still be committee chairmen in 30 years."[55]

This turf battle, however, was only a minor irritant as health care reform spiraled downward to defeat. In explaining the failure of reform, analysts instead emphasize factors such as the complexity of the main proposals, interest group opposition, and a lack of consensus about how to proceed (see chapter 7). Indeed, having five separate committees working simultaneously may have actually helped keep the reform process from ending during the spring of 1994, as committee after committee encountered difficulties building a majority, and finding a middle ground for the institution as a whole proved elusive. Overlapping jurisdictions can promote competition between committees, providing incentives for innovation as well as additional points of access into the lawmaking process.[56]

But there also was a downside to having so many committees consider comprehensive health care reform. Most important, the dispersion of jurisdiction probably made it more difficult for members and the public to make sense of the reform debate. It is difficult for the public to follow (and for the media to cover) an issue that is being considered simultaneously in five or more distinct arenas. If deliberations had centered on just one panel in each chamber, the dizzying array of alternatives may have narrowed earlier in the reform process, enabling the public and members of Congress to sort out the reform debate.

Rather than rely on the standing committees, the Speaker of the House could have appointed a temporary ad hoc panel to consider the

Clinton proposal and prepare a compromise vehicle for the floor. By using the standing committee system, Foley missed an important opportunity to help structure the national debate over health care reform and expedite the crafting of a compromise measure. A key advantage of an ad hoc panel is that preliminary deliberations on an issue can occur in one arena, helping members overcome the centrifugal forces of the committee system and better educate the public. Alternatively, the speaker might have designated one of the three lead panels as the primary committee of jurisdiction, and then sequentially referred that committee's report to the other panels, with strict time limitations. In the Senate, the majority leader also can appoint ad hoc panels to consider legislation but (unlike the House speaker) needs the approval of the full chamber.

In the end, no panel—standing or ad hoc—may have been able to develop a comprehensive, politically viable approach to health care reform in 1994. But with a more streamlined committee stage, at least the infeasibility of major change would have been apparent earlier in the process, providing members with the time necessary to consider and pass a more incremental measure.

Veterans Health Care

While comprehensive health care reform transcended committee boundaries, the less salient, less controversial, and more constituency-oriented jurisdictions in the health care arena are important for understanding policy outcomes. Of these panels, the two Veterans' Affairs Committees are the most active on health legislation. Together, they oversee the Veterans Health System (the VA), the largest medical care system in the nation. Treating more than 2.5 million veterans per year, the VA runs almost 300 hospitals and nursing homes in 50 states. According to one veterans advocate, "There really aren't too many congressional districts without a VA facility of some kind. . . . Only in the veterans arena do we run a miniature national health insurance system."[57] Although veterans bills affect the constituents of most members of Congress, they are less salient than major health care reform and are usually handled without controversy.

A range of influential interest groups represent the views of American veterans—groups such as the American Legion, the Veterans of Foreign Wars, the Disabled American Veterans, AMVETS, the Paralyzed Veterans of America, and the Vietnam Veterans of America. Rep. Gerald B. H. Solomon, chairman of the House Rules Committee, has described veterans as "one of the largest lobbies in Washington, as well they should be, because they represent one of the largest voting blocs."[58]

Members of Congress join the Veterans' Affairs Committees to promote goals of constituency service and reelection, and the environments of the committees are dominated by the main veterans organizations. Both panels conduct yearly hearings formally organized around the legislative agendas of these groups.[59] Not surprisingly, veterans organizations view the Committees as crucial advocates for their interests on Capitol Hill. For example, in a letter sent to key House reformers in 1993, the executive director of AMVETS urged that the House and Senate Committees on Veterans' Affairs not be abolished, because "These committees are invaluable in ensuring that the Department of Veterans' Affairs provides quality services to the nation's veterans."[60] According to the national commander of the American Legion, "The Veterans' Affairs Committees perform a tremendous service for those who have proudly served this great nation."[61]

Both the House and Senate Veterans' Affairs Committees have traditions of bipartisan decisionmaking. Current House Chairman Bob Stump observes that "[former Chairman Sonny Montgomery] and I are two of the closest friends. We've always done what's best for the veterans. We've always worked closely together and I expect that will continue [with Republicans in the majority]."[62] And although veterans bills in the House are often considered under suspension of the rules, without amendment, both the House and Senate Veterans' Affairs Committees are permeable to the views of committee non-members acting on behalf of the veterans in their districts or states.

The Veterans panels focus on veterans health issues, not as they relate to health issues in general, but as they relate to other veterans' concerns. By design, consolidating all veterans issues in a single jurisdiction enhances the ability of the groups to pursue their agendas. Senator John D. Rockefeller IV, ranking Democrat on the Senate Veterans' Affairs Committee, recognizes the point, as do other advocates for America's veterans: "If VA health care was under a committee dealing with general health issues, concerns about the [VA] system might well not be considered in connection with other VA benefits. . . . Our Committee looks at issues relating to service connection in the context of the potential impact of any new legislation on the [VA] health care system, a result that would likely be lost if the jurisdiction for veterans matters was divided among several committees."[63] Placing veterans issues in a single jurisdiction accentuates the linkages between these issues, but it also undermines broader efforts to formulated cohesive national policy in the *health care* arena.

Consider the matter of access to VA hospitals. For a number of years, the VA hospital system has had excess capacity, because of factors such as budgetary constraints, population shifts, and the aging of U.S. veterans. As many as one-third of the authorized beds in VA hospitals are unfilled, with underutilization particularly marked in rural areas. As a result, proposals have surfaced to open up VA hospitals to nonveterans to increase utilization and provide the demand necessary to support capital-intensive services such as surgery. However, key veterans groups have opposed integrating VA hospitals into the broader, nonveterans health care system, arguing that policy regarding VA hospitals should be based solely on the needs of veterans.[64]

In 1991, for example, the House Veterans' Affairs Committee conducted hearings about a proposed demonstration program aimed at opening up underutilized VA hospitals to nonveterans in rural areas, which often are medically underserved. According to one backer, the goal was to "better utilize the VA facilities that are there by providing some desperately needed health care to other citizens in [those communities]. And the irony of this is that . . . this may make those VA facilities more financially viable."[65]

However, the major veterans groups strenuously opposed the initiative, and it did not advance past the hearings stage. A spokesman for the Veterans of Foreign Wars testified, "Any kind of program that is a sharing . . . should be for the benefit of the veteran. . . . My membership would be much more receptive to opening [VA hospitals] up to the spouses and dependents of veterans than someone who possibly—well, is not a veteran for whatever reasons."[66] More generally, it has been difficult for Congress to consider changes in the VA hospital system from the perspective of broader health care goals. The main impediment has been the power of the various veterans groups. But their clout is reinforced by the structure of the House and Senate committee systems, where the two committees of jurisdiction mostly function as advocates for the veterans community.[67]

In short, the consolidation in a single panel of jurisdiction over programs affecting a particular constituency can have substantial consequences for policymaking. Such a committee will likely adopt a narrow, constituency-oriented approach to legislating, even when the underlying issue area is national in scope. The issues included in a committee's jurisdiction determine the constituencies that comprise its environment. These constituencies in turn shape the overall approach committee members adopt on their issues. As a result, jurisdictions that focus on the interests of particular groups have a relatively parochial perspective on policymaking. In the health care arena, such parochialism is most apparent on veterans issues but is relevant to the other federally managed health care systems as well.

Over the years, congressional committees with less visible, more constituency-oriented jurisdictions have been mentioned as potential targets for abolition. However, the interest group linkages that cause policy parochialism in the first place also make these committees politically difficult to dismantle. House Republicans were able to abolish the Committee on Post Office and Civil Service at the beginning of the 104th Congress, but the affected groups were mostly Democratic constituencies. Interestingly, House Republicans chose not to take on the jurisdiction with the largest federal health care system—the Veterans' Affairs Committee—because of opposition from America's veterans, many of whom vote Republican. Bypassing constituency-oriented committees with temporary panels or other ad hoc mechanisms is of little use, because the affected groups will simply shift their attention to the alternative decisionmaking arena. In short, while the policy impact of jurisdiction can be substantial for less salient, more constituency-oriented issues, addressing these problems through reform or ad hoc procedures is problematic.

Conclusion

Health policy probably will not dominate the Republican-controlled 104th Congress the way it dominated the Democrat-controlled 103d. A health care reform initiative is not included in the House Republican "Contract with America." And although Senate Republicans did include the topic on their list of campaign promises in 1994, the congressional agenda for the foreseeable future will mostly be driven by the more homogeneous and organized new majority in the House.

Still, the underlying problems of access, coverage, and cost that motivated and structured the health care debate in 1993–94 will remain. The medicare trust fund is still predicted to be insolvent within a decade, so the national respite from health care reform will be short-lived, no matter which party organizes Congress. In spring 1995, the House and Senate both passed budget resolutions that would require medicare savings in excess of $250 billion. As legislative attention returns to national health policy, how will committee jurisdictions affect congressional deliberations? Four main points merit special consideration.

First, health jurisdiction is widely distributed throughout the House and Senate committee systems. Almost all authorizing committees have a degree of health-related jurisdiction. Consolidating control over all of these issues in a single panel would not be feasible without creating a single "megacommittee" for domestic policy, undermining the congressional division of labor. A degree of jurisdictional fragmentation in health care policy is unavoidable.

Second, although health jurisdiction is dispersed, comprehensive reform measures fall primarily within the jurisdiction of two committees in each chamber. In the Senate, the Finance Committee has predominant jurisdiction, with the Labor and Human Resources Committee also playing a role. In the House, the abolition of joint referrals further concentrates jurisdiction over national health policy in the Ways and Means and Commerce Committees. If Republicans choose to push major health care reform, the measure will be salient and controversial—not the kind of issue where legislators defer to committee members. And Republican leaders will have the procedural prerogatives and informal tools necessary to counteract jurisdictional fragmentation in the standing committee system—if they choose to use them. In short, health jurisdiction is fragmented, but the key impediments to major reform are not jurisdictional. They arise instead from disagreements about policy, the complexity of the issues, and opposition from shifting portions of the interest group environment.

Third, jurisdiction matters more for the significant but less visible portions of the health care system that serve particular constituencies— veterans health care, for example. Fully integrating such programs into a cohesive national health policy is complicated by existing committee boundaries, which track the interests of affected groups. But the political costs to changing these jurisdictions are high.

Fourth, the early signs are that the new Republican majority in Congress will be less constrained by committee prerogatives, including jurisdictional lines. In the House, the committee reforms implemented at the beginning of the 104th Congress accelerated and reinforced long-standing trends away from committee autonomy. The abolition of joint referrals ensures that a primary committee will take the lead on complex health bills, which should reduce policy fragmentation and inter-committee conflicts over turf. Speaker Gingrich has also promised to use temporary panels and other ad hoc mechanisms when necessary to rationalize and expedite the flow of legislation. In the smaller, more informal Senate, jurisdictional boundaries are not determinative on major bills, no matter which party is in the majority.

The bottom line? For health care policymaking in Congress, committee boundaries still matter. But their importance varies by issue and probably will decline somewhat in the new Republican Congress.

Chapter 3

Budgeting and Health Policymaking

Joseph White

A NYONE WHO DOUBTS that congressional budget procedures and health policymaking are closely intertwined should consider the predicament of Robert D. Reischauer, director of the Congressional Budget Office (CBO) from 1989 to 1995.

As early as late 1983, while at the Urban Institute, Reischauer noted that Allen Schick's description of "the fiscalization of the policy debate" meant less attention was paid to what policy actually did and thus to its accomplishments or failures.[1] By 1994 Reischauer, as CBO head, had the power (through a statement about budget estimates) to determine whether crippling points of order applied to a given proposal. By expressing an opinion on whether revenues and spending should be considered on or off budget, he could, for example, define the Clinton health care plan's very nature, as "big government" or something else.[2]

Reischauer knew the effects of that power and dreaded it. He expressed that fear when he testified on February 8, 1994, before the House Committee on Ways and Means. In the "well over a hundred times" he had testified before Congress, he had normally "started with some customary remarks concerning how pleased I was to have the opportunity to testify." Yet, he added: "I did not start off that way today. I did not because I have considerable foreboding that the information contained in my statement and in the CBO report might be used largely in destructive rather than constructive ways—that is, it might be used to undercut a serious discussion of health-reform alternatives or to gain short-term partisan political advantage." No babe in the woods, he expected the CBO estimates would be used for these purposes, but usually after a while, "CBO's input has been put to use in constructive ways to shape better policy." In this case, Reischauer feared that would not be the case. A rare opportunity would thus be lost—the opportunity to "make America's health care system more equitable, more efficient, and less costly."[3]

Many forces killed health care reform, but surely the congressional budget process contributed to its death. The process affected the very terms of the debate, directing attention to arcane questions of scorekeeping instead of to the workability of policy. The budget process delayed the schedule of drafting and consideration again and again, first within the Clinton administration as it sought estimates for alternatives, and later in Congress as members waited for CBO to score (that is, to calculate the budgeting impact of) bills. One participant complained that policymaking became a form of simulation game, in which computer models displaced reality.[4]

Some may argue that the budget process is merely a tool and cannot be said to have an independent effect on policy; by analogy, it could be said that "reports don't kill policies, politicians kill policies." In practice, any tool can only be used for limited purpose. A gun, for instance, can kill people but not heal them. Is the budget process tool, then, more likely to be used to prevent sensible health care policy or to encourage it?

In assessing the effects of congressional budget procedures on health policymaking, this discussion must go beyond the 1993–94 reform issues, even though they are central to this book. The 1993–94 process may not be suitable for assessing any set of procedures. Any evaluation of procedure will depend on preferences about outcomes, and there is no issue on which those beliefs about goals varied more and with greater intensity than in health care reform. Indeed, one may question whether the recent battle can yield reasoned judgment about any aspect of Congress. No political system is prone to reform of 14 percent of its national GDP all at once. The sheer scope of the American health care system in particular—nearly $1 trillion—makes its reform comparable to restructuring one of the largest economies in the world. This is not ordinary politics.

To provide a more appropriate evaluation of congressional budgeting, I therefore will also consider the politics of reducing spending on federal health entitlements and of appropriating for health care discretionary spending, focusing on three themes. First, budget institutions are part of the division of labor in Congress and therefore shape the machinery through which policy is processed. Second, the budget process has an independent effect on policy, because those with authority within that process think about policy in a distinctive way. And third, the macropolitics of deficit reduction create opportunities for some kinds of coalition building for health care policies but inhibit others.

The Congressional Budget Process(es)

The federal budget process resembles the layers in an archaeological dig. The major layers consist of the following:

1. *A set of rules to prevent Congress from enacting, and inhibit the President from signing, legislation that would increase the federal deficit beyond the trend in "current law."*

These rules were created mainly in the 1985 Gramm-Rudman-Hollings Act, the 1990 Budget Enforcement Act (BEA), and the 1993 congressional budget resolution.[5] "Current law" refers to the spending that would occur or revenues that would be raised if permanent legislation such as tax law and entitlement authorizations were unchanged. In the case of annual appropriations, it refers to a fixed amount of money, called a "cap," legislated to limit discretionary appropriations for a number of years subsequent to a particular act. Thus the 1990 BEA created discretionary spending caps for FY91–95. The restrictions on further entitlement spending and on revenue cuts are called the "pay-as-you-go" or "paygo" rules. Both paygo and the limits on spending more than the caps are enforced by points of order that in the Senate can only be waived by an extraordinary majority of sixty Senators.

2. *The Congressional budget process.*

The House and Senate Budget Committees draft an annual budget resolution. This resolution's first function is to set limits on the new spending or revenue measures that can be reported by the various committees—limits that can be tighter but not looser than those in previous legislation, such as the 1990 and 1993 packages. The allocation to each committee is called the 602(a) or 302(a) allocation, for the section of law that creates the process.[6] If further reduction is desired, the budget resolution includes reconciliation instructions that specify the amounts, but not the manner, in which committees are supposed to report legislation to reduce the deficit. Reconciliation instructions have some dubious merit as moral suasion. More significantly, legislation that conforms with these instructions is packaged and debated under very restrictive rules that forbid filibusters on the Senate floor.

3. Authorizing legislation.

Authorizations set the basic rules of federal programs—the organizations, purposes, and authorities. In addition, much of federal health care finance is created by authorization legislation. Once created, unless there is some unusual provision for an expiration date, such legislation remains in effect unless new legislation is passed to change it. Thus if legislation is not reported to change the tax preference for employer-provided health insurance benefits, those benefits will grow or shrink in line with economic variables and employer behavior. Some spending programs, such as medicare part A, are authorized with "permanent appropriations."[7] Others, like medicaid, though they require annual appropriations, create entitlements in law that cannot be eliminated by simply failing to appropriate funds.[8] In both cases, then, the financial decisions are in the hands of the authorizing committees.

As C. Lawrence Evans explains in chapter 2, the division of authority over programs among committees differs between the House and Senate. In the House, the major committees are currently those on Ways and Means, Commerce, and Economic and Educational Opportunities. Before 1995, Commerce was called Energy and Commerce, and Economic and Educational Opportunities was Education and Labor. (In this chapter, I use the old names as needed to refer to these committees in past Congresses.) The key Senate committees are those on Finance and on Labor and Human Resources. For a study of health care policy and budgetmaking, Ways and Means and Finance are most important. This is not only because they have jurisdiction over the largest program (medicare) but also because, with all the revenues and the other huge spending jurisdictions, they are the dominant players in budget matters.

4. Annual appropriations.

The remaining programs, such as research efforts of the National Institutes of Health (NIH), medical services of the Department of Veterans Affairs, and public health efforts of the Centers for Disease Control and the U.S. Food and Drug Administration, require annual funding in appropriations acts. The House and Senate Committees on Appropriations have identical jurisdictions divided into thirteen parallel subcommittees. Appropriations must be renewed annually and must therefore run a gauntlet of congressional passage and potential presidential veto. They also must fit targets set by a budget resolution. The budget resolution's target can be lower but not higher than a previously legislated cap. The appropriations committees are required to divide their total among their thirteen subcommittees—the 302(b) or 602(b), allocation. Either bills or amendments that would exceed those allocations are subject to points of order similar to the paygo restraints.

Detailed review by the appropriations committees also allows for extensive intervention in the operation of programs. The actual level of intervention depends on many factors, such as the extent to which intervention can be attacked as political earmarking of funds that instead should be allocated by objective peer review. The need for annual appropriations makes such funding more vulnerable than either tax preferences or entitlements. At the same time, each of the bills (save perhaps funding for the District of Columbia) has something for almost everyone and will eventually pass in some form. In addition, the largest appropriated programs—health research and veterans' services—are extremely popular.

5. The president's budget.

Although not formally part of congressional procedures, the budget proposal submitted by the president at the beginning of each fiscal year is an integral part of congressional decisionmaking. It would be important if only as an indication of the preferences of the person who could veto legislation or appropriations, but its major function is more subtle.

Given that support for revenues generally falls short of demands for spending and that there is a political aversion to larger deficits, the presidential budget can help Congress meet its own targets in two ways. First, staff work by the Office of Management and Budget (OMB) or other offices can identify efficiencies in operations, thereby requiring less money for the same output. But much more importantly, when the president proposes either less spending for some program or a new tax, Congress can accept his proposal, blaming him for the pain. Or it can reject it and replace it with another; Congress would then get the blame for its own measure, but would also get credit for rejecting the president's. In return for this shelter against blame, Congress has given the president some initiative and ability to set the agenda.[9]

6. *Scorekeepers, which report on the budgetary implications of proposals and effects of legislation, thereby triggering the various rules referred to here, or merely adding authority to the arguments of one side or another in specific debates.*

The scorekeepers include CBO, the Congressional Joint Committee on Taxation, and the Executive OMB. OMB's scorekeeping controls the application of sequesters (automatic cuts in programs that must be implemented if legislation somehow sneaks past the various points of order). CBO scorekeeping controls application of these points of order. Joint Tax's scorekeeping provides the revenue estimates CBO is required to use, and thus application of the points of order to revenue measures.

This set of institutions creates an immense variety of possible interactions.

Deficit Reduction and Health Entitlement Policymaking

Periodically, demand for deficit reduction creates an understanding among politicians that they have to "do something" of a certain magnitude about the deficit. In search of ways to meet that target, if they had no preconceived ideas, they would look at recent trends and projections for programs to see what spending is the biggest part of the problem. Looking at data from OMB and CBO, they would see that medicare and medicaid are among the fastest growing and largest programs. CBO would have a series of possible medicare and medicaid cuts among the two hundred or so items in its annual volume of deficit reduction options.[10]

In the case of medicare, the major deficit reduction possibilities are 1) lower benefits to or higher contributions from elderly Americans; 2) higher payroll taxes; 3) lower payments to physicians; and 4) lower payments to other providers, especially hospitals. They are listed here in the order of least to greatest political plausibility, though numbers 1 and 2 are similar. Each involves powerful interests that Congress would not ordinarily attack.

If Congress is fortunate, then the president, seeing the same numbers, will propose some health care savings in his own budget. In the 1980s, Republican presidents tended to propose measures that would increase costs to elderly Americans. That enabled Congress to change the political question from "will some powerful group be hurt to reduce the deficit?" to "which powerful group will be hurt to reduce the deficit?" It should come as no surprise that Congress, instead of targeting older people, did hospital payment reform first, in 1982–83, and physician payment second, beginning with a fee freeze in the 1984 Deficit Reduction Act.[11]

In theory, Congress would adopt a budget resolution, and then the revenue committees and House Commerce would have to find ways to meet the reconciliation targets for medicare savings. In practice, targets have been enforced only when these committees already had a fairly good idea of how much they could do before the budget resolution was adopted.[12] The committees might have ideas generated by their own staff or in cooperation with federal bureaus, and they normally believe a target from the president gives them sufficient cover to go looking.

Because budgeting involves fundamental schisms between the parties, budget resolutions historically have been adopted nearly entirely along party lines in the House. The less partisan Senate occasionally passes a resolution with more minority support. The president has virtually no role in this. The exceptions are if he is of the same party as the congressional majority, or when a package is developed first in a "budget summit" among legislative and executive leaders, as happened in 1990. Then the budget resolution is simply the cover document for the package and is adopted at about the same time. Whatever the resolution's origin, its major function is to provide procedural protection that the revenue committees can use to bring unpopular deficit reduction bills to the floor with no chance of a filibuster and a presumption that something "must" pass.

The savings in any bill would be estimated by CBO for purposes of assessing compliance with the various rules and targets. When targets were solely annual, bills might create savings for one year but satisfy constituents by ending the savings (or even creating new costs) in the next year. That led to the adoption of three-year targets; bills would then sometimes have costs in the fourth and subsequent years.

This dynamic of scorekeeping, combined with the difficulty of forming a deficit-cutting coalition, made reconciliation bills an opportunity for medicaid expansions in the 1980s. The Republicans did not have the votes to pass a deficit reduction package without tax increases, but few House Republicans were willing to vote for a package *with* increases. Therefore every deficit reduction package needed substantial support from liberal Democrats. The chairman of the Energy and Commerce health subcommittee, Henry Waxman (D.-Ca.), pushed for somewhat bigger cuts to medicare providers to pay for expansions of access to medicaid. Between 1984 and 1990, there were seven expansions of benefits to pregnant women and children, and six of these were within budget reconciliation acts.[13]

Perhaps the most important expansion, enacted in 1990, "phased in coverage by 2001 of all children between age 6 and 19 in families with incomes below the federal poverty level."[14] In essence, children who were covered up to age 6 would not be dropped until age 19. These expansions are by no means the major portion of medicaid's cost growth; indeed, they were possible in part because they were relatively cheap. The fact that some were optional and that others were phased in also helped limit the visible costs. The last expansion would thus add another year of coverage each year: in the first to age seven, in the second to age eight, and so on. The first three years would provide only one-quarter of the ultimate expansion.

Budget procedures therefore not only provided the opportunity for coverage expansions in the 1980s but also determined their timings. Power politics—the fact that elderly Americans are even more influential than hospitals and doctors—determined that cost controls would be focused on the latter.[15] In any case, health care cost controls are likely to be highly technical. In the context of reconciliation legislation, they became the epitome of an inside game. In such circumstances, there is little opportunity for floor debate, and the health care measures are only a part of a much larger bill. As David G. Smith summarizes, "The substance of health policy was made through subcommittee micro-management and the budget reconciliation process."[16]

Inside players were further protected in the conflicts over hospital prospective payment and physician fee schedules by another aspect of budgeting. Budgeting put medicare cuts on the agenda each year. In the absence of structural reform, interest groups had reason to fear that Congress would, in frustration, adopt blunt cost controls—as it indeed did for hospitals in 1982 before adopting the prospective payment system (PPS) in 1983. Congress had also intervened substantially to create such a patchwork of physician payment restrictions that by 1989 significant sectors of the medical profession were willing to contemplate some kind of more coherent reform. Supporters of such reform could then threaten that, if it were blocked, they would take less "reasonable" measures.[17]

Last (but hardly least), the very definition of policymaking in terms of deficit reduction had to affect the behavior of interest groups. That does not mean that groups were generally disposed toward compromise. It does mean that, every few years, a reconciliation bill looked likely enough that some interests splintered off, each segment seeking to stick its erstwhile allies with the costs. The most dramatic example was the fragmentation among business interests in 1982, but the surgeons' pursuit of a separate deal in 1989 is another clear example.

Both budget processes and budget pressures therefore help to explain why a Congress that, with many more liberal Democratic members, could not adopt regulatory health care cost controls during the Carter administration ended up creating powerful new regulatory cost controls for medicare during the antiregulation Reagan and Bush administrations. Budgeting is not the whole story. For example, some Reagan administration officials saw the adoption of prospective payment as a competitive strategy, because more efficient hospitals would flourish with fixed prices.[18] But budgeting is nonetheless significant. Something had to be done—something to which scorekeepers would give credence; it had to be implementable in relatively short time frames to save money in the right years; and the coalitional structure of deficit politics meant liberal Democrats had to accept the measures.

The most basic reason for the relative success advocates of regulation had in the 1980s as opposed to the Carter years, however, is so obvious that it could easily be missed: public budgetary responsibility for medicare expenses already existed. Providers and hard-line conservatives oppose regulation of either public programs or the private sector. In the latter case, however, they could argue that regulation involved a major extension of federal activity and thereby ally themselves with centrist and moderately conservative politicians in opposition. In the former case, the same centrists already saw government responsibility in the form of the budget deficit. The providers could not argue against government involvement per se, because that would mean taking benefits away from people. This is much harder than resisting an expansion of benefits, especially when the attacked group (in this case, elderly Americans) is both powerful and popular. Regulatory cost controls must be more politically plausible when the government is already footing the bill rather than as part of legislation either to restrain costs for which the government is not paying (as in the Carter years) or to help pay for a major expansion of government responsibilities (as with the Clinton proposals).[19]

Deficit reduction efforts could also affect policies that use the tax code to influence health care. The most important of these is the provision that allows employers to treat the cost of health insurance for their employees as a business expense while not allowing the employees to report that benefit as income. Such "tax expenditures" have not been a significant portion of the reconciliation battles, probably because they affect an even wider constituency than does medicare. With rare and relatively small exceptions (such as gasoline taxes), revenue increases have been concentrated on groups that were not majorities and might be stigmatized (such as wealthy Americans and businesses).[20]

Budgeting for AIDS Treatment and Research

Medicare and medicaid entitlements are, along with tax expenditures, by far the federal government's largest financial commitments to health policy.[21] Yet discretionary spending on programs such as veterans' hospitals and medical research add about $30 billion dollars annually, a major activity in comparison with any other allocation other than social insurance.[22]

A wide range of social processes generates both demands for and constraints on this program spending. The government's response, however, is the result of conflict or cooperation among four forces: the authorization process within Congress; the appropriation process; the line agencies themselves; and the presidential agencies, such as the White House staff and OMB.

In this discretionary spending arena, the effect of budgetmaking institutions on the policy process raises two questions: whether Congress would act differently in appropriations than in authorizations, and how the two halves of the executive branch relate to the appropriations process. Appropriating differs from authorizing in certain fundamental ways:

—Authorizations for an activity frequently provide much more money than is appropriated, for two reasons. First, legislators can vote for (and presidents can sign) generous authorizations, pleasing the groups that would benefit, because the authorizations do not really spend the money anyway. Second, authorizations are considered separately and without a context of overall budget targets. Appropriations are considered at the same time and must be fit into targets, so the

Appropriations committees are forced to make trade-offs authorizers can avoid.

—Appropriations must be enacted annually, whereas authorizations normally are not.[23] Therefore, most parties in disputes about appropriations bills feel a greater need to compromise and "get a bill" than those in fights on even the same issue in authorizing legislation.[24] Most appropriations disputes also involve money, making the default compromise (that is, splitting the difference) evident to all participants.

—Some of the conflict about appropriations involves questions of administrative efficiency, such as how many workers (full-time equivalents, or FTEs) are needed to do a job. If efficiencies can be found, spending estimates can be reduced without consequences for beneficiaries. Sometimes few efficiencies can be made, but estimates can still be reduced without *immediate, visible* effects on output (for example, by deferring maintenance). The basic question for appropriators is "What do you *really* need?" Much of the process's dynamic involves subcommittees seeking the answers for each agency thus helping the subcommittees to best determine how to fit agency funding into the bill's 302(b) allocation. The subcommittee staff directors or "clerks" particularly rely on agency civil servants (usually called budget officers) to provide the answers. The president has power because he can threaten a veto. However, he cannot credibly use the threat of veto over too many issues within a given bill, and there are a lot of issues. The technical and administrative sides of the process mean that its nexus under normal circumstances is the relationship between subcommittee staff and agency budget officer.

—Appropriators are skeptics. They tend not to believe OMB's judgments.[25] They also do not believe the authorizers, because the authorizing committees are asking different questions than are appropriators. Both agencies and authorizing committees want to talk about the good a program will do; appropriators ask why these new inputs will yield new outputs. As one House Appropriations member put it, "There are three questions: Do we need it? Can we afford it? How'd we get along so long without it? It's much simpler." The appropriators are biased more generally against change than against new spending alone. A new need may be evident, and the focus on justifying changes in inputs may be used to oppose cuts as well as increases. In a clear example, one Reagan official's testimony was met with the skepticism of a Senate appropriator who noted, "The impression you give us is that somehow or another you have found a magic way of doing exactly the same thing that has been done years ago for two-thirds the cost." He did not support the cut.[26]

Some of the influence of budget processes on policymaking may be illustrated by briefly reviewing the federal response to the acquired immunodeficiency syndrome (AIDS) epidemic. At one level, AIDS is as unfair a test of the effectiveness of a decision process as the national health insurance battle would be. The federal government's difficulties with the supercharged politics of AIDS victimization and blame are also found within local and state governments. Even the most seemingly obvious failures (as with contamination of the blood supply) have occurred in very different political systems. A cure for AIDS continues to be as elusive as national health insurance.[27] Yet the pattern of use of budget institutions in shaping AIDS policy is still reasonably typical.

AIDS first emerged as a mysterious public health challenge, identified in the course of the routine public health surveillance: a mention in the Centers for Disease Control (CDC) *Morbidity and Mortality Weekly Report*.[28] CDC has a budget for investigating such matters; in the early years of the epidemic, no special action by Congress would have been expected in response.

As the mysterious disorder spread, however, Rep. Henry Waxman of Los Angeles, chairman of the authorizing subcommittee with oversight of public health matters, became convinced that the federal response had been inadequate. He held a one-day hearing in April 1982. Yet Waxman had no vehicle with which to force action, and it was not clear what should be done. The first direct action taken by Congress occurred in December 1982. Representative Edward R. Roybal, also from Los Angeles and a member of the Appropriations Subcommittee with jurisdiction over many of the major health programs, added $2.6 million to the CDC budget in a floor amendment to his Labor/HHS subcommittee's FY83 bill.[29] His chairman, William Natcher, accepted the amendment. This is rare, and it ordinarily means that the chairman and staff believe they did not know enough at the time they wrote the bill. During the Reagan years, the administration was continually demanding cuts in domestic spending, and the continuing resolution in which the FY83 Labor/HHS bill was included was no exception. In conference with the Senate, the House figure was reduced to $2.1 million.[30]

Roybal's initiative was the start of about five years in which the same story was repeated again and again, with institutional variations. AIDS was the exception that proved the appropriations rule—definitely a new problem that could justify new spending. A new and threatening disorder clearly justified, in the lingo of the process, a change in the program base. The administration wanted to cut or at least freeze domestic spending and therefore refused outright or cut agency requests for new spending within the executive budget process. Agency officials who testified to Congress on the need for new appropriations followed standard procedure and supported OMB's position. Either they said they had enough money, or they supported paying for AIDS allocations by cutting other parts of their agency budgets. The appropriators then had to figure out what was "needed" and how to provide it.

Of all the appropriations subcommittees, Labor/HHS, under the chairmanship of William Natcher, may have been most likely to follow the lead of agency officials in determining need. In health matters especially, the subcommittee tended to view NIH and CDC officials as nonpartisan experts. The Senate subcommittee was more willing to impose its own judgment but shared a desire to support the agencies. During this period the Republican leaders on those subcommittees, Rep. Silvio Conte and Senator Lowell Weicker, were as supportive as the Democrats. From the subcommittees' perspective, then, the problem was how to get the agencies to tell them what was "really needed."

Sometimes the administration would admit at the last minute that it needed more funds for AIDS, but claim they could be paid for if the appropriators would only allow a transfer from previously appropriated funds. Given the "right" numbers, the appropriators would then simply appropriate the extra money.[31] Sometimes the administration would refuse to forward a Public Health Service (PHS) request for more funds. In the most dramatic response, a memo from the assistant secretary for health, Dr. Edward Brandt, mysteriously found its way into congressional hands and was used to justify additions to the OMB request in 1984.[32]

By 1985 the extraction of the "right" number from the agencies had assumed a more common pattern. The administration was proposing budgets for the NIH in particular that did not resemble congressional preferences. Under such circumstances, appropriators ask administrators a question—"How much did you actually request?"—that is a matter of facts. OMB cannot forbid agencies to answer such inquiries. Appropriators would ask about AIDS just as they would about the

National Cancer Institute, and then fund something very close to the AIDS request.

Appropriators could do so only because the budget context allowed it. Although the Reagan administration was requesting large cuts in domestic spending, it also requested big increases in defense appropriations. The committee members' job was to stay within a target total for all spending, but they could do that by cutting the administration's defense figure and increasing the domestic allocation. The target was therefore not as tight as it would be in the 1990s. AIDS also still represented a relatively small program established in response to a new and frightening threat. There was overwhelming congressional support for action.[33] Funding scientific research on an unknown disorder could not be opposed by even the most gay-bashing conservatives.[34] The NIH in general has always been a congressional favorite, and the dynamic on AIDS funding simply replicated those for research on cancer and other dread diseases.[35]

But as the epidemic continued and AIDS policy and politics evolved, that dynamic would change. The agenda grew from epidemiology, research, and modest (and politically restrained) prevention efforts to include congressional debate about much more controversial issues— AIDS testing, a much larger public education effort, and the value conflicts inherent in those activities. Then as the program matured, AIDS evolved from a new emergency to an established problem, one that had to be compared with others in determining budget priorities.

In 1987, Congress was, as the *Congressional Quarterly Almanac* reported "Stalemated Over [the] AIDS Epidemic." One faction called for more public education and confidential testing, another for "routine testing of large groups . . . with names of those who tested positive for the virus [to be] reported to public-health authorities." Most members of Congress "were left sitting on the fence, if not hiding under it."[36] AIDS action had moved far beyond the appropriations arena. Whereas in earlier years the *Almanac*'s index included 3 or 4 lines on AIDS, in 1987 there were 27 separate categories.

From a budgetary perspective, Congress was not stalemated at all. It appropriated more than $900 million for FY88 within HHS for anti-AIDS activities—more than a $400 million increase. It also provided an extra $50 million in supplemental spending for FY87, including $30 million for purchase of the drug zidovudine (AZT) by the PHS for people with AIDS or who had tested positive for the human immunodeficiency virus (HIV) and who lacked insurance or medicaid coverage. But if the spending results reflected the same trend as before, for much the same reasons, the process involved much greater conflict. This was especially true regarding a Jesse Helms amendment to prevent education efforts that would "promote or encourage, directly or indirectly, homosexual sexual activities."[37] The same pattern of big increases but major controversy on nonbudget matters recurred in 1988.[38]

In subsequent years, Congress would pass new authorizations for special AIDS programs, such as the Ryan White Comprehensive AIDS Resources Emergency Act (PL 101-381). Federal spending in entitlement accounts would soar (outside the appropriations process) as medicaid became the AIDS payer of last resort. As the AIDS effort became routine, Congress would begin to worry about how it was being managed. This concern would lead to the creation of a separate Office of AIDS Research (OAR) within NIH in 1988, calls for an AIDS "czar," and in 1993 the granting of much greater authority to the OAR director within NIH. The 1993 NIH Revitalization Act (P.L. 103-43) gave the OAR director power to create an AIDS research plan, to submit a preferred budget directly to Congress (in addition to the administration's submission of its version), and to allocate the appropriation to the institutes within NIH.[39]

Throughout this evolution, the appropriators would behave like appropriators. They treated the Ryan White authorization as they treated most authorizations, and for the same reasons; by 1993, they had yet to approach full funding of that bill's programs.[40] Appropriators like to earmark projects to districts, but Natcher had long insisted that his bill was an exception. It continued to be so even when Senate appropriators fought hard for earmarks.[41] Yet appropriators still paid special attention to the effects allocations had on individual districts. As a result, one of their major concerns on Ryan White funding was which cities would qualify. Appropriators were especially concerned that new Ryan White funding not lead to cuts in established activities.[42] Before creation of the special "bypass budget" for OAR, the appropriators had already made a practice of getting the agencies' original requests on the record.[43]

By 1990 the appropriations committees had come to view AIDS as a high priority, but one large enough to be subject to tradeoffs. The NIH advocates within the committees worried that AIDS spending would constrain other research. The most fervent NIH advocate, Rep. Joe Early

(D.-Mass.), commented, "Five years ago we were not doing too much with AIDS or the [Human Genome Project]. Now funds are mushrooming for these two areas and are being taken from other places. . . . The rest of the research suffers."[44] Other members of Congress expressed that concern in the hearings. But they also joined with program administrators to build a record that emphasized the basic research value of AIDS work. This too reflected a programmatic evolution: the science of AIDS had opened new vistas in the study of immunology. In essence, AIDS research was redefined within NIH as a form of basic science with spinoffs in areas such as cancer and other diseases.[45] Early himself wanted more research money in general, not less for AIDS.

So did many other interest groups. But none of the health lobbies had the power to have much effect on the large-scale bargaining over budgetary caps that constrained appropriations from FY91 on. Within the appropriations process, advocates formed "302(b) coalitions" to ensure larger allocations to their favored subcommittees so there could be more for their programs. But these efforts too had little influence. The advocates were all fighting each other, all had reasonable cases, and the committee front office staff and chairmen were far more interested in what the subcommittee staff thought was "needed." Even a favorable allocation to Labor/HHS would succeed only in setting health advocates against education supporters (and, after the election of President Clinton, supporters of new job training initiatives). Presidents still tended to propose less for NIH than Congress would appropriate. Perhaps this is because they knew Congress would spend more, and presidents therefore view NIH as a cut they can make in their budgets without having to worry that it will actually be made.

Within the committees, appropriators worried, postured, decided, and punted back to the agencies their questions of relative priorities. Was AIDS receiving too much compared with cancer? The agencies generally said no.[46] Pediatric AIDS created a constituency whose claim could be doubted by no one, and both appropriators and non-appropriators pressed to ensure that enough was being spent on children. Others queried administrators about efforts to deal with the special problems of minorities (who were disproportionately diagnosed with AIDS). If truly controversial issues (such as what form educational materials should take) become attached to the appropriations, the committees try to settle the matter as peacefully as possible and get on with funding the programs.

The case of AIDS policymaking through appropriations is, in the end, typical. The exceptions prove the rules, and the rules are:

—Appropriators like to earmark spending according to districts. But they are not more prone to that activity in any meaningful way than anybody else in Congress; and when chairmen do not want to do it, they don't.

—Congress (including the appropriators) loves health research. It will be favored within any set of budget constraints, but the tightening of constraints in the late 1980s meant that allocations for such research began to grow more slowly.

—The appropriations process, even on AIDS matters, was relatively nonpartisan and agency oriented.

—The process favors the base, established programs over proposals for change. AIDS funding grew quickly because it was an addition; the committees refused to cut other spending to pay for it. The case for new funding to fight AIDS was exceptionally strong.

—Congress has the upper hand in appropriations, especially in setting priorities within a target. Health spending is, if anything, an extreme example of the power of Congress and the agencies vis-à-vis the president. That does not mean they always get their way—just most of the time.

—Appropriations must pass, and new activities often can be included under old authority. Stalemate is therefore less likely in the appropriations than the authorization process.

The election of 1994 is creating a different set of preferences within the Appropriations Committees. It will find them more willing to cut programs that were, after all, in a policy base constructed by a different ruling coalition. But the basic dynamics of the appropriations process will remain the same.[47]

Health Care Reform, 1993–94

Health care reform in 1993–94 involved a very different policy question: whether or not to expand the entitlement to health care significantly.[48] If Americans had been willing to pay potentially much higher taxes to provide universal coverage, there would have been no budget or political issue. But then there would have been no need for analysis. Given that taxes could not be automatically raised to pay for new commitments, there were four basic options.

First, the federal government could accept substantial risks of much higher spending (and increased deficits) than it would prefer. But it could not hide behind claims that there would be no deficit effect unless that were analytically defensible (that is, unless CBO agreed). Advocates could not propose even a small increase in the deficit because they would confront the paygo points of order, and legislation could then be blocked by forty-one votes in the Senate. It was unlikely that sixty senators would enthusiastically support any comprehensive reform that would actually control costs and guarantee coverage. Paygo meant that other Senators could use budget rectitude as an excuse for opposition. Therefore, even if the reform effort had remained popular, paygo rules would have been enforced.

Second, the federal government could create the entitlement but displace the risk of higher costs onto other parties. The most direct way to do this is to create a joint federal-state program with a capped federal contribution. The states could be given responsibility for cost control and, because their own budgets would be at stake, they would have sufficient incentive to try. (That is how the Canadian national government participates in health care finance.[49]) This option's failure to emerge in America is hard to explain.

Yet there are clear obstacles. The Canadian approach clearly makes health care a matter of government finance. But the Clinton administration's strategy was to keep insurance mainly in private (albeit heavily regulated) hands. In addition, a state-grant approach would move difficult questions of interstate transfers or equity to the forefront of the debate, where they might prove unresolvable. Within a framework of modest subsidies for private insurance, federal contributions made in addition to existing private collections might not be large enough to cause all states to participate. This problem can be solved only by moving away from private premiums to public finance, which brings everything back to square one.

The third option was to fail to provide (or fudge about providing) universal coverage. Coverage might be scheduled to expand over time as savings in existing programs are realized; consequently, if savings were not realized, coverage would not expand.[50] It might also be promised to all (or at least some more) Americans but would not be defined—a commission would decide later what benefits would be provided.[51] Following up on these options might have been politically safer for the Clinton administration, but it would have meant giving up on the basic goal of reform.

That left the fourth option: to limit federal fiscal exposure by proposing controls on national health care costs that CBO would believe. There was no point in sending up a proposal that would be out of order as written and that could be condemned for failing to meet a standard of responsible governance (that is, keeping to deficit targets). *Therefore, the congressional budget process, in the form of CBO scorekeeping, became a major factor in executive branch deliberations.*[52]

The most obvious effect was on the form cost control took in the Clinton administration's Health Security Act. The Democratic Leadership Council (DLC) faction within the party relied on "competition" alone to control costs. However, the Clinton administration proposed competition within an enforceable cap on national health care spending. That was in no way a breach of trust. Candidate Clinton's statement of health policy during the 1992 general election had specifically called for "annual budget targets."[53] Still, those statements had been made in campaign documents and speeches. The DLC faction could tell itself that, during policy drafting, the targets might become indicative rather than binding.

Given CBO's role, however, there was no way that the faction within the Clinton administration that disliked the budget caps could win. The caps were necessary because CBO would not give credence to estimates from managed competition advocates regarding how much money could be saved through their restructuring of the medical care marketplace. No responsible budget analyst could do so.

Budget analysts work from experience and through analogy. What have been the effects of similar changes under analogous situations? In estimating the effects of managed competition, CBO analysts first had to ask to what extent competition would move patients into systems of managed care. Second, they would have to estimate how much money various forms of managed care could save compared with the status quo. The data available could not allow for optimistic estimates, and CBO's judgments throughout the process would basically track those of other politically neutral analysts. Because much the same data would inform all analyses, some CBO studies had already been published, and there is enough communication among budget professionals that they tend to have some sense of what one another are thinking, Clinton administration designers knew that including an effective cap was imperative.[54]

The budget cap, unfortunately, was one of two provisions in the Clinton bill that made it anathema to the DLC faction. (The other, the employer mandate, was just as fundamental.) The Progressive Policy Institute issued a policy briefing condemning health care price controls as "A Cure Worse Than the Disease."[55] Under different circumstances, a Democratic president might have fudged the cost control issue. The president might have reasoned (probably correctly) that once the entitlement had been created, if the cost controls were ineffective, reluctant conservatives would have to accept budget caps or some other regulation. (Medicare had already provided an example of that dynamic.) But congressional budget procedures took away that option. President Clinton had to choose between paying for coverage or publicly abandoning it. Either way, he lost.[56]

Sponsors of other bills also had to deal with CBO scorekeeping. One of the subterranean battles in late 1993 involved Jim Cooper (D.-Tenn.), prime sponsor of the Managed Competition Act. Cooper attempted to get CBO to assume that the benefit package under that plan would be lean enough that the plan would pay for itself.[57] But in general, bill sponsors tended to avoid charges that their bills could not be financed by adopting other measures (such as some cross-subsidies in the Managed Competition Act) that, in protecting the budget, risked serious policy failures.[58]

Such strategies created CBO's dilemma. If CBO only issued opinions about the budgetary effects of proposals, it would seem to bless those that did the least and, in some cases, risked highly negative results. As Reischauer feared, CBO and the budget process would become weapons of use only to those who wished to prevent dealing with the health care policy problem. But CBO's standing to address other issues was shaky. No one expects CBO to attend only to the budgetary effects of proposals; its annual volume on reducing the deficit briefly summarizes the policy arguments against each option as guidance for those considering them.[59] Still, that is a far cry from providing a full-fledged policy analysis of each major health care proposal.

CBO's response may or may not have been strategic, but it was nonetheless coherent.[60] CBO reported both on budgetary effects and on effects related to budget issues: wider economic consequences and administrative concerns. Economic consequences included both total health care costs and the distribution of such costs. Administrative concerns included how each new system would be governed, whether the administrative steps required in a given proposal were practical, and how to account for each proposal's flows of funds.[61]

In its report on the Clinton administration's plan, CBO said a number of things that the administration did not want to hear. Where the administration estimated its plan would reduce the deficit by $38 billion in FY2000 and $59 billion in FY1995–FY2000, CBO estimated a $10 billion deficit increase in FY2000 and a combined deficit increase of $74 billion over the six-year period.[62] It raised a great many questions about the abilities of the government or other participants to gather the information needed to administer the Clinton plan's complex regulations.[63] CBO also advised that the spending of the plan's "health alliances" be considered part of federal spending.[64]

These reports, especially the deficit effect and the accounting, clearly embarrassed the administration. "With its decision that the Clinton plan's numbers don't add up," the *National Journal* reported, "the office gave ammunition aplenty to Republicans and proponents of other plans. And its treatment of the Clinton plan's mandated employer premium payments as part of the budget, rather than off-budget as the White House wanted, allows the GOP to roll out the T-word—a move that could pack big political punch."[65] Republican legislators had strongly pressured Reischauer to make the latter ruling. "I'm fully aware of the pressure that you're going to face," Senator Pete V. Domenici (R.-N. Mex.) remarked, "and we in the minority will surely not want to lessen that pressure."[66]

The detailed analysis in press reports could emphasize that, relative to the size of health care expenditure, the amount disagreed on between CBO and the administration was small. Yet the headlines of the articles that made these points carried a different message: "CBO Disputes Cost Estimates in Health Plan," or "A $133 Billion Difference of Opinion."[67] Reischauer let it be known that, in judging other plans, he would be more skeptical.[68] The text of the CBO report did not in fact "rule" that the administration's plan should be "on budget," and some Democrats claimed that how contributions were named should not matter.[69] Yet the report had to encourage the campaign to tar the Clinton plan as "big government," while CBO's disagreement had to add to an impression of administration dishonesty.

Despite various partisan suspicions, the best explanation of CBO's decisions is not that its leadership tried to balance partisan pressures but that CBO strove to follow norms of impartial analysis. The disagreements on spending were highly technical. The advice on budget classification was based on the understanding of CBO staff regarding precedents and on CBO's attempt to fit the case into those precedents. The Health Security Act was a square peg that CBO tried to fit into a round hole, and the classification advice was highly questionable.[70] That advice, however, fit the norms of budget staff: to follow precedent and to assume that advocates are looking for ways to do an end run around budget control, which should be blocked.[71]

Was CBO then simply a passive victim of the situation, hewing to analytic norms and thus torpedoing reform? Not quite. The broad sweep of CBO's analysis of the Clinton plan established a precedent that allowed it to perform similarly thorough analyses of the alternatives. The authors of the Managed Competition Act could not cry foul about CBO's criticism of that plan's administrative perversities—they had accepted the legitimacy of the broad analysis of the Health Security Act. If CBO had had enough time to analyze all the bills, its analysis might well have shown that the Health Security Act had far fewer weaknesses than those of the alternatives.[72]

But CBO was unable to transform its negative role as budget scorekeeper into a positive one as a source of analysis that would inform the debate and thereby (for believers in health care reform) make comprehensive reform more likely. Three reasons for this are most evident.

First, there were too many plans for CBO to analyze. Those whose plans escaped a CBO report—especially Senator John S. Chafee and his cosponsors—got a free ride: they could claim to be for a reasonable alternative without being subject to the same criticism. Because CBO had to make whichever plan seemed highest on the agenda its highest priority,[73] *advocates of minority positions avoided criticism, while the plans that seemed to have the most chance to pass attracted authoritative criticism from a nonpartisan and prestigious analyst.*

Second, the messages about the budget had to get more attention than warnings about administrative problems or destabilized insurance markets. Policy wonks might get the point of other CBO criticisms, but hardly anyone else would.

Third, the effect of criticizing a number of plans was not to inform comparison among them, but to weaken them all relative to the status quo.

The fervent advocates of any given plan would not change their minds in light of CBO's critiques; instead, they would merely dismiss the analysis as in some way biased. Thus Senator David Durenberger, a managed competition crusader, claimed that CBO Director Reischauer's estimates were not dynamic enough. "We're talking about changing behavior," Durenberger proclaimed, stating that Reischauer had "never met a medical market."[74] The public was not in a position to judge, and all the politicians needed was to be able to say they were for health care reform, but not one of those terrible other plans. As a result, CBO's analyses did not encourage compromise among advocates, whereas those reports could only make those who were neutral feel skeptical about doing anything at all.

Budget processes in general must be biased against creation of new government commitments. One point of any budget process must be to force attention to costs, an embarrassing issue that program advocates normally would prefer to avoid. The federal budget process of 1993–94 included particularly stringent procedures to force that attention—more stringent than any others in the history of the federal government.

In expanding the grounds of its analysis beyond purely budgetary scorekeeping, CBO's leaders tried to reduce the fiscalization of the policy debate. Yet under the circumstances, the grounds on which they could do other analyses, such as administrative complexity and uncertainty, only made the bills look worse.

None of these effects would have been significant if the public had been willing to pay the taxes to pay for care. Tax-based systems are much more administratively simple, pose far fewer regulatory complications, and can avoid deficits by setting the tax at the right level. Budget procedures were not enough, therefore, to prevent health care reform. If the political system were structured to allow only one or two alternatives, so that a debate comparing them were possible, CBO's more extensive analysis might have facilitated choice.

That is not necessarily grounds to condemn the budget process. The process does serve other values that many Americans consider very important. The policy disagreements were so deep and bitter that no one should believe the chance for success was ever great. It only seemed so compared with other times. Perhaps most important of all, the budget rules themselves reflect opinion—the panic about budget deficits. The power of that fear is even more important than the rules.

The Future

This book has been published within a changed world: a Republican Congress, for the first time in forty years.

The behavior of CBO scorekeepers under the new regime is not yet known. A new CBO director has been appointed, but what her values are and how she responds to pressures to favor the new majority's priorities will only be revealed over time.

We can be sure, however, that those in charge of the budget institutions will have Republican priorities, seeking to cut taxes and federal spending. Internal disputes over the priority of tax cuts versus deficit reduction do not matter from the standpoint of health care policy. Either way, health care spending is on the chopping block.

The fate of each particular program will depend partly on its own level of support and partly on the ways that the budgetary process provides opportunities for the new majority to force reductions yet avoid blame. In this context the first thing to note is that budget resolutions can fudge the details a bit, as expressed in the immortal words of former House Minority Leader Robert Michel as he sought votes for Reagan's 1981 plan: "Geeminnie Christmas! When are you guys going to recognize that this is only a budget resolution? It doesn't cut anything! It's all assumptions! If you've got problems, write 'em down and send 'em to me. We'll take care of them later!"[75]

Second, the politically best way to cut spending is to force someone else to make the necessary proposals. Therefore, Congress wants to force the president to make as many proposals as it can. From Congress's perspective, that's the point of the president's budget. Third, of course, Republicans will prefer to cut programs that serve Democrats more than Republicans. Finally, the Republicans will probably view Clinton's budget policies as, by definition, a liberal base from which they must be able to cut.

Given these guidelines, the budget process suggests certain strategies. Discretionary spending at the end of 1994 was defined by caps frozen at about $547 billion through FY98. A budget resolution calling for reconciliation to lower those caps, probably in stages, seemed inevitable. For the first year, the new majority probably will be able to think of enough spending reductions that it really wants to perform. In subsequent years, the president will be required to make proposals to meet the targets and will therefore get much of the blame.

If this analysis is correct, we can expect medical research, which is popular with Republicans as well as Democrats, to be relatively protected for the most part in the first year. Other health care programs—especially any that involve federal payments for activities that states might be deemed capable of undertaking (such as CDC surveillance)—would be seriously threatened. In subsequent years, the squeeze should be so severe as to even lead to cuts (in real terms at least) in NIH, but much larger cuts in some other programs (such as personnel for meat inspection).

On the entitlement side, the new Congress may consider cutting programs for poor people over slashing middle-class programs. On the health care front, the simplest approach would be to cap the federal contribution to medicaid and claim that states, given more flexibility to manage medicaid patients' care, will be able to save enough to avoid harm to their own budgets. Governors may not like this. But many of them have asserted that they could save money if given flexibility, and cutting medicaid has fewest political costs for a Republican Congress, so some such cap is at least an obvious tactic.

Any entitlement changes as well as new discretionary caps would be part of a reconciliation bill, thereby avoiding any Senate filibuster and providing the spending cuts necessary to pay for a tax cut and avoid the paygo points of order.[76] Medicare cuts could also be included in that package. Yet the new majority's basic problem will be how to make sure that the president signs the tax cut and reconciliation bill, which means they will want the bill to be as popular as possible. Medicare cuts might give the administration the excuse it needs to veto.

If larger spending cuts are needed than can be provided from discretionary caps and slashing programs for poor people, the Congress is therefore most likely to enact some form of entitlement cap. It is hard to design such a cap sensibly. If it includes specific automatic cuts, then it will be opposed by the groups targeted by that threat. The alternative is to give the president wide discretion or require that a proposal be made that would be voted on by Congress. This latter strategy seems more promising, because (like the discretionary caps), it would force the Democratic president to propose cuts and thereby lose the ability to attack the Republican Congress for making them. The most significant obstacle to this entitlement cap maneuver would be if CBO did not believe the savings.

Once any set of caps is in place, *removing them will be subject to the paygo points of order.* Forty senators could block change. Even a new

Democratic president with a Democratic majority in 1997 might not be able to reverse the constraints—or, at the least, would have to pay the political price of raising taxes to do so.[77]

If this analysis is correct, medicaid and discretionary programs are in trouble no matter what. Reconciliation provides a vehicle to enact cuts that might otherwise be filibustered. But the bigger problem is political: the president could veto the bill, but only if he wanted to seem to favor poor Americans over their middle-class brethren. The problem is budget preferences more than budget process.

The fate of medicare is harder to predict. Will CBO give credit for caps, thereby providing cover to the new majority by forcing the president to propose medicare cuts? If the budget can be used to hide or displace blame for the effects of budget cuts, they can be made much more easily. The enactment of broad caps on discretionary spending already has shown the attractiveness of such strategies. Even the Clinton administration in its FY96 budget proposed extending a freeze on discretionary spending, a tactic that must squeeze appropriated health programs but does not admit as much. In May 1995, it remained to be seen whether either the new CBO director or a clever maneuver would help the Republican Congress overcome public objections to slashing medicare.

Chapter 4

How Health Policy Information is Used in Congress

Mark A. Peterson

THE SUMMER OF 1991 brought one of the now ubiquitous examples of how the technical complexities of modern policymaking have transformed the way Congress makes decisions. In the late 1980s, during the second stage of reforming how the medicare program pays providers for their services, Congress enacted a new fee schedule for reimbursing physicians as part of omnibus budget legislation. No longer were physicians to be compensated on the basis of their "customary, prevailing, and reasonable rates." Instead, payment for the various treatments doctors administer would be based on an elaborately developed resource-based, relative-value scale (RBRVS).

The RBRVS related all treatments to one another based on the time, cognitive requirements, and supporting resources associated with them. This scale, when multiplied by a specified dollar conversion

This chapter derives from a health care policymaking project made possible by the generous support and activities of many institutions and individuals. My appreciation is extended to the American Political Science Association Congressional Fellowship Program; Senator Tom Daschle, as well as Rima Cohen and Peter Rouse of his staff; Thomas Mann and the Governmental Studies Program at the Brookings Institution, where I was a guest scholar; and the Faculty Aide Program and the William F. Milton Fund at Harvard University, along with the Dirksen Congressional Leadership Center, the Caterpillar Foundation, and the Graduate School of Public and International Affairs at the University of Pittsburgh, which provided financial assistance. Special thanks are owed Ranjan Chaudhuri, a most dedicated research assistant, for gathering the information about congressional support agencies.

factor, would yield payment rates for each treatment in a given year. The new payment methodology would raise reimbursements for primary care services while reducing the rates associated with some specialties. With the addition of a feature called volume performance standards, the RBRVS would also bring greater budgetary oversight to physician payment under medicare. Organized medicine had determined that cooperating with these changes was in its interest; the American Medical Association worked closely with Congress and the Health Care Financing Administration (HCFA) to design the new system.[1]

Implementation was scheduled for January 1, 1992. On June 5, 1991, HCFA announced the Notice of Proposed Rulemaking (NPRM), its proposed regulations for implementing RBRVS, and the sparks began to fly. The final legislation enacting the new medicare fee schedule, OBRA 1989, specified that it was to be budget neutral for the first year—the introduction of RBRVS would not change overall medicare expenditures for physicians in FY1992. But HCFA was concerned that reduced reimbursements had always motivated physicians to increase their volume of work—a behavioral adjustment that would counter some of the cost-saving potential of reduced rates. Because many reimbursement rates were to be cut under RBRVS, the agency expected doctors performing those services to do more of them, thereby increasing the program's costs. To maintain budget neutrality, HCFA concluded that the conversion factor for the first year had to be cut enough (3 percent) to compensate for an expected 50 percent behavioral offset. Physicians were outraged, believing that the Bush administration was using the implementation of the medicare fee schedule as a hidden strategy for further budget reductions. This would have violated both the dictates of the law and the spirit of cooperation that had generated the new payment methodology.

What was Congress to do? On the one hand, physician associations geared up a massive lobbying campaign to challenge the implementation rules proposed by HCFA. What physicians want has traditionally been given a good deal of credence on Capitol Hill, and this expression of their collective outrage could not be easily ignored. In addition, as so often happens during periods of divided government, the Democratic majorities in the House and Senate had reason to be suspicious of the analysis generated by an agency directed by Republican presidential appointees. Perhaps there was an empirical basis for the complaints the doctors made. On the other hand, the issue was so complicated and posed such serious financial implications that it was difficult for Congress to judge who was right. A few years earlier, it might have been impossible to know, but this Congress had a new instrument to aid its decisionmaking. As part of the Consolidated Omnibus Budget Reconciliation Act of 1985, Congress had established the Physician Payment Review Commission (PPRC) to assist it and the Department of Health and Human Services in the creation and oversight of fee schedules. The PPRC—composed of physicians, health economists, and specialists in employee benefits, public health, and a variety of health-related fields, and supported by a staff of professional health care specialists—thus gave Congress the capacity to assess HCFA's conclusions independently and analytically.[2]

In its 1991 *Annual Report to Congress*, the PPRC identified two core problems with the HCFA calculations. These findings were based on a review of the extant literature in the field, the PPRC's own multivariate statistical analysis of medicare data, and computer simulation models of physicians' revenues that would probably be generated by different fee adjustments.[3] First, the new medicare fee schedule included both decreases and increases in fees. Would the latter result in some physicians performing fewer services, thus lowering costs in those areas? The answer was ambiguous; only one study existed that made any effort to determine the effects of elevated rates, and it used 1970s data from a single state. Second, although the general estimate of a 50 percent behavioral offset could be analytically supported in the aggregate, there was considerable variation by specialty and treatment. An across-the-board reduction in the conversion factor would not be well targeted to actual behavioral patterns. The PPRC concluded:

> The Commission recommends that a volume offset amounting to a 1 percent [instead of HCFA's proposed 3 percent] reduction in fees be included in the 1992 budget-neutrality calculation. Analysis of expenditure changes suggests that some volume response is likely. However, the size of the fee changes in 1992, the presence of large increases in fees, and the potential for changes in assignment behavior all add uncertainty to the actual 1992 offset. In this situation, it seems sensible to use a lower figure than that suggested by the 50% offset assumption. The smaller offset recommended here provides some protection against overly high Medicare outlays without un-

duly penalizing physicians. Additional changes in volume will eventually be dealt with through the VPS [volume performance standards].[4]

The PPRC granted Congress analytical capacity that it otherwise would not have had to put some leverage on HCFA in drafting the final rules for implementation. In the House, for example, legislation that would prohibit HCFA from decreasing the conversion factor due to any behavioral adjustments attracted cosponsorship from more than half the body. Given weight by the PPRC's assessment, congressional objections had to be viewed as more than overly sensitive responsiveness to special interest grumbling, an all too present feature of the legislative process. Ultimately, HCFA proceeded with an adjustment, but not of the magnitude originally indicated (although still higher than the PPRC recommended).[5]

In 1965, Congress had enacted the original medicare and medicaid programs—which have since become the largest publicly financed health insurance system in the world—with virtually no internal institutional capacity to evaluate their effects and little external expertise to call on. As Henry Aaron has noted, social science analyses of the Great Society period tended to *follow* the implementation of policies rather than presage their consequences.[6] In health care policy, these rapidly growing federal forays into financing services helped spawn health services research and the analytical techniques that play such a significant role in judging today's policy options.[7] Leaps of faith are no longer possible, nor are they necessary.

Just how far does this information revolution and the demands for it extend in congressional policymaking? Reforming the health care system, which constitutes one-seventh of the U.S. economy and is a leading employer in the private sector, is one of the most complex policy ambitions imaginable. But it is not the only policy question for which legislative judgments call for massive amounts of information. Modern postindustrial economies and the politics associated with them put previously unheard-of demands on political institutions. The externalities of private action, such as industrial pollution, are more apparent than ever and invite a public response; collective goods like public health emerge as enduring political issues; and the trade-offs made while dealing with prevailing social and economic challenges may result in zero-sum resolution and conflict.[8]

What kinds of information are required to design and assess policy initiatives in this setting? How can anyone be certain that information in this extraordinarily tangled environment of substantive and political issues is both workable and legitimate? Is the story about reformulating physician reimbursement and PPRC an anomaly, or is it representative of important ways in which Congress has changed, institutionally and procedurally, over the past two decades? Does Congress get the information that it needs, and if so, do its members actually use this information to deliberate rationally about policy? In the end, has Congress been knowledgeable about the policy decisions it must make? Finally, what are the implications of the latest round of institutional reforms advocated by the new Republican majority in Congress?

In this chapter, I explore these issues primarily in the context of the recent debate over national health care reform. Congress as an institution has recently been well poised to generate and exploit a vast range of informational resources. This has sometimes been accomplished quite ably, and even in ways potentially superior to the efforts of presidents and executive officials. But all information systems depend not only their design but also on the incentives for their use. Our national legislature, quite naturally, remains a decidedly political institution. The latest round of the health care debate revealed just how much information—even sophisticated policy analysis—is subordinate to far more powerful political purposes. Republican efforts to trim congressional excesses by reducing Congress's own analytic capabilities will likely only enhance the power of politics over information.

Coping with Uncertainty

From the perspective of a member of Congress, each decision about a piece of legislation introduces two potentially threatening sources of uncertainty: the political and the programmatic.[9] In a legislature with comparatively weak party organization (at least in contrast with the Westminster model of parliamentary government) and significant electoral independence (both among its members and from presidential politics), reliance on cues from party leaders or the executive branch is insufficient.

Before casting a vote, therefore, members of Congress must first come to relatively autonomous, knowledgeable conclusions about how their actions will be perceived and interpreted by those in the political arena. These are the individuals who can influence or directly affect the support legislators receive within their electorates, among core constituencies, or inside the Washington community. Members of Congress also want to arrive at what Sir Geoffrey Vickers termed "instrumental judgment"—knowledge that permits assessment of the effects that different legislative options are likely to have on actual policy outcomes, such as availability and affordability of health care services.[10]

I consider it reasonable to presume that many members of Congress are motivated by a commitment to improving the quality of life of their constituents and the public in general. They want to be able to predict which policy approaches will work and which won't. Even if legislators are only "single-minded seekers of reelection," however, they are compelled to try to resolve programmatic uncertainty. Their constituents make electoral decisions based on factors such as how government action has affected the state of the economy, the quality of the schools, or the fairness of the health care financing system. Legislators will want to understand the precise linkages between the policy choices they make and the actual effects of enacted laws.[11] Of course, the broader, and more complex the policy issue being addressed, the greater the difficulty (especially for the nonspecialist) in coming to sound programmatic conclusions.[12] Although the motivation may or may not be political, for such a judgment to be beneficial to any legislator, it must be grounded in the use of information free of preemptive bias.

Members of Congress intent on crafting policy options of their own (or simply wishing to choose among those introduced by others that minimize their own political and programmatic uncertainty) need to develop three distinct types of knowledge, built on the various information streams that enter the congressional arena.

ORDINARY KNOWLEDGE. To guard against being swayed by dry abstractions that risk distancing them from their electoral base and the sentiments of the average citizen, legislators must tap into their reservoir of *ordinary knowledge*, "the perspective and attitude formed through everyday observation and interaction."[13] This flows from implicit popular assumptions about individual motives, fairness, and government capabilities and represents a broad understanding of how the world works and how events can be explained. Ordinary knowledge is "unsystematic and biased" and thus "highly fallible."[14] Based more on gut instinct than on reasoning, it nonetheless serves as a reality check and exploits common sense in judging the verisimilitude of complex policy plans. It also gives the policymaker a way to anticipate how the general public would understand and react to various policy formulations. Successful innovations are rarely those that run counter to what strikes people as sensible or reasonable.

During the 102d Congress, for example, Senator Jesse Helms (R.-N.C.) used Senate consideration of a variety of appropriations bills to pursue amendments that would have altered federal policy towards those infected with the human immunodeficiency virus (HIV), the virus that causes acquired immunodeficiency syndrome (AIDS). One such amendment stipulated that health care providers who were HIV positive and who conducted invasive procedures with patients without the patients' knowledge could be subject to substantial fines and imprisonment. Despite pleas from various knowledgeable sources (including Dr. William Roper, the Bush administration's director of the Centers for Disease Control) based on existing epidemiological evidence, and a strenuous countercampaign launched by Senator Ted Kennedy (D.-Mass.) and his staff, the Helms amendment passed the Senate overwhelmingly. With regard to AIDS, fears based on ordinary knowledge could overpower guidance from the scientific community. One senator who (surprisingly) voted in favor of the Helms amendment, against the strenuous objections of his staff and of "expert" advice, had highly personal reasons associated with his own ordinary knowledge: a family member was about to enter the hospital for major surgery. For someone confronting this situation, the precautions in the Helms amendment just seemed to make sense. That is how most senators thought their constituents would react politically.[15]

DISTRIBUTIONAL KNOWLEDGE. No elected official—either the advocates of policy change or the protectors of their own electoral self-interest—can ignore the consequences that policy options could have on affected interests. They need to cultivate *distributional knowledge*, what David Price calls "particularistic knowledge" that "comprises the needs and interests of particular groups and communities [and] incorporates knowledge about the effects of existing and prospective policies on those groups and communities."[16] This requires garnering information about both the impact of the policy options and the intensity of the response to them from the relevant organized (and presently unorganized) interests, stakeholders, and constituencies. This is especially true when there are distinct and identifiable winners and losers. Having such knowledge in and of itself does not suggest that policy alternatives reflect the distribution of group influence, but it is instrumental in building coalitions and balancing policy effectiveness with the perceived legitimacy of government action.

The final stage of reforming how medicare paid providers involved incorporating reimbursements to hospitals for capital costs (which had previously been retrospective) into the new prospective payment system (PPS) implemented in the mid-1980s to finance the operational side of hospital care. Instead of retrospectively reimbursing hospitals for the claimed costs associated with treating a medicare patient (the procedure introduced when medicare was enacted), under PPS a hospital prospectively receives a fixed payment for the bundle of treatments generally associated with the particular diagnosis related group (DRG) in which a patient is coded.

Because of the enormous technical complexities and political divisiveness associated with the issue, payments for capital costs were originally excluded from PPS.[17] In the Omnibus Reconciliation Act of 1987, however, Congress specified that the executive branch would have to find a way to include capital costs in PPS by FY1992. When the HCFA responded with its proposed plan in 1991, numerous distributional concerns were raised. The definition of "new" capital, the structure of the transition rules, and the nature of the data used to calculate hospital costs had highly differential implications for hospitals. These depended on various factors: how far along they were in their schedules for current capital projects, how many beds they had, what their markets and patient mixes were, and whether they were located in urban or rural settings.

The American Hospital Association (AHA), among others, made computer software available to hospital administrators that helped them calculate the impact of the proposed regulations on their individual institutions. Members of Congress and their staffs received a considerable amount of mail and many visits from representatives of constituent hospitals and trade associations. The distributional consequences of PPS (especially the negative ones) were forcefully stated. Because the success of this reform, like the others in medicare, depended on overall provider support and legitimacy within the hospital industry, Congress paid close attention to these distributional effects. The Senate, which "overrepresents" states with smaller populations, was especially attuned to geographic interests.[18]

POLICY-ANALYTIC KNOWLEDGE. As the preceding illustration implies, reducing programmatic uncertainty requires *policy-analytic knowledge*, "policy research [that involves] systematic inquiry, typically using the tools of analysis, into the objectives and effects of government programs." Allen Schick notes that "policy research strives for objectivity. . . . [It] generally values data that can be expressed statistically and that are free of bias or subjectivity."[19] This often involves the search for conceptually and empirically derived lessons from past experience or from other settings, such as the states and other nations.[20] These attributes, at least as they are formally expressed, pose policy-analytic knowledge as quite the opposite of ordinary subjective knowledge. Instead of common sense or intuition, it relies on what Karl Popper terms "the method of science," with "bold conjectures and ingenious and severe attempts to refute them" based on the principles of "testability, falsification, tentativity, and the importance of methods over results."[21]

There are three types of research that generate policy-analytic knowledge in policymaking.[22] The most common, documentation, involves "gathering, cataloging, and correlating facts that depict the state of the world." Analysis reveals "what does and does not work and explain[s] why." Prescription is least likely to be compelling, but the "unveiling of an appealing strategic model . . . can be one of the most significant contributions of research to policy."[23] Whichever type of research advances the policy-analytic knowledge of representatives and senators, it gives them the capacity to mitigate programmatic uncertainty. In the process, they may reconsider assumptions (especially those associated with ordinary knowledge) and check the credibility of positions articulated by interests whose orientations are reflective of distributional knowledge.

Without the use of highly sophisticated studies of physician practices and the cognitive component involved in treatment delivery (such as those conducted by Dr. William Hsiao at the Harvard School of Public Health) or the program evaluations done of existing PPSs for hospitals (such as New Jersey's), Congress quite simply would not have been able to enact the physician and hospital reimbursement reforms of the 1980s.[24] The programmatic uncertainties would have been too overwhelming. It is also unlikely that health care reform would have risen so high on the agenda during the early 1990s without comparative trend analyses of international health care expenditure data document-ing just how expensive the U.S. system is relative to its economic com-petitors.

Ordinary knowledge, distributional knowledge, and policy-analytic knowledge rely on quite different types of information and represent sometimes contradictory dimensions of a policy problem and its possi-ble solutions. In a system of representative government, however, it is difficult to imagine Congress drafting and enacting public policy that retains its legitimacy and that also has a fair chance of fulfilling its stated objectives unless there is some synthesis of these three categories of knowledge.

Availability of Information

The need to mitigate political and programmatic uncertainty among members of Congress suggests why a market for such information has emerged on Capitol Hill. The generic demand for information is appar-ent; but what of the supply? In the recent health care reform debate, did members of Congress, individually and collectively, have access to the information they needed to acquire ordinary, distributional, and policy-analytic knowledge?

Numerous potential sources of information for legislators address particular sorts of uncertainty, whereas others are more diverse in their contributions. Table 4-1, which combines the dimensions of the two categories of uncertainty and the three types of knowledge, offers gen-eral examples of various entities and activities that could generate the information those in Congress need to become knowledgeable.

It should come as no surprise that Congress is an institution well primed to acquire ordinary knowledge relevant to both political and programmatic uncertainty. The frequent travel back to the district or state, the numerous town meetings, the innumerable letters and phone calls from constituents prompting intensive constituency service, and the near-permanent campaign all provide forums and opportunities for representatives and senators to derive fairly precise impressions of what people want politically and what government involvement they think makes sense. Especially when the issues are salient to the public, legislators are likely to be most responsive to the ways in which ordi-

TABLE 4-1. *Examples of Sources of Information for Members of Congress*

Nature of uncertainty	Type of knowledge		
	Ordinary	*Distributional*	*Policy-analytic*
Political	Personal experience Home travel Letters, calls	Lobbyists Political action committees Political advisers	Opinion surveys

Programmatic	Personal experience
	Home travel
	Letters, calls
	Media
		Lobbyists
		Interest group
		  research
		Constituents
			Executive agencies
			Interest group
			  research
			Consulting firms
			Specialists
			Think tanks
			Universities
			Congressional
			  agencies:
			CBO, GAO, OTA,
			CRS, ProPac,
			PPRC, Joint Tax

nary people think.[25] In addition, members of Congress, as both politicians and policymakers, also naturally develop personal perspectives about politics and policy nurtured by their own day-to-day experiences. Despite all the recent attacks on Congress for being out of touch, few members are actually much removed from ordinary knowledge, however they choose to respond to it.

Although comparative data across issues and over time are not available, there is every reason to believe that representatives and senators interacted with their constituents in myriad forums on health care reform as much as any Congress has on any other issue. During the 102d and 103d Congresses, health care reform was on the agenda at many open-door meetings (some solely on that topic) and generated innumerable letters and phone calls. As one might expect of ordinary knowledge, however, health care reform was also subject to enormous confusion, misunderstanding, and distortion by the public. This resulted in something much closer to what Daniel Yankelovich calls "mass opinion," marked by "inconsistency, volatility, and nonresponsibility," rather than "public judgment," with the opposite attributes.[26] With respect to health care, most people "haven't thought through all the consequences of their opinions."[27] A recent study commissioned by the National Institutes of Health found that only one-fifth of Americans had adequate information about scientific terms and procedures; nearly two-thirds wanted to be well informed about health matters, but less than one-third thought they were.[28] In this context, it is not surprising that even in October 1993 only about one-fifth of the public or less understood the meaning of managed competition or health alliances, or were even knowledgeable about health care reform in more general terms. Such a lack of understanding breeds a certain mercurialness. Witness President Clinton, who watched support for his plan (as measured in the *Washington Post*-ABC News poll) fall from 67 percent when the plan was announced in September 1993 to 44 percent five months later.[29]

The point of this discussion is not to cast judgment on the quality of public opinion but rather to note what it communicated to elected representatives regarding ordinary knowledge about this terribly complex subject.[30] Policy legitimacy—a program's acceptability to the public—is always of concern in a representative system and is probably essential to successful implementation, and the actual experiences of constituents can both motivate and inform policy debate. Yet what matters most to elected officials is what ordinary knowledge reveals about the likely political consequences of their choices.[31] That gets reinforced by the information provided to legislators by trusted political advisers, as well as by representatives of important organized interests in the home districts and strategists for political action committees who study the political landscape of various constituencies.

In addition, with regard to any issue, Congress is particularly well equipped to receive whatever information about political and policy implications organized interests wish to disseminate. During the health care debate, few in Congress lacked perspective on the distributional consequences of various reform options, especially as interpreted by stakeholder groups. Just as Ira Magaziner, Hillary Rodham Clinton, and other members of the President's Health Care Reform Task Force met on hundreds of occasions with group representatives, so, too, the schedules of most Hill staffers and the legislators themselves were filled from 1990 on. These meetings included discussions of health care reform issues, individual appointments with lobbyists, informal coalitions, or get-togethers with constituent members of the associations in Washington for their annual legislative conferences. Because of the salience of the emerging reform debate, lobbyists seized almost any opportunity to exchange intelligence and send signals. For example, during a 1991 meeting on other issues with Senator Tom Daschle's staff and lobbyists for a variety of small business associations, the representative of the National Federation of Independent Businesses (NFIB) asked us in casual conversation whether the senator was considering cosponsoring Majority Leader George Mitchell's play-or-pay health care reform initiative. In the course of the conversation, she made it clear that regardless of NFIB's respect for Daschle, the moment he endorsed anything resembling an employer mandate, several thousand pieces of mail would go out from NFIB to all its member small businesses in his home state of South Dakota. Thousands of similar exchanges were held throughout Capitol Hill over the course of the reform debate.

Of course, the accretion among members of Congress of both ordinary and distributional knowledge intended to alleviate political and policy uncertainty did not depend solely on anecdotal information from constituents and lobbyists. Modern analytical techniques played an important role in assembling and presenting information far more persuasively. The almost daily national opinion polling by various media outlets and survey research firms, as well as public testimony at congressional hearings by opinion experts, let members of Congress know what the sentiments of the nation's voters were at any given moment, as interpreted by the pollsters. As a result, legislators gained perspective on the apparent political viability of different reform options. In addition, prominent leaders in developing legislative initiatives (such as Pete Stark, then chairman of the Health Subcommittee of Ways and Means) received tailored, detailed analyses of public opinion trends on health care from prominent analysts in the field, such as Robert Blendon of Harvard University's School of Public Health.[32]

Those interests with a particular stake in reform tracked the public mood as well. The American Association of Retired Persons (AARP) hired The Daniel Yankelovich Group to conduct sophisticated studies of public opinion based on survey instruments and focus groups.[33] The Employee Benefits Research Institute, funded by businesses concerned about effects on employee benefits, presented "The EBRI Poll" conducted by Gallup.[34] The Health Insurance Association of America (HIAA) assessed public opinion by commissioning its own polls. It actually sought to transform congressional impressions of constituent concerns by broadcasting the infamous "Harry and Louise" advertisements in targeted areas, thus raising questions about the Clinton health care reform plan.[35] Some polls even surveyed the attitudes of other influential stakeholders—for example, the Metropolitan Life Insurance Company, which hired Louis Harris and Associates to produce "Trade-Offs and Choices: Health Policy Options for the 1990s."[36]

The distributional consequences of possible reform options (either directly stated or implied) were also widely analyzed by affected groups, and their interpretations were communicated to Congress. Studies were produced by (among numerous others) NFIB, EBRI, and the employer Partnership on Health Care and Employment, which commissioned the Consad Research Corporation to generate the report "Jobs at Risk."[37] These studies assessed the potential negative impact on jobs and employment of employer mandates, including the mechanism by which most insurance coverage would be financed in the early pay-or-play schemes, President Clinton's Health Security Act, or Senator Mitchell's last initiative introduced during the summer 1994 floor debate. The tobacco industry provided estimates of the jobs that would be lost because of the proposed increase in levies on tobacco, a commonly suggested method of raising federal funds to expand insurance coverage. Employing the analytic capabilities of Lewin/ICF (now Lewin/VHI), a major Washington health care consulting firm, the Federation of American Health Systems, which represents for-profit hospitals, assessed the impact of various types of regulation on hospital finances.[38] The American Society of Internal Medicine, a physicians group, provided a detailed description of "the hassle factor"—the administrative burdens of the existing system—that affects doctors and patients.[39] These are just a few examples of the scores of sometimes slick, often expensive, and typically data-dense analyses sponsored by groups concerned about how they would be affected by reform.

What is new about the grasp Congress has on ordinary and distributional knowledge is the frequency and level of sophistication at which such knowledge is generated. Thirty years ago, almost no one had the resources to take the pulse of the American public (or specialized segments of it) on a frequent basis. Nor had focus groups yet been effectively exploited to test and reinforce messages put forth by proponents or opponents of the many approaches to reform. Further, although (as Tocqueville reminded us) American society has always been prone to association, never before have so many varied interests been formally represented in Washington.[40] The change in the distribution of group types, with more sustained mobilization of cause-oriented citizen organizations, has changed the character of many policy arenas quite dramatically.[41] The realm of health care reform is no exception. There has been an explosion of groups representing diverse segments of the health care market as well as both nonprofit-sector associations and citizen organizations joining many of the long-established labor unions, all prepared to challenge the assumptions and analyses of many other stakeholders.[42] For every report, newsletter, fax, or videotape sent to members of Congress by the American Medical Association (AMA), the American Hospital Association (AHA), HIAA, NFIB, and all the other representatives of medicine, insurance, and business, there was a corresponding flood from the AARP, the National Council of Senior Citizens (NCSC), the Consumers Union, Citizen Action, Families USA, the National Association of Social Workers (NASW), Physicians for a National Health Plan (PNHP), Public Citizen, the Communication Workers of America (CWA), and United Auto Workers (UAW), as well as their compatriots among consumer groups, progressive health care providers, liberal religious coalitions, and labor organizations. The data could not be taken simply at face value. But during the last health care reform debate, Congress was certainly not kept in the dark about what ordinary people thought or how organized or geographic constituencies would be affected.

A second change from thirty years ago, however, transformed far more as Congress tackled the highly complex and momentous issue of health care reform. As has been mentioned, health services research was not sufficiently developed to have much impact on congressional thinking about the proposals that became medicare and medicaid. Capitol Hill had to rely on more rudimentary information from organized interests, the executive branch (which was also relatively limited in its ability to analyze health issues), and a few academic specialists. It had almost no capacity to generate policy-analytic data and analysis on its own or to fairly judge information from external sources. Beginning in the early 1970s, however, an analytical revolution was under way both off and on the Hill. This gave Congress the potential to be the best informed and most knowledgeable legislature in the world, and one almost akin to the public bureaucracy in this regard.[43]

Of course, Congress always had access to the increasingly sophisticated analyses generated in or supported by executive agencies. These included the Department of Health and Human Services, the Office of

Health Planning and Evaluation, HCFA (which oversees the management of medicare and medicaid), and the Agency for Health Care Policy and Research, in addition to the Office of Management and Budget (OMB) and the Department of the Treasury. Armed with computerized simulation models of the health care sector and the U.S. economy, private consulting firms provided both interest groups and members of Congress with the means to assess the impact of various plans, including financing schemes and benefits packages. Senator Bob Kerrey, for example, contracted with Lewin/ICF to analyze the major reform bill, S. 1446, that he introduced in 1991.

A growing number of specialists located in think tanks and universities were also purveyors of analysis and frequent visitors to the Hill. They appeared at formal committee and subcommittee hearings or closed meetings of the respective party caucuses, met with individual members of the House and Senate or their staffs, and attended forums like the Senate Democratic Policy Committee's off-the-record Thursday lunches. Their scholarship regarding health care reform was also readily available through conferences conducted near Capitol Hill, including the ongoing George Washington University Health Policy Forum, as well as special symposia, such as "Beyond Medicaid: Building a Health Care System for the Ages," sponsored by Generations United in July 1991. Various journals, including *Health Affairs* and the *Journal of Health Politics, Policy and Law*, which are directed at both academic and policymaker audiences, published articles relevant to the debate.

What Congress did for itself analytically, however, is what is most noteworthy. As the legislative agenda grows to include issues of greater complexity and of significance to even broader segments of the population, legislators confront ever-increasing levels of programmatic ambiguity. They therefore have an enhanced interest in creating incentives for Congress to develop policy expertise. Keith Krehbiel assumes that legislators are judged by their constituents according to changes in their lives that result from the actions of their elected officials in the legislature.[44] For their own protection, representatives and senators must understand the link between the policy choices they make and the outcomes of those choices. But there is great uncertainly about that relationship:

> Other things being equal, legislators would rather select policies whose consequences are known in advance than policies whose con-

sequences are uncertain. Under conditions of relative certainty, legis-lators can plan and make the most of credit-claiming. . . . Under conditions of relative uncertainty, however, surprise and the pros-pect of embarrassment lurk beneath any policy choice. Implicit in this risk-aversion assumption about legislators as individuals is a more commonly articulated view about the legislature as a collective en-tity. A well-designed legislature is a producer, consumer, and repos-itory for policy expertise, where "expertise" is the reduction of un-certainty associated with legislative policies.[45]

Because legislators can benefit individually and collectively from information that reduces this uncertainty, they agree to rules, proce-dures, and institutional features that encourage development of the requisite substantive knowledge. As the electoral fortunes of legislative incumbents depend more on their own actions than on the generic attractiveness of their parties, the urgency of acquiring such expertise increases for each member of Congress.[46] Observers who witness con-gressional sensitivity to group interests and distributional issues are obviously not mistaken, but the demand for other kinds of information also influences congressional behavior and institutional design.

That imperative can be seen in how Congress has allocated itself staff resources. Between the mid-1960s, when Congress was battling over health insurance for elderly Americans, and the late 1980s, just before the most recent reform debate began in earnest, enormous numbers of staff (many of them trained in public policy schools) were added to the congressional payroll. Consider the four main committees with juris-diction over health care reform in the House and Senate. In the House, from 1960 to 1985, the staff of the Energy and Commerce Committee grew from 45 to 162 and that of the Ways and Means Committee from 22 to 99. During the same period the Senate Labor and Human Re-sources Committee staff rose from 28 to 127, while the Finance Commit-tee staff increased from 6 to 54.[47] After the Democrats recaptured the Senate in the 1986 election, Labor and Human Resources Chairman Ted Kennedy (D.-Mass.) abolished the committee health subcommittee (to keep control at the full-committee level) while maintaining a large health policy staff led by Dr. David Nexon.

The Democratic health policy staff of the House Ways and Means Committee offers a profile of the analytical and professional capabilities of the modern Congress.[48] In 1994 they advised Representative Pete

Stark, chairman of the Health Subcommittee, Representative Dan Rostenkowski, the committee chairman, as well as Majority Leader Richard Gephardt on health reform. The health policy staff's leader was David Abernethy, who has a master of public health degree from Yale and seven years of experience working on health planning and hospital cost regulation in the New York State Health Department. James Reuter received his doctorate at Johns Hopkins and was previously employed at the Congressional Research Service (CRS). Patricia Neuman had worked with the Senate Aging Committee and earned her doctorate at the Johns Hopkins School of Hygiene and Public Health. Lisa Potetz brought long experience from previous positions at the Senate Finance Committee, the Congressional Budget Office (CBO), and the Prospective Payment Assessment Commission. Ellen Magini was a lawyer and Eric Trupin a child psychologist. Stark, their primary boss, suggested: "They have no equal in any federal agency or any committee on Capitol Hill. No one in the United States is more familiar with, or has been more active in designing, the health care reform package." Even a senior official—a Republican at the Health Insurance Association of America—while recognizing that these staffers "are people of strong views," nonetheless characterized them as "hardened professionals [who] probably know more about health than any other group of people on Capitol Hill. . . . These are the best people I have ever worked with. They know the issues. They know the law."[49] From my personal experience in the early 1990s, I know the Finance Committee health staff was similarly capable. These are the types of people who understand the substantive issues and can synthesize and employ the most sophisticated policy analysis in the health reform debate.

Such analytically competent committee staffs were, of course, not available to every member of Congress, especially those not serving on the committees or subcommittees of jurisdiction. But the professional staffs working in House and Senate personal offices grew as well. They were also assisted by the resources of the CRS, a branch of the Library of Congress, which itself has served the Hill since 1800. CRS is a major resource for all congressional offices, invigorated as an instrument of policy research by the Legislative Reorganization Act of 1970. It now "conducts seminars on specialized topics for members and staff, analyzes issues before Congress, undertakes legal research, maintains automated databases, prepares digests and summaries of bills, furnishes questions for committee hearings, engages in policy analysis, and gathers factual and statistical information." By the mid-1980s, its staff of Ph.D.s and other professionals processed 430,000 requests for information from members and their staffs.[50] The CRS protects the confidentiality of all requests, so it is impossible to know how many requests and of what kind were made by legislators during the health care reform debate. Yet it unquestionably played a significant role in helping to educate Congress on the issue's complexities.

The 1970s in general saw Congress's own in-house analytic capabilities invigorated and dramatically expanded. The increase in professional staff and the reorganization of the CRS helped Congress process analytical material; the creation of new institutions permitted Congress to generate original research and analysis. As noted in other chapters in this book, one of the most significant developments was the creation of the CBO, mandated in the Budget and Impoundment Control Act of 1974. CBO, a haven for those of technical minds and nonpartisan disposition, employs advanced methods of data collection and analysis. It was designed to provide support to the new budget committees in the House and Senate, as well as the existing appropriations and revenue committees. CBO estimates what course federal expenditures will take and determines spending and revenue implications of pending legislation (a process called scoring).[51] During the budget wars with President Richard Nixon, CBO was meant to give members of Congress a capacity to independently judge fiscal and economic matters. It would thus serve as a check against the increasingly suspect estimates announced by the Office of Management and Budget in the executive branch, which had become more and more politicized to serve the president's own strategic needs.[52]

But more than dry numbers are involved. CBO also passes judgment on how certain policy options are to be treated—for example, stipulating that federally imposed employer mandates to finance health care coverage by requiring employers to pay premiums to government-sponsored health insurance purchasing cooperatives be treated as "on budget" items because of their semblance to taxation—and whether or not they are likely to fulfill their stated objectives.[53] In the 103d Congress, the twenty health analysts at CBO, along with its director Robert Reischauer, served to "highlight inconvenient facts" and "speak truth to power."[54] Noting CBO's impact on the search for a politically viable and substantively workable solution to the nation's health care problems, Representative Jim McDermott (D.-Wash.), sponsor of the single-payer bill in the House, commented, "Each individual group would think that they'd discovered a new route to China. And they'd go down to Bob Reischauer, and he'd say, 'No, boys, you can't go that way. It's all ice up there.' "[55]

CBO is "supposed to function as a careful, wary superego in the Congressional psyche."[56] Congress can now take the measure of its own psyche and not rely on anyone else.

The General Accounting Office (GAO) dates back to the Budget and Accounting Act of 1921. However, its responsibilities and resources as a congressional agency were also partially recast in the 1970s. In the past GAO was largely a "green eye-shade operation." It was headed by the comptroller general and its purpose was to ensure that the use of federal funds was in accord with the law. With the addition of the Program Evaluation and Methodology Division and the hiring of policy analysts throughout other units, GAO became more active and proficient in providing policy analysis requested by congressional committees.

In 1974 Congress also established the Office of Technology Assessment (OTA), which includes the division of Health, Education and the Environment. Like GAO, OTA worked in close association with congressional committees. But its specific mandate was to conduct large-scale, often long-term studies of technological issues and their likely economic, social, and political impact. "Technology" was rather broadly defined by OTA. Its multidisciplinary staff of about 150, subcontracting with specialists in universities and other settings, produced policy-analytic reports in a variety of policy areas.

Two additional congressional analytic support agencies were added in the 1980s, both with direct implications for health care policy. As Congress considered reforming the ways in which medicare reimbursed hospitals and physicians, it once again was concerned about having to rely on the executive branch for information and analysis during a period of divided government. This time, the worry was the responsiveness of the HCFA. As part of the 1983 legislation establishing a new PPS for hospital services under medicare, Congress established an independent body, the Prospective Payment Assessment Commission (ProPAC), to provide the legislature with independent advice about ongoing implementation of PPSs. ProPAC was "to buffer decisions from direct political pressures and to provide an independent and expert perspective."[57] Two years later (as described in the opening of this chapter), Congress created a similar entity, the PPRC, to help guide the development and implementation of the new resource-based relative-value scale (RBRVS) payment methodology for physician services covered by medicare.[58] Both commissions are composed of prominent health policy specialists, selected by the director of OTA, who have full-time positions in universities, the medical community, and other nongovernmental settings.[59] Each commission's work is assisted by a relatively small coterie of professional analysts with advanced degrees. In subsequent years the commissions pursued the study of issues more broadly than their original mandates might imply. The analytical domain of ProPAC, for example, expanded in 1989 with the explicit approval of Congress when it began "surveying and commenting on the status of hospitals, the health care industry as a whole, and the quality of care in America."[60]

During the most recent health care debate, these congressional agencies—CRS, CBO, GAO, OTA, ProPAC, and PPRC—furnished Congress, its members, and their staffs with an extraordinary amount of independently derived policy analysis pertinent to a multitude of issues associated with assessing and drafting health care reform. Table 4-2 presents summary characteristics of some of this material for selected agencies from January 1990 to September 1994. CRS is excluded from the tabulation, because most of its transactions with congressional clients are confidential and no public records are available. Nonetheless, it is worth emphasizing that CRS produced literally scores of continuously updated documents that are publicly available, including reports to Congress (such as "National Health Expenditures: Trends From 1960–1989," "Controlling Health Care Costs," "Characteristics of Nursing Home Residents and Proposals for Reforming Coverage of Nursing Home Care," and "The Canadian Health Care System") and issue briefs (including "Health Care Expenditures and Prices," "Health Insurance," and "Mandated Employer Provided Health Insurance").

These publications, which were prepared by specialists, typically summarized and synthesized the policy analysis literature as well as pending legislation, and often supplied detailed bibliographies of source material. I have also excluded ProPAC from table 4-2, because I was unable to compile as complete a record of its publications. The data in table 4-2 reflect my best judgment about the types of reports and other documents that could have been useful to members of Congress and their committee and personal staffs as they drafted health care

TABLE 4-2. *Reports Relevant to Health Care Reform by Issuing Congressional Agencies, January 1990–September 1994*

Topic	GAO[a]	OTA	CBO	PRRC
Performance of existing federal programs				
Medicare	32	1	3	12
Medicaid	20	1	0	5
Veterans Administration	17	0	0	0
Department of Defense/CHAMPUS	6	0	2	0
Federal Employees Health Benefit				
System (FEHBS)	4	0	0	0
State programs (non-medicaid)	22	1	0	0
International/other nations	14	5	0	1
Private insurance				
Employer-provided benefits	10	0	1	0
Other	15	2	2	2
Pharmaceuticals	13	2	1	0
Long-term care	21	0	0	0
Managed care	11	1	5	1
Malpractice	8	2	0	6
Health care reform (assessment of				
options, implications)	21	8	8	2
Published in 1993–94	92	28	13	5
Total	166	37	24	19

Sources: Library bibliographic search, library databases, and materials obtained from the General Accounting Office, the Office of Technology Assessment, and the Physician Payment Review Commission.

a. GAO issued 2.9 relevant reports per month, 4.4 during 1993–94. In addition, it offered testimony at committee hearings on 23 of the reports, and separate testimony on another 33 occasions unrelated to specific reports. GAO also transmitted eight substantive letters to Congress. The total number of reports, separate testimony appearances, and letters for this period is 207.

reform legislation and evaluated bills introduced by others. Sometimes a report's relevance is obvious (for example, GAO's June 1991 report, "Canadian Health Insurance: Lessons for the United States," or OTA's September 1993 report, "Benefit Design in Health Care Reform: Patient Cost-Sharing"). But other studies not specifically addressing health care reform could also be beneficial. Any GAO, OTA, or PPRC assessment of RBRVS under medicare, for example, would be extremely pertinent to anyone drafting legislation that would affect how physicians are paid in a reformed health care system.

Reading reports from congressional agencies—before even turning to the executive branch, consulting firms, interest groups, and scholarly publications—would obviously have kept health policy staffers rather busy. GAO, the largest of the support agencies, had the most prodigious output, generating 166 relevant reports related to health care during the roughly five-year period, including 92 reports during that last two years alone—overall, about 3 relevant reports a month. GAO personnel also presented more than 50 topics in testimony before congressional committee and subcommittees, including 33 on subjects other than those covered in specific GAO reports. OTA was the next most prolific agency, with a total of 37 reports, followed by CBO with its 24 analytical publications (produced in addition to its general work scoring specific health care reform bills). The much smaller number for the PPRC is somewhat misleading; its major publication, an annual report to Congress, was usually a document several hundred pages in length that covered a wide range of issues.

Table 4-2 also offers some perspective on the subjects covered in reports issued by the congressional agencies. A thorough analysis was done of existing federal programs, all of which would be affected by health care reform and many of which involve practices that could well affect consideration of reform options. Medicare received the most attention, but GAO also frequently reported on the Federal Employees Health Benefits Program (FEHBP)—a program that arguably offered some insight into the workings of the managed competition model, and which some reform proponents considered a means for expanding insurance choices to the general population.[61] Health policies in the states, beyond the medicaid program, were also subject to considerable study, as were the health care systems of other nations. The private insurance system (including employer-provided benefits) and long-term care also naturally attracted much attention. Major issues such as managed care, medical malpractice, and pharmaceuticals were also much investigated, often by a number of congressional agencies. As the health care reform debate heated up, it is also not surprising that these agencies were asked by committees and subcommittees to examine various questions raised about health care reform itself. This resulted in 21 reports from GAO, 8 each from CBO and OTA, and coverage by the PPRC in its 1993 and 1994 annual reports.

As the Clinton administration began to formulate a health care reform plan, Donna Shalala, the Secretary of Health and Human Services, "declared that the Administration would 'corner the market' for health policy experts by recruiting the best ones to work in Washington."[62] However well the administration may have succeeded in its aggressive recruitment strategy (and it is worth remembering that a significant number of those experts who labored in the working groups of the President's health care reform task force were in fact leadership, committee, subcommittee, and personal office staff from Capitol Hill),[63] Congress also had access to extensive, sophisticated policy analysis, much of it produced in house. The executive branch could not corner the market. At the PPRC some years before, for example, "The diversity and quality of experts on the commission matched or exceeded the policymaking expertise in the executive branch."[64] By the early 1990s, Congress had experienced two decades of structural changes. These had increased the electoral independence of representatives and senators; decimated norms of apprenticeship; dispersed power among numerous subcommittees with overlapping jurisdictions; increased the professional staffs of committees, subcommittees, and individual members; and established the legislature's own policy-analytic agencies. Congress had become an institution characterized by *"informed entrepreneurialism* [italics added]."[65] Legislators on and off committees of jurisdiction could and did become active policy advocates, introducing their own initiatives after often being well versed in at least some aspect of the policy-analytic debate. In addition, each committee and subcommittee with jurisdiction over health care had the professional wherewithal to arrive at decisions based on policy-analytic knowledge.

These institutional changes had in many respects fragmented Congress, making coalition building more unpredictable and difficult. For reasons to be discussed later in this chapter, the new availability of analytic information could not serve to unify the disparate legislature in and of itself. Nonetheless, unlike any time previously, Congress in the aggregate had emerged as a potentially serious analytical competitor to the executive branch. During the same period, the presidency had also changed institutionally. It is now conceived in a way that favors the political bias of the sitting president and threatens the long-term institutional competency of the president's support agencies. In an effort to be seen as a more successful policymaker in a highly contentious political environment, each chief executive has sought greater responsiveness to their personal needs and perspectives from executive institutions, especially those within the Executive Office of the President, such as OMB.[66]

Although executive policymaking and its use of information may now be more accommodating to the perceived needs of individual presidents, that very process left members of Congress disenchanted about the quality of information they could obtain from executive agencies. Congress reacted by establishing its own analytical capabilities, which are responsive to its needs. But because of partisan and jurisdictional divisions within the legislature, rather than politicizing the generation and flow of information, Congress actually developed agencies whose reputations and futures were built on supplying relatively objective, nonpartisan expertise. To establish themselves on the Hill, secure their position in the policy process, and protect their budgets and autonomy, these agencies had to demonstrate to all committees (which were often fighting jurisdictional battles) and to members of both parties (who were commonly locked in partisan embroilments) that the information they supplied was reliable, nonpartisan, and favored no particular interests. Each agency established somewhat different rules to meet that objective, but all had generally succeeded in earning the reputation they desired.[67] In the process, they achieved something else that was quite important: The analytic resources that function as a check on the executive branch also provide Congress with the means to "test the empirical claims of the interest groups."[68] Indeed, in their efforts to influence the policy-analytic knowledge of Congress, organized interests have had to hire their own specialists, support their own research offices or institutes, and present data and analysis as persuasive as other readily available sources.[69]

Information Use in Congress

Ascertaining that Congress had many sources of information of all three types available to it does not offer much evidence that the information was used intelligently or that it actually contributed to the advancement of knowledge. A more difficult methodological problem than trying to determine the extent to which policymakers used relevant information in arriving at policy decisions (especially in ways other than simply to fortify their own initial assumptions and biases) can hardly be imagined. Because members of Congress confront political and programmatic uncertainty when making decisions, it is safe to conclude that they make a serious effort to assuage uncertainty: *Some* kinds of information are indeed used. It is also probably safe to conclude, however, that elected officials are most apt to pay attention to signals from their constituents and from interests that could have some relevance to their electoral fortunes. Because of potential criticism about parochialism (that is, worrying more about their constituencies than the national interest) and indebtedness to special interest (particularly the moneyed variety), legislators may be consciously influenced by their evolving ordinary and distributional knowledge even more than they care to publicly admit—and they are willing to admit quite a lot. For the purposes of this discussion, given the nature of Congress as a legislature with geographically defined constituencies, a relatively fragmented and individualized electoral process, and internal political party organizations with few disciplinary sanctions, the vast body of information associated with ordinary and distributional knowledge probably was readily exploited during the health care reform debate.

The more interesting question is whether Congress demonstrated any willingness and capacity to enhance its policy-analytic knowledge and apply it in a policy area whose political and substantive dimensions were complex and of awesome consequence.[70] This particular question is no less challenging than the more general one. For one thing, there may be no concrete evidence of the impact of specific examples of policy analysis in bill writing, deliberation, or votes, yet such impact could still be quite significant. The body of policy-analytic work could—over time and in relatively subtle ways—have influenced policymakers' assumptions or beliefs, or what they are willing to accept as meaningful information. Carol Weiss, a leading student of how information is used by decisionmakers, describes this as the "enlightenment model" of the influence of policy-relevant research, the primary way in which analytical studies affect decisionmaking in any political environment.[71] "Not here the imminent decision, the single datum, the weighing of alternative options, the shazam!"[72] Rather, as Brookings economist Henry Aaron has suggested, "Analysts not familiar with the government decisionmaking process are surprised and often shocked by how small a direct contribution research makes. In fact, the contribution of the social sciences seems to be not so much specific information and conclusions as a perspective, an encouragement to evaluate programs in terms of their demonstrable effects. . . . The analyst can help raise the standards of admissible evidence; they can enrich and deepen understanding of the complexity of problems and the unintended consequences of action."[73]

Political scientist Lawrence Brown describes a similarly amorphous but no less important contribution of analytic information: "Research assists policy less by offering definitive answers to questions under debate than by improving the quality of debate; less by inventing the elusive idea whose time has come than by shaping the temper of the times in which policymakers review the long parade of ideas proffered by proponents of various intellectual persuasions."[74] Helping to ask the right questions, enhancing the perspective used to judge an advocate's position, elevating the caliber of debate, and invigorating the standards of evidence are decidedly important effects.[75] They are also difficult to track.

Even when members of Congress make explicit use of information that must have had its origin in policy-analytic research (such as citing statistics or evidence for causal relationships), it is difficult to know where it came from or how it informed even the individual using it. "Decisionmakers often absorb research information without clear marking of its origins. They merge what they learn from research with information derived from a variety of other sources."[76] Congressional bills, "dear colleague" letters, floor statements, correspondence, and speeches violate every academic norm of attribution and citation. Plagiarism is a high art form in the legislative arena. Before long, it becomes difficult to determine where a statistic first saw the light of day: in a GAO report, in an interview with a specialist reported in the newspaper, as a back-of-the-envelope estimate calculated by a lobbyist, or as an educated guess casually tossed out by a "knowledgeable" constituent (such as a hospital administrator) at an open-door meeting with a member of Congress. Once in a senator's "dear colleague" letter, that statistic may reappear in another's floor statement. How much influence it will have on the judgments of others in either case cannot be determined. Still, it may nonetheless be fruitful to this discussion to offer some perspectives on the impact that policy analysis has had on the legislative process and on the health care reform debate.

One reasonable conclusion is that Congress's own analytic agencies have not been ignored. According to Robert Pear of the New York Times, "Lawmakers continually cite the [GAO's] findings in deciding whether to create, abolish, cut or revise programs. . . . Congress follows more than half of [GAO's] suggestions for legislative action"[77] Close, scholarly study of particular support agencies also tends to reveal both general and specific effects on the legislative process. For example,

Thomas Oliver concludes that the Physician Payment Review Commission "performed a variety of functions and exerted substantial influence over physician payment policies in the nation's health care system. . . . The PPRC helped Congress establish an agenda for physician payment reform and set it into law despite initial resistance from the executive branch."[78] After being responsive to the information needs of individual members, presenting committee hearing testimony, and participating in congressional retreats (such as the one organized by the Ways and Means Committee in the spring of 1989), the PPRC "emerged as a regular source of technical assistance" for the three committees with jurisdiction over medicare—the Ways and Means Committee and the Energy and Commerce Committee in the House, and the Finance Committee in the Senate.[79] The dramatic impact of CBO scoring on congressional deliberations needs no reiteration. As a general proposition, therefore, Congress has acted with greater policy-analytic knowledge than would have been the case without these particular agencies. It is therefore more policy-analytic in its orientation in the 1990s than prior to the 1970s. That does not mean that policymaking is any easier. Especially in an era of severe financial constraints, knowing the precise details of the budgetary implications of policy options as they can best be estimated can in fact paralyze legislative action.

To pursue this issue with respect to health care reform would require the transcripts of every markup session of the subcommittees and committees with jurisdiction over the issue (or at least the five most prominent ones: Ways and Means, Energy and Commerce, and Education and Labor in the House; and Labor and Human Resources, and Finance, in the Senate). In addition, transcripts would be needed from the private working sessions of every leadership, committee, and personal office involved in generating legislative options. Yet no one can know to what extent specific suggestions about what to include in bills and the decisions made about them were pursued with regard to pertinent policy analysis.

Because in 1994 the Senate held the first serious floor debate on health care reform in the nation's history, the *Congressional Record* can be examined for indications of how policy-analytical materials entered these most public of deliberations. For the period from May 1 to August 15, 1994, when reform was discussed most intently (the debate increased in intensity on August 9th, when Senator Mitchell introduced his version of the Health Security Act), I identified the individual references each speaking senator made to specific identified sources of policy-analytic information (most of which fall into the "documentation" and "analysis" categories identified by Lawrence Brown and discussed previously). Given the significance of costs associated with reform plans and their potential impact on employment and the economy, it is not surprising that reports and assessments from CBO were referred to frequently by both Democrats and Republicans. CBO studies were independently cited 37 times. On four additional occasions CBO estimates or conclusions were specifically challenged by senators on the floor. Reports from GAO were identified 11 times. Other government sources include one reference each to analyses performed by the Joint Committee on Taxation and the Joint Economic Committee, two to work by the Health Care Financing Administration, and one to a study by the Council of Economic Advisers. Analyses reported by think tanks, policy institutes, foundations, consulting firms, and university specialists almost matched the number of references to CBO, 36. Within that category, Lewin/VHI received five mentions and EBRI four. Studies sponsored by interest groups such as NFIB and the U.S. Chamber of Commerce generated nine favorable cites and one challenge. A single professional journal, *Health Affairs*, was also noted once. In addition, many senators made extensive use of a variety of statistics—for example, on the economic standing of uninsured Americans, or on comparative infant mortality rankings—without specifying a source. At least in the forum of public debate, almost all of these references to policy-analytic information could easily be identified as efforts to give credibility to long-held (and probably previously held) positions, and to make these positions more attractive to the public. Few assumptions were reassessed and few minds changed.

Policy analysis is not just window dressing, however. Delving below the surface of congressional debate would reveal a reasonably influential and practical role for policy-analytic knowledge. I cannot document evidence of that assertion throughout Congress. But I can illustrate it through my own experience as a legislative assistant on health policy in the office of Senator Tom Daschle (D.-S.D.) in 1990–91 and subsequently, and informally, as an unpaid consultant. From December 1990 to April 1992, Daschle, a member of the Finance Committee, collaborated sequentially with two of his Senate colleagues—first John Danforth (R-Mo.), until his involvement with the nomination of Clarence

Thomas to the Supreme Court, and then Harris Wofford (D.-Pa.). They developed a comprehensive health care reform initiative, which ultimately became S. 2513, the American Health Security Plan, which Daschle introduced with Wofford on April 2, 1994. The crafting of that bill is, at least in part, the story of the role policy-analytic knowledge plays and a reflection of the modern Congress. It is also a long story, so I will simply highlight a few relevant points here.

By December 1990, after years of increasing study, Senator Daschle concluded that something had to be done about the American health care system. A few months earlier, while on a trip abroad, Daschle developed a friendly relationship with John Danforth, a Republican member of the Finance Committee with whom he had essentially no previous contact. Informal communications between the staffs of the two offices coincidentally revealed that Daschle and Danforth shared similar concerns about the direction American health care was taking and the nature of government involvement in it. Both believed that the skyrocketing costs of the health care system had to be brought under control. After some initial discussions at the staff level, Daschle and Danforth agreed to launch a joint effort to explore relevant health care issues and educate themselves on the problems and their possible solutions. They recognized that they might individually come to rather different conclusions, and they therefore avoided any commitment to cosponsor legislation that might ultimately be introduced.

The staffs of the two offices began by outlining a schedule of meetings for the senators that would be fully briefed by the staffs working in concert. The first session was intended to set some parameters by engaging Daschle and Danforth in a discussion of two broad approaches to organizing health care financing: the single-payer model (exemplified by the Canadian system, with public financing of a private delivery system) and the all-payer model (often identified with the German system and its largely private financing and delivery systems, governed by expansive government rule setting and regulation). The staff read extensively about these two systems and prepared background memos for the senators. The meeting itself was effectively a seminar with substantial give and take. John Iglehart, editor of *Health Affairs* and a student of the German health care system, was the point person on the all-payer option; Theodore Marmor of the Yale School of Organization and Management, an expert on Canadian health care, presented the single-payer perspective.

As a result of that meeting, Daschle and Danforth agreed to explore (without making any commitments) the development of a reform plan that would be generally consistent with core elements of the single-payer design, because of its potential for simplicity of administration and effective cost containment. What followed were innumerable meetings at the staff level and a series of sessions with the senators to make tentative decisions about specific dimensions of the plan. These dimensions included structure and responsibility of federal institutions, administrative responsibilities and procedures intended for the states, mechanisms for raising revenues to fund the system and establishing health care budgets at the federal and state levels, mechanisms for allocating payments for services to practitioners and institutional providers, role of patient cost-sharing, scope of the benefits package, efforts to expand the availability of providers in underserved areas, changes in the domain of medical malpractice, effects of the emerging reform plan on existing federal programs, and others. After Danforth's departure, the process continued with Senator Wofford and his staff. For each of these issues, the staff paid close attention to a considerable body of policy analysis. This was in addition to the information we received in the normal course of business from GAO, CBO, OTA, and CRS reports, committee hearings, routine meetings with lobbyists, newsletters, and other sources. A few examples illustrate the way we collected and used this information.

Throughout the process we were engaged in ongoing informal discussions with a number of health policy specialists (and read much of their work). They included Theodore Marmor; Uwe Reinhardt, health economist at Princeton's Woodrow Wilson School; William Glaser of the New School for Social Research, who has conducted detailed field research abroad and written extensively about the structure of health insurance and provider payment mechanisms throughout the world; Judy Feder, then director of the health policy program at Georgetown University and former executive director of the Pepper Commission; and Daniel Callahan of the Hastings Center. We gathered basic data about the existing health care system and current expenditure patterns from the chief of the National Health Accounts Branch in HCFA and gained some analytical perspective about financial issues from the economists on the staff of the Joint Tax Committee, as well as the health policy staff of the Senate Finance Committee. The Office of Legislative Counsel in the Senate, which drafted the bill's actual language, furnished the perspective of its experience.

For specific issues we turned to additional analytical resources. Cost sharing by patients, for example, is a complicated issue. It is colored by often firmly held preconceived notions about the incentives and health care outcomes produced when patients are required to pay out-of-pocket for some part of costs associated with their medical care. In preparation for the meetings on this issue, the staff read, assessed, and debated the most important studies on this subject conducted in the United States (such as the well-known RAND experimental study) and Canada.[80] Discussions were also held with people like Cathy Hurwit, legislative director of Citizen Action, a group opposed to patient cost-sharing; Theodore Marmor, who held a similar view; as well as representatives of provider groups in both Washington, D.C., and South Dakota, who tended to favor it. On the basis of all this information, the senators decided on very low patient-cost sharing provisions, with none for preventive services.

Medical malpractice is an even more controversial area, with sharply drawn lines between contending forces, such as the AMA and the American Trial Lawyers Association (ATLA). We met with both. We also gathered as much information as we could about state-level experience with malpractice reform and examined the Harvard Medical Practice Study of New York.[81] Given the political divisions and analytical conflict in the field, we chose to draft a provision that would motivate more state experimentation with a variety of alternatives to existing tort law that were identified in the literature.

The CRS, at our request, provided three kinds of particularly important analytical assistance. First, we were interested in designing a Federal Health Board to oversee the reformed system that would have as much independence as possible from the political pressures in Congress. To that end, we proposed a mechanism by which the Board would submit its proposed budget—both projected expenditures and premium levels—to Congress each year. Congress could only vote it up or down but could not amend it. CRS legal experts provided us with the assurance (and with the support of a legal precedent, the unanimous 1989 U.S. Supreme Court opinion in *Skinner* v. *Mid-America Pipeline Company*) that Congress could constitutionally grant such a broad delegation of authority, even taxing authority, to an executive agency as long as it provided sufficient guidelines.[82] Second, CRS specialists furnished us with a memorandum that described in detail the federal tax provisions currently financing health care services and the revenue losses produced by various health care-related tax expenditures. The memorandum also assessed the tax implications of various reform options. Third, a second lengthy memo from CRS identified all of the myriad existing federal health care programs and how they might be affected by various approaches to reform.

Policy analysts were, of course, not our only source of information. Views, impressions, expertise, and ideas were also solicited from many groups, which expanded both the policy knowledge of the enterprise and its sensitivity to distributive (and political) concerns. For the specific purposes of discussing health care reform and the outlines of the emerging bill, staff-level meetings were scheduled with Citizen Action, the Consumers Union, and Public Citizen (all well versed in national health insurance issues); the NCSC and the AARP (long-term care); the AMA, the American Nurses Association, and the Medical Group Management Association (physician payment); the AHA and the FAHS (hospital payment); the National Governors' Association, the National Society of State Legislators, and the Association of State and Territorial Health Officials (state financing and administration); Group Health Association of America (role of managed care); the NFIB (role of small businesses); insurance companies (role of insurance carriers); the National Association of Community Health Centers (delivery in underserved areas); and the ATLA (medical liability); along with other associations. Phone calls, faxes, and correspondence with these and other organizations supplemented these more formal sessions. So did the ongoing discussions with staffs in other offices in both the House and Senate who were also immersed in health care reform. Daschle also formed the South Dakota Health Advisory Group, composed of doctors, insurance agents, hospital administrators, business and labor leaders, and others involved in health care. He hoped to benefit from their expertise, enhance his knowledge of their interests, and build support for reform in his home state.

It is worth noting that this bill writing project was managed within the confines of personal offices, not committee staffs. Most of the other health care leaders in Congress (such as Senator Ted Kennedy, then chairman of the Labor and Human Resources Committee, and Representative Pete Stark, then chairman of the Ways and Means Committee's Health Subcommittee), had far greater experience and staff resources at their command. However, the Congress of informed entrepreneurialism makes it possible for small Senate offices, even those of freshmen (as Daschle was at the time), to be serious players in writing complex legislation.[83] The Daschle staff who contributed to the reform bill changed some over time but would score high on any measure of professionalism. The staff was anchored around Daschle's top permanent health aide, who received a master's degree in public policy at Princeton's Woodrow Wilson School, had studied under Uwe Reinhardt, and had some experience working at HCFA. As an American Political Science Congressional Fellow on leave from Harvard, I brought the skills and perspectives of a quantitatively trained political scientist with a doctorate from the University of Michigan. A Robert Wood Johnson Congressional Fellow (the chief of surgery on leave from the University of Washington Hospital) succeeded me. Two Presidential Management Interns (PMIs) also participated—one with experience at the National Institutes of Health, the other in public health. Daschle's tax counsel had a law degree from the University of Virginia and previous experience in corporate law. John Danforth's two primary legislative assistants on health care policy had received law and divinity degrees, respectively, from Yale University. His tax counsel left the Hill before the project was complete to become a law professor.

This group of people had the background and skills that equipped them (given the time and opportunity) to locate, synthesize, and use the results of policy-analytic research. They helped draft a bill that reflected reasonable lessons drawn from that research, as well as from the imperatives of ordinary and distributive knowledge. The senators and their staffs who wrote the legislation knew that the bill, as drafted, would never itself be enacted into law. Rather, it was intended to influence the health care reform debate. Whatever parts of the bill might be incorporated in legislation reported out of committee and passed on the floor would, we understood, reflect the collective policy-analytic expertise of many offices; the highly experienced professional staffs of the Finance Committee, among others; and the impact of full CBO scoring and evaluation.

Explaining the Use of Policy-Analytic Information in Congress

Thus far two general conclusions about the use of information in Congress can be made. First, information that promotes ordinary and distributional knowledge has a strong and efficacious effect on the Hill.

The important caveat should be added, however, that because not all interests in American society enjoy organized representation or resources proportional to their scope (E. E. Schattschneider's notion that organization is the "mobilization of bias"), distributional knowledge in particular is not based on complete information about the allocational effects of policy choices.[84] Second, information that nurtures policy-analytic knowledge among congressional decisionmakers is neither absent from nor inconsequential to the legislative process. How influential it has been, however, may be impossible to ascertain.

At the end of the 103d Congress, health care reform had died a rather ignominious death; no workable compromise could be found that would draw the sixty votes necessary in the Senate to fend off a potential (and likely) filibuster. Not so many months earlier, most observers—including many journalists, experts on the politics of health care, and representatives and senators themselves—had confidently believed that Congress would do something significant to transform the health care system.[85] So what produced the defeat? Senator Phil Gramm, the conservative Republican from Texas who worked assiduously to thwart the reform plans, would argue that the demise of health care reform speaks well of the policy-analytic process. People had learned, appropriately, that the problems cited were not so significant and the advertised remedies were unworkable. However, most participants would not conclude that the negative results of Congress's deliberations were the product of applied policy-analytic knowledge. Indeed, many specialists on health policy and the political process would argue that the entire health care debate—on and off the Hill— was enlivened more by unsubstantiated fears and sound-bite strategies than through careful, empirically grounded appraisals of the health care system's conditions or the competing options for reform. Identifying and adhering to standards of admissible evidence (a function often associated with policy analysis in political discourse) had hardly occurred.[86]

If policy analysis is as readily available to members of Congress as it seems to be, and if policy-analytic knowledge has a plausible, demonstrable, and yet problematic role to play in congressional policymaking, factors that may either promote or inhibit the use of such information in the legislative process need to be examined. Three such factors come readily to mind: the congruence of messages representatives and senators receive from different kinds of information, the incentives they have to pay attention to information, and the capacity they have to use information appropriately.

When John Kingdon studied how members of Congress decided how to vote on legislative issues, he concluded that most followed a "consensus mode of decisionmaking."[87] As much as possible, each legislator voted in ways consistent with the positions held by others in his or her "field of forces," including constituencies, other members who served as cuegivers, and the president (if of the member's party). When there was no conflict within this field of forces (which was the case for almost half the votes sampled) members of Congress had no difficulty deciding how to vote.

A similar process is at work regarding the influence of information.[88] If the information members of Congress received was consistent across the three domains of ordinary, distributional, and policy-analytic knowledge, then making judgments would be easy. In this sense, policy-analytic information is not ignored. However, its value and impact derive from its confirmation of what seems to make sense in more conventional ways. One overriding criticism of the Clinton health care reform plan, for example, is that however well the design might have worked if it had been implemented, it violated—or was too easily perceived to violate—basic dictates of comprehensibility and common sense.[89] Policy analysis did not square with ordinary knowledge, at least as the former was publicly presented. For an issue where every dimension defied ready understanding or simple options, and for which the stakes for so many organized interests were so high, it comes as no surprise that conflicts between policy-analytic information and the other types of knowledge went against the advice of experts.

Policy-analytic knowledge is likely to have the greatest impact and to be most resistant to the countervailing pressures when the experts themselves agree.[90] Despite the common language of academic authority, there was certainly tremendous variation in the analytical integrity of the innumerable studies that addressed some dimension of health care reform. But much of the deliberation in Congress had an aura of dueling policy analysis reports, each of which presented conclusions that ultimately depended on the quality of the assumptions that guided the analysis. Assumptions about how the economy and individual behavior would respond to policy changes varied widely, and none were so firm as to be universally adopted. As a result, one study would demonstrate sizeable loss of jobs because of employer mandates, while another would reveal the significant financial savings gained by businesses that already offered employees health insurance coverage. Sometimes the same report would be cited by different members of Congress to substantiate opposing claims. Perceived ambiguity in analytical results naturally diminishes the impact of policy-analytic knowledge. In this context, it is not surprising that "There are moments in this final phase of the health care struggle when people yearn, just a little, for the old leap-of-faith days of policy-making, before the Congressional Budget Office was tallying up the costs, the risks and the impact on the deficit of every good intention."[91]

The relative importance among the types of information available to Congress depends, of course, to some extent on the incentives senators and representatives have to emphasize one kind of knowledge over another. External incentives—the need to win reelection or to secure a reputation within the Washington community—are likely to work against policy-analytic knowledge when it is incongruent with others. In the extreme, "The overriding imperatives in legislatures (accommodating diverse interests) . . . relegate the rational contributions of research and analysis to peripheral consideration. . . . Social science research does not enter a benighted world that is bereft of understanding and direction. It is not a beam of light in a dark room. It is more like a candle in a lighted room."[92] (Often, a brightly lit room.) The goal of reelection almost always comes first with members of Congress—defeat in the electoral arena spells defeat in all others as well. They therefore have every incentive to give more weight to the ordinary knowledge associated with public opinion (no matter how specious or lacking in "public judgement,") than to policy-analytic knowledge, no matter how unambiguous it might be, at least when the issues involved are of considerable interest to their constituents. Health care reform, one of the most salient issues of our time, was also one on which the public was particularly ill informed. Constituents were poorly served by the media, which focused on the campaign aspects of health care reform rather than the substantive issues.[93] This lack of public understanding led to the Robert Wood Johnson Foundation's decision in May 1994 to grant NBC $2.5 million to produce a two-hour uninterrupted television program to inform the public on issues associated with health care reform, plus another $1 million for promotion—all of which was probably too little, too late.[94]

Internal incentives—those induced by factors within Congress itself—also affect the role of policy-analytic knowledge. Persuasive cases have been made that the desire to ensure good political and good policy outcomes creates incentives for members of Congress to seek ways to overcome policy uncertainty, including rewarding institutional development of expertise. Legislators want all kinds of information. In recent years they have collectively been diligent about gathering policy-analytic information and establishing the institutional means for Congress to expand on such knowledge. The evidence from the congressional agencies is impressive. Yet the question of how information is used still remains. Legislators want it. They make sure massive amounts are available. But do they do anything with it?

The other institutional changes of the 1970s, mostly in the House—the proliferation of subcommittees, the subcommittee "bill of rights" that gave each more autonomous leadership and independent staff resources, and the growth of personal office staffs—"created a new and effective constituency for incremental innovations in health policy and for research to assess their potential effects."[95] Recall the Daschle story, and the opportunity for nonincremental innovation. These analytical resources have made members more like "enterprises," less dependent on leaders internally as well as on organized interests or the executive branch externally.[96] The institutional decentralization of Congress has therefore both heightened the congressional need for policy analysis and greatly expanded the clientele for it.

At the same time, however, in many policy areas institutional dispersion also diminished the role of policy-analytic knowledge in helping shape legislative decisions. "Outside of budget preparation, legislators lacked an institutional mechanism to integrate policy and undertake major initiatives in lieu of presidential support. The ironic outcome of the expansion of staff resources was that Congress acted less as a collective institution and more as a collection of institutions, with subcommittees setting themselves up as the overseers of policy. When there was overlapping jurisdiction . . . this dispersion of power and authority threatened the capacity of Congress to act as a whole."[97]

All sources of policy-analytic information have even more ports through which to enter the congressional arena. Whatever lack of consensus exists in the disparate field of analysis is amplified by the diverse claimants for legislative jurisdiction. Several committees in Congress and innumerable subcommittees asserted authority over some aspect of health care reform. Each had the ability to acquire the analytic information needed to justify its positions (House committees with some jurisdiction included Ways and Means, Energy and Commerce, Education and Labor, Judiciary, Post Office and Public Service, Armed Services, Natural Resources, Veterans' Affairs, and Rules).[98] Congress was probably never so well informed or so knowledgeable about the intricacies of the health care system; nor was it ever so debilitated by the discordant chorus of analysts favored by various legislators. On narrower issues such as medicare policy, the PPRC and other entities could and did promote coherence where little had previously existed. But no single congressional support agency or external source of analysis could command dominion over the entire health care system.[99] The open, competitive system of presidential-congressional government in the United States, in contrast with far more centralized and parliamentary systems in many western democracies, also means that the civil service in the executive branch cannot perform this function.[100]

Suppose for the moment that Congress had both the external and internal incentives to exploit the vast body of policy-analytic information available to it. Would it have the capacity to use it? Capacity can be thought of in a couple of ways. The first, quite simply, has to do with time. Given the way Congress has been organized, could it process, synthesize, and appropriately apply whatever policy-analytic knowledge it has at its disposal? With regard to individual members, the answer is decidedly no. There is simply no opportunity to do the vast amount of reading and thinking required. Former Senator James Buckley of New York put it this way: "There is only one thing to say about [the reading load] and that is that it can never be done. The amount of reading necessary to keep a Senator minimally informed on matters of maximum importance is always double that which [he or she] can possibly accomplish in the time allotted."[101]

Members of Congress, of course, are not alone. They have their staffs, frequently professional and activist, both in their personal offices and for committees. They can call on the CRS to help summarize and synthesize analytical materials. These resources are a member's (and the institution's) only hope, but they have their own practical limitations. Congressional staff are also overwhelmed by the workload and the volume of reading. Congressional aides, especially those on the far smaller House staffs, are typically responsible for a number of issue areas. The structure of their workdays—consumed by meetings with lobbyists and constituents, committee and subcommittee hearings, and responsibility for following floor proceedings, and rocked by unanticipated events—leaves precious little time to do any reading (much less thinking) in a sustained and serious manner. In addition, although staff unquestionably add to the ability of members of Congress to incorporate policy-analytic knowledge in their decisionmaking, trust and confidence can extend only so far and can only add so much. "There are only 535 members of the Congress; only 100 Senators. Each member will delegate important political judgments to only a few, in some instances only one or two, trusted staff members. As a result, the ultimate consideration, distillation, and value judgments about all of the research and policy analysis presented to the Congress concerning all of the major issues of government must be made by a few hundred individuals in the Senate and perhaps less [sic] than a thousand in the House."[102]

For most representatives and senators, what they did about health care reform (either in drafting their own legislation, voting in committee markup sessions, or anticipating how to vote should the issue come to the floor) was among the most important decisions they had to make in the 103d Congress, and perhaps in their careers. These choices, which also required a careful balance of ordinary, distributional, and policy-analytic knowledge, were not going to be left up to even the most sophisticated assistants. The analytical task could not thus be easily segmented and allocated among many legislative aides to synthesize the mountain of health care policy analysis.

Even if there were time enough to read the policy-analytic materials, members of Congress require a second capacity: the ability to make sense of them. As social science research has become increasingly arcane, with more complex research designs and technically advanced quantitative methods, the analyses it produces risk being beyond the understanding of even reasonably intelligent and educated legislators. Study authors may strive to ensure readability, but most denizens of Congress would be unable to judge the quality of the interpretations that authors give to their results. If anything, the electoral process in the United States favors those candidates with the common touch, not the manner of the intellectual or sophisticate. Policy wonkism, like Bill Clinton's, is the target of biting jokes, not mass approval.

Here, too, congressional staff can provide invaluable assistance in compensating for their bosses' lack of analytical expertise, up to a point. The more staffers have the requisite professional training in analytic work and the longer their experience in a policy area, the more proficient they become as thoughtful readers of policy research (if they can find the time). These attributes describe committee staffs more than those in personal offices and apply more to aides in the Senate than those in the House, where noncommittee staffers are typically younger and often fresh out of college.

Even professionally educated legislative assistants, such as lawyers, may lack the background to assess the more esoteric policy-analytic work. For example, when we were assessing the proper role of patient cost sharing when Senators Daschle and Danforth were engaged in their joint health care reform effort, I discovered that some of my colleagues who were not trained in policy analysis had considerable difficulty reading, comprehending, and evaluating the RAND study. The nature of the experimental design and the use of multivariate regression analysis to model the effect of cost sharing on utilization and medical outcomes (hardly the state-of-the-art in research methodologies) was virtually incomprehensible to them. Because some of the conclusions of this study seemed to be contrary to those of the Canadian studies we had also surveyed, the ability to read these reports critically was important. In my experience, not many staffers outside of the committees or the support agencies would be able to do so. They are much better consumers of research that descriptively documents the state of the world than they are of analyses that test and explain causal relationships.[103]

However, congressional staff (including the professionally trained assistants in personal offices, but primarily the committee staff and analysts within the support agencies) at least make it possible for Congress to collectively attempt to balance ordinary, distributional, and policy-analytic knowledge in ways that the members themselves could not on their own. As illustrated in table 4-3, members and staff bring quite different perspectives to the legislative process. By the nature of the political lives they lead, their backgrounds, the character of interactions they have with other participants in the process, and the time constraints they face, most members of Congress probably rank high in acquiring information linked to ordinary knowledge and are reasonably well versed on the distributional effects of policy choices. Few, however, have well-developed policy-analytic knowledge. Only those representatives and senators who have the intellectual capacity and interest as well as the long tenure of experience in a specific policy domain are likely to gain a firm grip on policy-analytic information, if only vicariously. To the extent that the seniority norm for selecting

TABLE 4-3. *Likely Differences in Levels of Knowledge among Members of Congress and Congressional Staff*

	Information Knowledge		
	Ordinary	Distributional	Policy-analytic
Members	High	Medium	Low (usually)
Staff	Low-Medium	Medium-High	High (potentially

committee chairs and ranking members brings such individuals into leadership roles (often a dubious proposition), Congress's policy-analytic capacity is enhanced.

There is no law of congressional behavior that dictates that staff will be any different from the members they serve. The array of issues about which members must make decisions, the onslaught of constituency business, and the relatively limited resources members are allocated for hiring staff lead to a recruitment process that brings many young, often inexperienced people into staff positions of considerable responsibility. Sometimes congressional staff, especially if they are novices deluged by information, bring to mind the old story about the blind leading the blind. Nonetheless, the nature of staff work makes it likely that there is at least some difference in what staffers emphasize compared with their bosses. Because almost any member of Congress seeks ways to over-come programmatic uncertainty and to project some mastery over leg-islation, even the greenest of legislative assistants has an incentive to develop some policy expertise. The ready availability of information, the unsolicited onslaught of materials of analytical relevance, and the press of hearings that require preparation and briefings all facilitate the education of staffers. Learning policy on Capitol Hill is akin to learning a foreign language through the most intense immersion in the country itself. It may take a while to get rid of the novice's accent, but a level of fluency is achieved quickly. Several years ago a particularly bright new Senate staffer, fresh from an Ivy League law school, sat through a long meeting of the Senate Rural Health Care Caucus. Analysts from OTA were presenting early results of their study assessing how to ensure access to medical personnel in rural areas. At the end of the briefing, the new staffer turned to a more seasoned colleague and whispered, with trepidation, that he did not understand anything that had just been said. (This is certainly understandable; for one thing, the alphabet soup of health care acronyms takes time to absorb.) A few years later, the same staff member was deeply immersed in the complexities of a previously unimaginable range of health care subjects.

The more staff members are given the incentive and granted the opportunity to work on detailed legislative issues, the more likely they are to become knowledgeable about policy analysis. The constant stream of meetings with lobbyists is also likely to promote their distributional knowledge. But judging how much ordinary knowledge congressional staff have is less certain. Everyone, of course, comes to any job with prior assumptions and gut-level reactions to events, but the ways in which those assumptions are reinforced varies. Personal offices that hire legislative correspondents to process mail from constituents free the legislative assistants of this burden. In the process, this gives them more time to assimilate policy-analytic information and to invigorate the institution's overall analytic capacity. However, it also intensifies differences in informational orientation between members of Congress and their policy staffs. In those settings where legislative assistants must handle constituency missives as well as policy, aides are less likely to lose sight of the balance between ordinary and policy-analytic knowledge that their bosses must necessarily achieve. Letters from the home district and visits by constituents serve as important reality checks. In either case, committee staffs and personal office legislative assistants act as funnels (and ultimately narrow conduits for information). They communicate this highly distilled material from an environment saturated with policy-analytic information to elected officials with even less time or capacity to become analytically competent.

Congress and Information, with Thoughts on the 104th

Congress is a supremely political organization, as any legislature in a representative democracy must be. The perspectives of citizens and those of organized interests cannot be ignored, no matter how contrary they might be to the insights generated by professional policy cognoscenti. It should therefore come as no surprise that policy-analytic knowledge is often overwhelmed by politics informed by ordinary and distributional knowledge. The role of analytic information in practice is thus all too frequently to lend credibility and argumentative force to positions previously identified as the result of bias, hunches, and ideology.[104] As Larry Brown puts it, "A wide range of intervening variables extraneous to the merits of issues—constituency demands, partisan promises, ideological biases, interest group preferences—invade and generally conquer the policy process."[105] Ideology is the foundation of that construction, and the "core values respond mostly to experience and very little to information."[106]

In the political world, the principles of objective inquiry associated with policy-analytic information are apt to be weakened. "Information in organizations is not innocent," as James March notes.[107] Politicians and their aides are deeply rooted in partisanship, ideology, and politics, and they give credence to information that is on their terms. Their beliefs, perhaps based only on personal experience or false impressions, came to be viewed by them as objective appraisals of reality, even when they are contradicted by more reliable data.[108] In the legislative arena, therefore, the risk is that one coalition challenges another in a "dialogue of the deaf." Information may only serve to identify the interests at stake and motivate those interests to take action, including using policy-analytic information to support long-established positions.[109] Even social learning—the process by which policymakers derive meaningful policy lessons from previous experience and other settings—can be distorted by the thick predispositional bias that permeates political institutions.[110]

The limits of objectivity extend beyond the impact information can have in explicitly political arenas such as Congress. Knowledge itself "is made and remade by people in particular political situations; it is, in the sociologists' useful metaphor, 'socially constructed.' "[111] Health services research, for example, could be motivated by various approaches, including concerns about social conflict or the promotion of collective welfare. Instead, it has come to be dominated by what Daniel Fox calls the "economizing model," which focuses on health financing and delivery as a "sector of the economy" generating "benign externalities." The best solutions are therefore to be found in a proper mix of highly technical incentives and disincentives.[112] Much of the analytical work directed at health care issues is subsumed in the free market orientation of American society at large. According to Robert Evans, "The free market is not preferred because it achieves other objectives, whether of cost, quality, or access; it is *itself* the objective, and whatever emerges from the market is right. . . . This normative position, as a number of observers have noted, is not merely intellectually isomorphic with religion, it *is* a religion."[113] Policy-analytic knowledge quite understandably has its greatest impact when its information base rests on assumptions congruent with the values and beliefs of the policymakers to whom it is directed.[114] Challenges to these assumptions, however rigorous, are easily dismissed.

No one should ever expect that Congress, even when organized through informed entrepreneurialism, would fulfill a policy analyst's dream. Nor should it: Choices about ideological and partisan orientation are largely what elections are all about. We should have quite different expectations about the role of information (especially social science research) in any legislative debate. Policy-analytic knowledge should not and cannot supplant the normal political process but rather should enrich it.[115] There is considerable evidence from the attempts at health care reform that such improvement has occurred, as well as confirmation that there is still room for progress.

After CBO issued its "good news/bad news" report on President Clinton's Health Security Act, the *Washington Post* published an editorial that expressed hope about the prospects of an analytically informed Congress: "The administration fears the political uses to which the agency's report on the president's health care plan will likely be put. Our own sense is that, if the report is read instead of being mined for sound bites, it could serve to depoliticize the debate instead. Rational discourse does that."[116]

The *Post's* editorial board was more optimistic than it should have been. The work done by CBO, I believe, did improve the quality of congressional deliberations, even as it made them more difficult. But its report, and many others, were mined for political purposes. Minority Leader Robert Dole immediately proclaimed on the floor of the Senate that the CBO assessment "confirms what many of us have been saying all over the country for the past several months. The Clinton plan calls for multibillion dollar doses of deficit spending and government control." This was stated despite the fact that CBO verified the future savings that the administration program would produce and spoke of government budgeting rather than government control.[117] Indeed, a few days later in an op-ed piece in the *Washington Post*, Democratic Senator Jay Rockefeller countered that CBO had given credibility to the president's claims that his plan would move toward universal coverage, preserve choice, ensure cost containment, and expand jobs.[118] Nonetheless, as Robert Blendon noted, Republican and conservative opponents of reform recast the CBO analysis to support the notion that Clinton was proposing a "big government plan."[119]

However unfortunate these dueling interpretations of CBO numbers might be, consider the alternative. Suppose CBO was not engaged in nonpartisan evaluation of legislation . . . or that GAO, OTA, PPRC, and ProPAC were not around to conduct well-respected policy analyses and evaluations of existing programs . . . or that congressional commit-tees, the bill-writing entities of Congress, lacked professional staff with the training and perspective to make sense of analytical work generated on and off the Hill. In such an environment, ordinary and distributional knowledge would go unchallenged, and debate would be subject even less to the discipline of distinguishing fact from fiction. For example, in the course of his vociferous opposition to any reform plan that involved measurable government intervention, Senator Phil Gramm often repeated stories that were not verifiable. These included his empirically refuted claim that the Johns Hopkins Medical Center, like others around the country, had a high patient load of wealthy exiles from countries with socialized medicine.[120] Without the institutional changes in Congress that have promoted professionalization of staff and establishment of analytical capabilities, such homespun tales might have been granted even more clout than that provided by ideological conviction.

The new Republican majority in Congress, capturing both houses for the first time since Dwight Eisenhower gained the White House, is naturally enthusiastic about its opportunity to reshape federal policy and the broader course of events. After four decades in the minority, the Republican majority in the House developed a well-honed sense of some of the deficiencies in that institution, such as the excess fragmen-tation that complicated the task of coalition building. Most students of Congress, and even many Democrats, support Republican reforms to reduce the numbers of committees and subcommittees and to minimize the individualistic character of the congressional establishment and reinvigorate its partisan organization.[121] Entrepreneurialism may be yielding just a bit to more "responsible" majoritarian governance.[122]

Other "reforms" already engineered or under consideration by the Republican majorities, however, quite directly threaten the analytical maturity that Congress has achieved, and thus its capacity to act in a manner imbued with policy-analytic knowledge. In their effort to trim the size of the congressional bureaucracy, the majority has cut commit-tee staffs—the analytical and legislative workhorses of the institution—by one-third, while leaving the personal staffs untouched. It is the personal staffs that give individual members greater access to analytical information but that also allow them to promote their independence from party and other coalitions by forging direct, often particularistic ties to their constituencies. If staff are to be cut in the interest of reducing the Hill's structural bulk and fragmentation, then the axe should fall in the personal offices, not in the committee rooms.

Also under threat at this writing are prime analytical support agencies. OTA may be eliminated altogether, while GAO, the most prolific of congressional agencies, could lose up to half of its budget.[123] Evisceration of ProPAC and the PPRC, with their relatively tiny budgets, may follow. Perhaps more than any other institutions (including executive agencies and think tanks), the analytical arms of Congress have earned reputations for nonpartisanship and objectivity. If they are abolished or severely cut back, Congress becomes even more fertile territory for those wishing to promote unchecked ordinary and distributional knowledge, or politically tainted analysis presented in the guise of academic language.

Another challenge to the Hill's recent analytic ascendance is that many Republicans want to compel CBO analysts to use "dynamic" scoring in appraising tax reduction proposals.[124] CBO currently makes rather conservative judgments about the behavioral effects of tax cuts and their contributions to productivity and job growth. The more apparent revenue losses from tax cuts are given greater weight than the revenue increases prompted by any economic expansion that the tax cuts might stimulate, which are difficult to predict. Just as the responsiveness of OMB to the political needs of sitting presidents lowered the esteem in which that budget office was held, so too dynamic scoring, favored by conservative supply-siders, risks damaging the analytical reputation of CBO.

Finally, if term limits are ultimately implemented, the demise of Congress's analytical capacity will be complete. Members themselves would no longer gain enough policy experience to make reasonably independent judgments of their own, and it is uncertain to whom they would be responsive. Only if policymaking in a complex society is best left to relative amateurs heavily influenced by their own biases and particularistic interests (a highly implausible proposition) will the aggregation of all of the reforms initiated in the 104th Congress prove beneficial to the governance of America. If, on the other hand, a responsive and effective legislature is one capable of balancing the sometimes contradictory impulses of ordinary, distributional, and policy-analytic knowledge, then these challenges to the analytical core of Congress are cause for concern.

Chapter 5

Congressional Oversight of Health Policy

Mark V. Nadel

Quite as important as legislation is vigilant oversight of administration.

Woodrow Wilson[1]

IN THE 1960s it may have been true, as political scientist John F. Bibby maintained, that oversight was "Congress's neglected function."[2] By the 1990s, however, it had become a dominant one. In 1993, for example, the House Subcommittee on Health and the Environment held 103 hours of investigative and oversight hearings, compared with only 35 hours of legislative hearings and markups combined.[3]

As the federal government has increased in size, complexity, and reach, the incentives for Congress to conduct oversight have likewise increased. One reason for those heightened incentives, according to Joel Aberbach, is the growth of government itself. "When those in Congress began to believe that the citizenry was increasingly burdened by government size and complexity, or even disenchanted with government per se, then there was a shift in the relative payoffs of endeavors such as creating new programs compared with overseeing those already established."[4]

Divided government has also changed the nature of oversight. Congress and the president have always vied for effective control of the executive agencies of government. But when one party controls the

The author is with the U.S. General Accounting Office. The views expressed here are his and do not necessarily represent the opinions of GAO.

legislature and the other the executive branch—as was the case from 1981 through 1993 and with the election of 1994 is once again—congressional distrust of executive branch actions magnifies and oversight intensifies.

Perhaps an even more important explanation of the increased use of oversight is money—or the lack of it. In the face of a continuing struggle against a massive federal budget deficit, now further constrained by budget rules that militate against spending on new programs, legislative work on existing programs is usually the only substantive game in town. Moreover, it is often a zero-sum exercise, as Allen Schick has observed, because politics has become more partisan during a time of relative scarcity. As a result legislators seek to exercise as much influence as possible over the administration of programs.[5]

Thus oversight has moved beyond simply monitoring the operation of federal programs and exposing fraud, abuse, and mismanagement. Those functions are still important, but even more important is Congress's increasing use of oversight as a policymaking tool. Oversight has become the vehicle through which Congress retains some power over the myriad choices—many of them involving policymaking—that are made in implementing any federal program. That is as true in the health policy arena as in any other policy area.

The Changing Nature of Oversight

Broadly defined, oversight is the legislative branch's formal and informal review of the executive branch's implementation and operation of programs and policy. Since its creation, Congress has always exercised oversight. But the function was not formalized until passage of the Legislative Reorganization Act of 1946, which required House and Senate committees to undertake "continuous watchfulness" over the programs and agencies within their jurisdiction.

The Congressional Research Service (CRS) has outlined eight distinct goals of oversight.

—Ensure administrative adherence to congressional intent

—Improve the efficiency, effectiveness, and economy of governmental operations

—Evaluate program performance

—Prevent executive encroachment on legislative authority

—Investigate alleged instances of poor administration, arbitrary action, abuse, waste, dishonesty, or fraud

—Assess agency or individual ability to manage and accomplish program objectives

—Review and determine federal financial priorities

—Ensure that executive policies reflect the "public interest."[6]

Oversight through Appropriations

In the past, the appropriations committees were considered the foremost instruments of congressional oversight.[7] According to Richard Fenno, the House expected its Appropriations Committee to "engage in oversight of administration. The Committee is expected to keep itself and the rest of the House informed on the way in which executive agencies use the money granted to them and, indeed, to influence the use of public funds in ways prescribed by law."[8]

The oversight function of the appropriations committees stems from their responsibility to examine and pass on budget requests of the administration, and the decisions of the committees are conditioned on their assessment of the agencies' proposed budget as indicated by past performance. But as more and more of the federal budget is consumed by mandatory spending for legal entitlements or other federal obligations, the reach of the appropriations committees is correspondingly shortened.

By 1994 about two-thirds of the federal budget consisted of mandatory spending programs, and the rate was even higher for health programs. Congress had discretionary authority for only $24 billion, or less than 10 percent, of the $256 billion spent on federal health programs in 1994.[9]

Most government health programs have vital missions with powerful constituencies and congressional champions and with responsibilities that often far exceed the resources provided by their appropriated funds. The appropriations committees thus can do little more financially to agencies such as the Food and Drug Administration (FDA) and the Centers for Disease Control than influence them at the margins.

Yet even with static or declining appropriations, the committees still have considerable power over program initiatives and emphases. Appropriations bills often contain specific instructions on how funds must be spent, and the committee reports accompanying these bills also include such directives. Unlike bills, these "nonstatutory" directives are not legally binding, but agencies usually treat them as if they were.[10] For example, the FY1993 House Appropriations Committee report stated: "Within the total provided for Title II [comprehensive care programs—Ryan White AIDS programs], the Committee intends that 10 percent be retained by the Secretary for special projects of national significance. The Committee intends that no less than 50 percent of the set-aside be used to continue the dental reimbursement program for dental schools and postdoctoral dental education programs for the costs incurred in providing oral health services to HIV[human immunodeficiency virus]-positive patients."[11]

Legislation through Oversight

Because of budgetary constraints, bold new programs driven by federal spending are increasingly a memory. The whittling down and eventual demise of President Clinton's health reform plan is more testimony to that reality than an exception to it. Therefore, Congress has tried to achieve its policy ends by shifting functions and costs to the private sector (through regulation) or to state and local governments (through mandates) or by changing existing programs and agency administration (through oversight). Since the change in party control, however, unfunded mandates have been proscribed and regulation is out of favor, leaving oversight as a more prominent means of policymaking.

When legislators deem that admonitions to agencies have been insufficiently heeded, oversight often results in amendments to existing legislation. Oversight hearings preceded ten of the fourteen bills reported by the House Commerce Health Subcommittee in 1993, for example.

Most major federal programs must also be reauthorized periodically. Under these so-called sunset provisions, the programs or agencies are supposed to go out of business if Congress does not pass a reauthorization. Although that rarely happens, sunset provisions do build oversight into the legislative process. "We require reauthorization to keep the agencies on a short leash—to make sure that there will be oversight," one staff member explained.

In recent years, Congress has increasingly written requirements for studies of specific problem issues directly into legislation. Senate and

House committees, for example, have long been concerned that several small grant programs for medical education were not achieving the objective of increasing the number of doctors practicing in minority and other underserved communities. Consequently, the 1992 reauthorization of these programs required an evaluation of their effectiveness before the next reauthorization.

In this era of tight budgets, recognized oversight jurisdiction confers influence over policy and is now a key component in exercising power in Congress. As a result, oversight itself has become the prize in debates over policy formulation. Several committees asserted jurisdiction over health reform legislation, for example, and a major reason for the competition could be viewed as committee chairmen trying to stake a claim for future oversight jurisdiction. That motivation was at the heart of a *New York Times* editorial attacking the medicare-centered reform plan proposed by Ways and Means Health Subcommittee chairman Pete Stark: "It comes as no surprise that [Stark's] idea of health-care reform is to shove as many Americans as possible into Medicare, making him czar over an industry as large as the Italian economy."[12]

Techniques of Oversight

The basic techniques of oversight in the health arena are the same as they are in any other policy area—informal staff contact with executive branch personnel, member contact with executive branch personnel, hearings, and the use of various support agencies to perform evaluations of program and policy operations.

The most frequently used oversight technique is staff communication with agency officials.[13] Such contacts range from routine casework for constituents to meetings where staff probe for more information about particular agency actions, upbraid executive branch personnel for shortcomings, or pursue policy goals.

Hearings are perhaps the most visible technique of oversight and in fact are often carefully orchestrated to maximize media coverage. Committee chairman use hearings and any press coverage to try to shape public (and congressional) perception of an issue or problem. Hearings also provide a public forum at which to hold agency officials accountable for their actions.

Congressional Oversight Agencies

Congress also makes frequent use of several agencies it has created to conduct investigations and evaluations of programs that legislators and their staffs have neither the time nor often the expertise to do on their own. The largest of these agencies is the General Accounting Office (GAO), which issues about 900 reports a year; in 1993, 100 of these reports covered health topics. The other support agencies are the CRS, the Office of Technology Assessment, and the Congressional Budget Office.

A congressional committee usually requests a GAO study because it suspects or has already uncovered a problem. GAO personnel can examine agency documents, systematically interview agency officials and others, and generally delve deeper and provide far more detail and verification than committee staff can.

The offices of inspector general, the audit and investigative agencies established by Congress in all the major Cabinet departments during the 1970s, are another important oversight tool. The inspector general's office in the Department of Health and Human Services (HHS), for example, not only looks at financial and management issues within the department, but also investigates fraud and other abuses in the medicare and medicaid programs. Inspectors general are unique in that they are part of the agencies they oversee but also report to Congress.

Special Health Support Agencies and Oversight of Medicare

Health policy oversight is distinguished from oversight in other policy areas by two agencies that Congress created in the 1980s specifically to conduct detailed studies of health financing issues and make recommendations. The Prospective Payment Assessment Commission (Pro-PAC) was set up in 1983 to recommend changes in medicare hospital payment policies, while the Physician Payment Review Commission (PPRC) was established in 1985 to devise more effective and less costly methods for paying physicians.

Medicare was enacted in 1965 to provide medical care for elderly Americans. It has two parts: part A, hospital coverage financed through payroll taxes; and part B, supplementary medical insurance, primarily for physicians' services, financed through modest monthly premiums paid only by enrollees and through general revenues. By the early 1980s medicare was growing more rapidly than any other federal health program. For ten years Congress had struggled in vain with rising medicare costs. Finally, in 1982 it directed HHS to develop a new prospective system for paying hospitals. Rather than reimbursing on the basis of costs, HHS devised a system that would pay hospitals on the basis of patients' illnesses, which are categorized into hundreds of diagnosis related groups (DRGs). Congress adopted a modified version of HHS's initial plan in 1983 and created ProPAC to advise Congress and HHS on updating the system. Not only had congressional oversight led to legislation, but ultimately the change in policy was shown to have come reasonably close to achieving its objectives. Medicare costs continue to escalate, but recent studies have found that the prospective payment system (PPS) that Congress pushed on the administration restrained the growth of spending without seriously affecting access or quality of care.[14]

Although part A accounted for most of the medicare expenditures, part B was also of concern because it was growing at a faster rate than part A. After the Reagan administration ignored congressional requests to develop reform proposals for part B, Congress temporarily froze physicians' fees in 1984. In 1985 the Democratic Congress, reflecting its distrust of the Reagan administration, exercised its oversight by creating an agency, the PPRC, to recommend new methods for determining physician payments and payment levels.[15] In 1988 Congress further charged the PPRC with the task of recommending policies to hold down the increasing use of procedures.

The PPRC substantially influenced congressional decisions about physician payment policies. Originally, some members of Congress had flirted with the idea of adopting a PPS for physicians similar to that used for hospitals. Instead in 1989 the PPRC recommended a physician fee schedule based primarily on resource costs, rather than on "customary, prevailing, and reasonable" fees. This resource-based, relative-value scale (RBRVS) tends to increase the compensation of primary care physicians and decrease fees for procedure-based specialty practices.[16] Following hearings, Congress enacted legislation requiring the Health Care Financing Administration (HCFA) to adopt RBRVS for part B of medicare.

The PPRC and ProPAC are unique among congressional oversight tools. As John Iglehart has observed, "The PPRC has quickly become the most important influence on the direction that Congress pursues in changing Medicare's physician-payment methods."[17] The PPRC and ProPAC do not initiate oversight, but instead respond to the policy directions set by Congress. Nonetheless, because of their ability to conduct focused research, these two specialized agencies have expanded the oversight reach of the congressional health policy committees. The success of these agencies in assisting Congress would seem to be confirmed by the inclusion in the short-lived Medicare Catastrophic Coverage Act of 1988 of a similar organization to monitor prescription drug prices.

Setting the Oversight Agenda

Apart from subjects dictated by a reauthorization schedule, there is no science in picking targets for oversight in the health policy arena. In addition to reauthorization, evidence of scandal or malfeasance, a policy or funding crisis, or ineffectively run programs are the most common factors triggering an oversight investigation. But almost all possible factors that convince members and staff to pursue one topic rather that another are at work. These range from personal experience, to complaints from companies that regulators are unfairly favoring their competition, to reports from whistle-blowers. One veteran staff investigator related how a friend had a "horror story" regarding the price of a medical device that she needed. That led to an inquiry into one company and then into the pricing structure of an entire industry under medicare.

Medicare and medicaid are almost continuously the objects of oversight. Beyond the basic issues of program design, congressional oversight has focused on the quality of service beneficiaries receive and whether providers are enriching themselves, legally or otherwise.

Oversight of the medicare program is conducted in an environment suffused with the political power of its beneficiary group. Because there is little political appetite in Congress to even appear to erode benefits for elderly Americans or to seriously increase their share of the costs, oversight of medicare focuses either on fraud, program administration, or on more fundamental problems of cost control. All the medicare oversight hearings held in 1993 by the program's two most active oversight subcommittees focused on issues such as payment rates for laboratory services and end-stage renal disease (the question usually is whether payments are *too* high), as well as questions concerning medicare's effect on hospital finances.

Local and regional considerations spur many congressional oversight investigations and hearings, particularly when there is conflict among states and regions regarding the distribution of federal funds or when they fear that they will be disproportionately harmed by federal action. Health oversight is not often propelled by such parochialism, but it does occur. Members may seek an oversight investigation or hearing, for example, of reported problems in the way a state is handling medicare claims payments.

In another example, when he was governor of New York, Mario Cuomo frequently and vociferously complained that the federal-state formula for medicaid assumes New York is richer than it is and therefore shortchanges the state in the distribution of federal medicaid funds. New York Senator Daniel Patrick Moynihan requested a GAO study, which confirmed that New York was underfunded, but no action was taken.

One respect in which health oversight has been unique is the importance of gender issues. Women demonstrated their growing political influence in 1990 when the Congressional Caucus on Women's Issues teamed with the House Commerce Health Subcommittee to ask GAO to investigate whether adequate numbers of women were included in National Institutes of Health (NIH) medical studies. Staff members of the caucus had evidence that most large-scale longitudinal studies sponsored by NIH included only men, which raised questions about whether the results of the studies could be safely applied to women. GAO evaluators quickly determined that NIH had not been following its own guidelines about including women in such studies. With the GAO information in hand, the Health Subcommittee held a hearing to increase the issue's visibility as well as to call NIH officials to account. A repentant NIH pledged to adopt GAO's recommendations. The episode, which garnered considerable publicity, eventually resulted in legislation creating an Office of Research on Women's Health at NIH.

The same members of Congress subsequently asked GAO to study the gender composition of clinical drug trials sanctioned by FDA. Similar problems to those at NIH were found, and FDA changed its procedures. Equal and appropriate treatment of women has also been the focus of investigations and hearings conducted by the House and Senate Veterans' Affairs Committees.

Changing the Agenda: How the Parties Differ

With the change to Republican control of Congress, oversight became less freewheeling and entrepreneurial. Particularly in the House, the overall legislative agenda was driven by the leadership, and committee chairs have had far less latitude in setting the oversight agenda than was the case before 1995.

The change of party control was accompanied by a marked change in the agenda and focus of oversight and emphasizes oversight's policy dimension. There has always been a broad range of issues for which oversight has been bipartisan. In hearings on issues such as the national organ transplant system, drug abuse, and health care fraud, there is no discernable partisan split. However, the onset of Republican control starkly illustrates that oversight is ultimately a vehicle for Congress (or at least the majority) to influence the implementation of policy. This can be seen in oversight of FDA and of the medicare and medicaid programs.

Food and Drug Administration

Differing attitudes toward federal regulation have long characterized the two major parties. Although it is difficult to find anyone who will say a kind word about regulation in 1995, in the past oversight of FDA usually examined whether the agency was acting with sufficient efficiency, aggressiveness, and speed in dealing with identified problems. For example, in the 1980s a committee staff investigation and a series of GAO reports and related hearings charged that FDA was lax in monitoring the safety of medical devices. As a result, legislation was enacted in 1990 expanding the reach of FDA in this area. In the 1980s, thirteen major new laws were passed (most resulting from oversight hearings) that likewise added to FDA's regulatory responsibilities.

Because a number of leading Republicans have been critical of FDA for being *too* aggressive and burdensome, it is not surprising that oversight activities under Republican leadership more forcefully represent the perspective that the FDA stymies innovation and takes too long to approve drugs and medical devices. In opening a series of hearings on FDA in 1995, Senator Nancy Kassebaum (R.-Kan.), chairwoman of the Labor and Human Resources Committee, noted: "The regulated industries, as well as many patient advocacy groups, have increasingly come to see the agency as a barrier to rather than a partner in innovation." With the exception of the FDA commissioner, all the witnesses echoed that viewpoint.

Medicaid

Since at least the 1980s, powerful leaders in Congress have used their health oversight authority to protect two large but very different constituencies: those who receive medicare and those who receive medicaid.

Congressional overseers of medicaid, the health insurance program for poor Americans funded jointly by the federal and state governments, have used their oversight powers to expand program eligibility and to protect existing benefits. Claiming that the program was not reaching enough poor people, the proponents of expansion used a variety of opportunities to extend benefits to new categories of recipients. A provision of the Omnibus Budget Reconciliation Act of 1989, for example, extended medicaid coverage to young children in households with earnings up to 133 percent of the federal poverty line.

The major policy thrust in medicaid in the mid-1990s is the attempt by state governments to require that beneficiaries be enrolled in managed care programs. Medicaid has been the fastest growing part of state budgets since the mid-1980s, and the states have sought desperately to hold those costs down. Under managed care plans, health maintenance organizations or other physician networks are paid a monthly rate for each enrollee rather than being reimbursed for services rendered. Officials in Tennessee, Ohio, and other states argue that such plans can better control costs and even improve access for poor Americans, who often have trouble finding doctors who will accept the low reimbursement offered by most medicaid programs. To run a managed care plan, each state must first get a waiver from federal medicaid officials; the states are seeking to make the waiver automatic.[18]

Congressional overseers—particularly Democrat Henry Waxman, former chairman of the House Commerce Health Subcommittee—have been leery of such efforts. They are skeptical about routinely forcing poor patients into managed care programs composed entirely of medicaid beneficiaries or other low-income people, and they oppose easing the waiver process. Despite the budgetary burden on the states, the Children's Defense Fund and other advocates for poor people argue that more federal oversight would be needed because managed care plans have an incentive to provide less service—that is primarily how they save money. Medicaid payment rates to doctors and hospitals are already lower than private rates, and medicaid beneficiaries typically lack the sophistication and clout to protest inadequate care. "The poor are already underserved," Waxman once said. "We don't have to force them into plans where doctors are paid not to serve them."[19] Just as Waxman and others used oversight to expand medicaid, they have used oversight activities to prevent the erosion of benefits.

The shift to Republican control, however, brought a sea change in the agenda of oversight. The driving force behind such oversight has become the implementation of managed care plans and budgetary issues. Although hearings have not been devoid of concern for beneficiaries, there is now far greater concern for the budgetary plight of the federal and state governments. The biggest change of all is the move to convert medicaid to a finite block grant, which is being pushed by congressional Republicans. This would substantially diminish federal involvement with the program (other than writing the checks) and consequently would decrease congressional oversight on behalf of the beneficiaries.

Is Oversight Systematic?

One of the key criteria for assessing Congress posited by the Renewing Congress Project is a legislative agenda. "Congress needs to have the ability to set priorities and, every bit as significant, to act on them with reasonable coherence, predictability, and dispatch," Mann and Ornstein wrote.[20] It is therefore reasonable to ask whether congressional oversight is systematic. Are oversight priorities established for each session? Are major programs reviewed periodically? Is there coordination across the oversight agendas of the various subcommittees, at least within a single committee?

The common perception is that oversight is not systematic but instead focuses on the scandal of the moment, with congressional attention jumping from one issue to the next with no clear strategy or priority. In some ways that is a valid criticism of oversight in the health policy arena, but in others it is not.

Even though the quantity of oversight has increased, the process is still short of the comprehensive and strategic review considered ideal by some scholars.[21] Oversight may be an integral part of the policymaking process, but that process is political. Even when committee chairmen, for example, set out an oversight agenda at the beginning of a new Congress, that agenda serves the chairmen's political needs and policy preferences.

Furthermore, there has been little coordination of oversight among committees within a chamber and almost none between the House and Senate. Until Newt Gingrich reasserted the power of the Speaker of the House, the House and Senate leadership offered little if any input in shaping oversight priorities, and there was little jurisdictional control. Subcommittees of the House Small Business Committee, for example, have held hearings on women's health programs and on FDA's pharmaceutical regulation. As a result, administrative agencies spent a great deal of time and resources responding to similar demands from several different congressional committees. (During the 102nd Congress, for example, FDA was summoned to appear at seventy hearings before eighteen separate committees and subcommittees.)

The change of party control in the House after the 1994 elections could lead to more systematic oversight. Because the Republicans have a more centralized leadership structure than the Democrats and the number of committees has been reduced, the Republican leadership has an opportunity to conduct more focused oversight with less duplication of effort than prevailed under the Democrats.

Even if that does not come to pass, oversight has been more systematic and constructive than a review of oversight hearings alone might suggest. For one thing, the increased use of periodic reauthorization not only forces oversight, but also helps to establish a framework for committees' oversight and legislative agendas. Periodic reauthorization may not compel attention to the most pressing issue or to the weakest points of program implementation, but it does at least require staff to attend to the programs to be reauthorized.

Moreover, congressional staff members carry on a continuing dialogue with agency officials on a large number of issues. Veteran staff members in particular know the programs and the agencies quite well. They might not produce the same list of oversight targets that a comprehensive, criteria-driven review of all programs in a specific policy area might yield, but neither is the list likely to be scattershot or trivial.

Additionally, the support agencies greatly amplify the surveillance by Congress. For example, three or four staff members spend most of their time on FDA issues, but GAO alone issued nine reports on the agency in 1992. Neither GAO nor the HHS inspector general provides comprehensive oversight of the public health and health financing agencies, but they do offer a scope of coverage that allows Congress to study more issues in depth than would otherwise be possible.

Nor does health policy oversight concern itself only with less important issues. Indeed, medicaid and medicare have been subject to such intense and extensive oversight that Congress has been criticized for being too intrusive. During most of 1994, for example, GAO was conducting eighteen reviews involving the HCFA's implementation of the two programs.

How Effective is Health Policy Oversight?

It makes no difference, of course, how systematic oversight is if it has no effect on policy. Effectiveness cannot be precisely measured, but congressional oversight in the health policy arena has substantially affected both program policy and implementation. The medicare PPS and the revised physician fee system are primary examples of this.

Oversight has also led to myriad less comprehensive changes in health programs. Although the budget reconciliation process may not receive high marks for careful deliberation, the almost-annual bills have become the most common vehicle for following up oversight with legislation. Among other things, the 1993 budget reconciliation act adjusted the medicare prospective payment rate for rural hospitals, directed how HHS should calculate payment rates for skilled nursing facilities, set payment limits for durable medical equipment, and extended the ban on physicians' referring patients to facilities they own.[22] All of these changes were part of a continuing oversight process characterized by staff studies, GAO reports, PPRC recommendations, and congressional hearings.

Oversight and Health Care Reform

Although oversight leads to continual changes in existing programs, it played only a minor role in the ultimately futile struggle to enact health care reform in 1994. The Clinton administration's proposed plan basically ignored the results of previous congressional work on health care, opting instead for new structures and an untested strategy. Congressional hearings were held on relatively peripheral issues such as medical education, private long-term care insurance, and state capacity to regulate insurance. But Congress's nearly two decades of overseeing cost control efforts under medicare were swept away by a tidal wave of negative hyperbole about bureaucracy and government control of health care. Only the House Ways and Means Committee reported out a health reform bill providing new coverage through medicare—an approach that never had much chance of passage in the House, let alone the Senate.

Thus, both the administration and most members of Congress rejected an approach to health care that, whatever its other merits, was based on a program that had been reviewed and amended as oversight produced better ways to control costs. Indeed, toward the end of the reform debate citizens' groups lobbying legislators wore T-shirts that said "No Government-Run Health Care"—as if medicare and the Department of Veterans Affairs simply did not exist. If the health care reform debate is a guide, it would appear that the politics surrounding passage of any major new program can easily swamp any factual analysis derived from congressional experience and oversight.

Oversight in a Republican Congress

Under the Republican presidencies of Ronald Reagan and George Bush, congressional Democrats, hampered by budget constraints and suspicious that the Republican administrations might be lax in enforcing health programs they did not agree with, turned from initiating new public health programs to overseeing the ones that had already been enacted. Even after the Democrats gained the White House in 1992, Democratic legislators were still wary of executive branch implementation. Thus congressional staffers who were unhappy during the Bush administration with HHS monitoring of federal funds used by the states for drug abuse treatment were no more trusting under the Clinton administration. Although some have criticized this level of scrutiny as micromanagement, it is often not management but policy that drives the oversight.

In an era of tight spending constraints, it is this disagreement over policy choices that increasingly is at the heart of oversight. Just as the line between politics and administration has long been regarded as artificial, it is time to recognize that oversight is part of the policymaking and implementation process and that Congress is a partner in that process. The political earthquake of 1994 in no way changes the basic purposes and functions of oversight. Indeed, so long as Democrats hold the White House, the Republican Congress is likely to step up its use of oversight to rope in executive agencies and programs in pursuit of its own policy objectives.

Part Two
Health Policymaking

Chapter 6

Congress's "Catastrophic" Attempt to Fix Medicare

Julie Rovner

Courage is a commodity that shows its face from time to time on Capitol Hill. I don't think this is one of its greater moments.
          Senator John D. Rockefeller IV, September 1989[1]

THE TWENTIETH CENTURY has seen a raft of case studies on how a bill becomes a law. But the saga of the 1988 Medicare Catastrophic Coverage Act provides one of the few case studies on how a bill becomes a former law.

At first glance, the brief life and publicly humiliating demise of the catastrophic costs law is an overwhelming warning for any Congress considering overhaul of a health care system that will affect *every* American, not just the 35 million elderly and disabled people who participate in the federal medicare program. The warning is that it is easy to expand benefits, but you better make sure those who will be getting something new are also willing to pay for it.

The conventional wisdom on the ill-fated Medicare Catastrophic Coverage Act is that it was all a big mistake. Congress passed it overwhelmingly in 1988. But financially secure senior citizens rebelled when they realized they would have to pay for expanded benefits they felt they did not need. A chastened (or perhaps cowed) Congress backed down and repealed the law just over a year later.

In fact, the conventional wisdom oversimplified the complicated political dynamic, and in the process, the moral of the story—that Congress is enslaved by the political power of elderly voters—came out wrong. The real story of the rise and fall of the Medicare Catastrophic Coverage Act sends several ominous messages about the state of the Congress and our political system, but the power of the senior citizens' lobby is not one of them. Those who lived through this nightmare instead learned a lot more about the power of direct mail, the ease of manipulating the public with information that is simply wrong, the resistance recipients of federal entitlement programs feel toward change, and the lack of knowledge Americans have about programs that so directly affect their lives.

The efforts of the media and backers of the law to simplify what was a necessarily complex construct probably doomed the program more than anything else. More often than not, attempts to make the program fit a twelve-second soundbite or six-line paragraph led to mistakes that would have been comical had they not so directly led to the law's downfall. Take, for example, a 1988 news story in a Myrtle Beach, S.C., paper stating that under the law, all senior citizens would have to pay an amount equal to the lesser of $800 or 15 percent of their income. (In fact, less than half of medicare beneficiaries would have been required to pay a surtax of the lesser of $800 or 15 percent of their federal income tax liability—and less than 6 percent would have paid the top amount.) In light of such "innocent" mistakes, no wonder people misunderstood and became upset. And small wonder that groups that make their money by fomenting fear among elderly Americans rushed to fill the information gap.

The catastrophic costs law also represented the first major piece of social legislation passed by Congress in the "pay-as-you-go" (or paygo) budget era. In other words, for the first time Congress sought to expand benefits for some by explicitly making others pay for them. Of course to some extent this is always true—all federal money comes from the taxpayers in some fashion. But in the era of massive budget deficits, it became necessary to spell out for all to see exactly who would provide the funds. In this case, the payers—relatively well-off elderly Americans—screamed bloody murder.

Another faulty conclusion is that Congress's willingness to back down so readily in the face of the resulting onslaught showed how out of touch members of the House and Senate were with the public. In fact, the startling turnaround illustrated even more clearly how hypersensitive members are to voters' complaints. Indeed, Congress folded rather than fight to convince misinformed constituents that the law would actually be a good deal for them.

The story of the rise and fall of the Medicare Catastrophic Coverage Act has important implications for the continuing debate over health care reform. Both intimately affect people's life and death decisions about their health care. Both deal with highly complex subjects, both financial and medical; both involve multijurisdictional trips through the Congress that heighten the ability to raise roadblocks and further confuse the public; and, perhaps most significantly, both force the Congress into decisions that will adversely affect at least some interested people. Indeed, the ignominious fate of the catastrophic coverage law did not so much foreshadow Congress's inability to pass any health reform bill in 1994 as much as it contributed to it by reminding members how politically perilous redistribution schemes are.

About Medicare

Understanding the story of "catastrophic," as the law came to be called by those who designed it, first requires a brief understanding of medicare, the federal health insurance program for elderly and disabled persons that the law sought to expand.

Medicare has two parts. Medicare part A, officially the HI (hospital insurance) program, helps pay the costs of inpatient hospital and limited nursing home, home health, and hospice care. Like social security, part A is financed by a payroll tax of 1.45 percent of income paid by both employer and worker on all earnings.[2] Anyone age 65 or older who is eligible for social security or railroad retirement benefits is automatically eligible for part A coverage. Those under 65 who receive social security disability payments (or railroad retirement disability) become eligible for part A after a 24-month waiting period. Anyone over age 65 who is not otherwise eligible may purchase part A coverage. The 1994 premium was $245 per month. Under a special program created by Congress in 1972, about 200,000 people who need kidney transplants or renal dialysis because of chronic kidney disease are also eligible for part A coverage.[3]

Medicare part B, formally the SMI (supplementary medical insurance) program, is an optional program that helps pay for doctor and other outpatient medical expenses. About 25 percent of part B costs are covered by premiums ($41.10 per month in 1994) that for most beneficiaries are deducted from social security checks. The remaining three-fourths of the program is financed from general federal revenues. Part B is available to anyone age 65 or over, regardless of eligibility for part A, and also to those under age 65 who receive part A coverage. Nearly all medicare part A beneficiaries (about 98 percent) also take the optional part B coverage.[4]

Although medicare in some ways resembles most private health insurance plans, any analyst unfamiliar with its origins will see at once that the program has no internal logic. That is because, like so many other government programs, medicare's structure was dictated by political compromise. Part A, the compulsory social insurance portion, was pushed from the beginning by Democrats who sought a broader government role in providing health care to those who lacked it. (In 1965, before the enactment of medicare, only an estimated 56 percent of elderly people had hospital insurance.)[5] The voluntary part B, based on traditional indemnity insurance plans common at the time, was pushed primarily by Republicans who wanted to stave off national health insurance, as well as the American Medical Association, which branded any broad-scale government involvement in the health care system as "socialized medicine." House Ways and Means Chairman Wilbur Mills ensured political support sufficient to enact the measure by combining the two (along with a third proposal, to create the joint federal-state medicaid program for poor people).[6] That produced a program that made political sense but was otherwise quite confusing—an element that would come back to haunt policymakers during the fight over the catastrophic coverage law.

Why Catastrophic?

Two separate dynamics, one policy and the other political, spurred the movement of the Medicare Catastrophic Coverage Act through Congress.

The policy dynamic had been obvious for some time—although medicare seemed to resemble many private insurance plans, it lacked the key financial protection common to virtually every other form of health insurance: a cap on out-of-pocket costs beneficiaries could be expected to pay for covered services. Typical indemnity insurance plans require beneficiaries to pay a deductible before insurance kicks in (usually $100 to $500). They then require coinsurance (10 to 30 percent of bills for covered services) but usually impose a limit on the annual amount policyholders must pay in such cost-sharing (typically $1,500 to $5,000).

Medicare, in contrast, had no such limits. In fact, the sicker a person was, the more he or she was required to pay, particularly for hospital care. Both before the catastrophic coverage law and since its repeal, after a hospitalized patient pays a separate hospital deductible ($696 in 1994), medicare pays all the remaining costs for 60 days. Patients who remain hospitalized after that time (or who reenter the hospital less than 60 days after discharge from the hospital or a medicare-covered nursing home stay) must pay coinsurance for the next 30 days ($174 per day in 1994). Patients whose "spell of illness" exceeds 90 days get a 60-day "lifetime reserve," which requires a copayment that is higher still ($348 per day in 1994). After 150 days (or 90 days if the lifetime reserve was exhausted previously), medicare ceases coverage altogether for hospital care. Under part B, patients must pay an annual deductible ($100 in 1994), after which the program pays 80 percent of the medicare-approved fee for covered services for the remainder of the year. There is no limit on the coinsurance beneficiaries may be required to pay. Thus, a patient with $50,000 in covered outpatient costs (not an implausible amount in these days of outpatient surgery and other advanced treatments not requiring hospitalization) would be left with a bill for 20 percent of that amount, or $10,000.

Medicare also lacked (and still lacks) other coverages common to most private insurance. One of the biggest lapses is its failure to cover costs of outpatient prescription drugs, even though (some would say because) elderly people use significantly more in the way of such drugs than the rest of the population—three times the rate of those under 65.[7] Designed expressly as an acute-care program, medicare also includes little coverage of preventive care, such as routine physicals and most screening procedures. (Since 1990, however, some preventive services, including influenza vaccines and mammograms to detect breast cancer, have been added.)

Of course, the biggest gap in coverage, and the one that would ultimately help bring about the downfall of the catastrophic coverage law, was medicare's failure to pay for long-term custodial nursing home care. Although medicare does include a limited nursing home benefit, beneficiaries must meet stringent eligibility tests. As a result, in 1988 medicare paid less than 2 percent of the nation's nursing home bill.[8] And as both supporters and opponents of the catastrophic coverage law were quick to point out, long-term care was by far the leading cause of catastrophic medical costs for elderly people. Of the over-65 population who spent more than $3,000 out-of-pocket for medical care in 1985, more than 80 percent of the funds went to finance nursing home stays.[9]

One of the principal sources of confusion surrounding the catastrophic coverage effort from the start was defining just what word "catastrophic" was supposed to modify. Policymakers seemed perpetually confused over whether the problem was the illness itself or the cost of treating it. In fact, the issue all along was cost, not the type of illness. Indeed, while a broken leg might be considered a minor financial burden for a wealthy medicare beneficiary, the expenses associated with it could well be catastrophic for a person living solely on social security benefits. Indeed, the legislation itself, in the words of the Ways and Means Committee report, "would protect medicare beneficiaries from catastrophic *expenses* [emphasis added] associated with covered hospital and physician services."[10]

Analysts defined catastrophic medical costs according to two main criteria—a money threshold for unreimbursed out-of-pocket costs regardless of income (generally in the $2,000 to $4,000 range), and out-of-pocket expenditures that exceeded a specified percentage of a person's annual income (generally 5 to 10 percent). According to the Department of Health and Human Services (HHS), elderly people were more than two and a half times as likely as those under 65 to have catastrophic medical expenses.[11]

Another factor driving the policy side of the debate was how quickly out-of-pocket medical costs were rising for the medicare population. The American Association of Retired Persons (AARP) noted in 1987 that elderly Americans were paying roughly 15 percent of their income out of their own pockets for medical care—the same percentage people over 65 had paid for health care before the enactment of medicare.[12] The House Ways and Means Committee noted that in 1986, 7 percent of elderly Americans spent 25 percent or more of their income on medical care. Noting that nearly half of older Americans had incomes below $10,000, the committee wrote, "Paying twenty-five percent of a $10,000 income on medical care is truly catastrophic."[13]

But perhaps the most controversial element on the policy side was that only a minority of elderly people were actually at full financial risk from the gaps in medicare coverage. In 1988, an estimated 62 percent of medicare enrollees had some private insurance to supplement medicare.[14] Much was privately purchased "medigap" insurance expressly designed to plug the holes in medicare coverage. About one-third of medicare beneficiaries had coverage provided by employers or former employers, some but not all of it specifically designed to supplement medicare.[15] Another 10 percent of medicare beneficiaries were covered by medicaid, the joint federal-state health plan for poor Americans, which protected *them* from virtually all out-of-pocket medical costs. Thus, only about 27.5 percent of medicare beneficiaries were technically subject to financial catastrophe due to a medicare-covered illness.[16]

Opponents of the catastrophic costs legislation argued that it would effectively eliminate the medigap market, which was working well. But supporters pointed to studies showing numerous abuses in the medigap market (which would lead to separate legislation in 1990). They noted that the federal government could provide the same coverage at far lower administrative cost than the private sector. Nevertheless, the effect on the medigap market and on those Americans with their own supplemental coverage (particularly the estimated 23 percent of beneficiaries who had some or all of their supplemental coverage subsidized) would remain a bone of contention throughout the effort to pass and later to repeal the catastrophic coverage law.

The political imperatives that drove the catastrophic coverage law were considerably more simple: elderly Americans were a well-organized and powerful political bloc that voted in higher proportions than their younger counterparts.[17]

Ronald Reagan had lost significant standing among elderly people with his proposed social security cuts in his controversial 1981 budget—an unpopular move the Democrats capitalized on in the 1982 elections.[18] In 1985 administration officials were therefore looking to mend some fences even as they were seeking new domestic initiatives. The specific idea came at the instigation of Otis R. Bowen, a physician and former Indiana governor who became HHS secretary in December 1985. Bowen had chaired the 1984 Social Security Advisory Council that made such a program one of its principal recommendations.

Reagan officially launched the effort in his 1986 State of the Union message. Buried about two-thirds of the way through—between a call for welfare reform and an urge to the youth of America to resist the temptations of illegal drugs—were these words: "Further, after seeing how devastating illness can destroy the financial security of the family, I am directing the Secretary of Health and Human Services, Dr. Otis Bowen, to report to me by the end of the year with recommendations on how the private sector and government can work together to address the problems of affordable insurance for those whose life savings would otherwise be threatened when catastrophic illness strikes."[19]

Bowen enthusiastically fulfilled the president's directive and on November 20 unveiled his proposal. The secretary's Private-Public Sector Advisory Committee on Catastrophic Illness actually addressed the needs of three separate populations—elderly people who required lengthy hospitalizations; elderly people who required long-term, non-hospital care; and the under-65 population at financial risk for catastrophic medical expenses. But it was only Bowen's proposal for the first group—to extend medicare's hospital coverage and put a $2,000 out-of-pocket cap on part B coverage by adding $4.92 monthly to the optional part B premium—that caught on.[20]

The Road to Passage

President Reagan did not formally endorse the Bowen plan until February, after much hand-wringing within the administration, particularly from more conservative advisors who complained about undercutting the private medigap market. But by then it was clear that Congress was ready to go ahead with or without a formal administration proposal. By late January, four separate committees—House Aging, House Ways and Means, Senate Aging, and Senate Finance—were already holding hearings on the subject of catastrophic costs legislation.

It was not hard to figure out why Congress was so eager to get off to a quick start. The 1986 election had given the Senate back to the Democrats for the first time since 1980. In the House, new Speaker Jim Wright (D.-Texas) was similarly inclined to leave a legislative legacy. After six years of retrenchment under Reagan and the conservatives, the Democrats were eager to get back to pushing their agenda, rather than simply defending existing programs from dismantlement. Ways and Means Chairman Dan Rostenkowski said as much on the House floor during the initial debate on the bill: "The President's interest in the issue and endorsement of the Bowen proposal provided Congress with the unexpected opportunity to make long overdue improvements in the Medicare Program. Improvements that, a few months earlier, virtually no one would have thought possible."[21]

But the problems Democrats had with the president's plan were more than just political. Those at the highest risk for financial catastrophe were elderly people of low to moderate income (since the poorest would be covered by medicaid). But those were the very individuals who would have been most hurt by a flat increase in the part B premium—a classic regressive tax. Noted Rostenkowski, "In fact, some of the same low-income elderly who currently cannot afford private medigap policies would not opt for the new coverage contained in the president's bill because they could not afford the additional premium."[22]

And then there were those who wanted to use this opportunity to do as much as possible. In that regard, the single most important individual was not Bowen, Reagan, nor Rostenkowski, nor even any member of the various committees that would ultimately oversee the legislation. It was Rules Committee Chairman Claude Pepper (D.-Fla.). An unreformed New Deal liberal, as chairman of the House Select Committee on Aging in the late 1970s Pepper had exposed all manner of scams against America's senior citizens. Indeed, it was a series of hearings demonstrating how elderly Americans were being sold duplicative and worthless insurance to supplement medicare that led Congress to first attempt to regulate the medigap market in 1980.

Although most Democrats and many moderate Republicans were lauding the Bowen plan as an important starting point for efforts to improve medicare, Pepper remained unmoved. "The President calls this a giant step forward," he said upon hearing of Reagan's formal endorsement of the Bowen plan. "This isn't a step taken by a giant, it's one taken by a pygmy."[23] In March, Pepper testified before a Ways and Means Subcommittee hearing: "Isn't it time we dealt with this problem in a comprehensive way? If we pass up this opportunity, we may not come around to this again for another 20 years."[24]

And what Pepper thought counted for a lot. As chairman of the powerful Rules Committee, he had the ability to determine not only which amendments would be offered on the House floor, but also in what order—often a key determinant of the outcome of a floor fight. A man who had served a total of 40 years in the Senate and then the House, Pepper was beloved by elderly Americans and revered by members of both houses of Congress. As if that were not enough, more than a few members of Congress literally owed Pepper their jobs. In 1982, the then 81-year-old Pepper crisscrossed the country for endangered Democrats to stir up support among elderly voters. This tour prompted the political director of the Democratic National Committee to call him "the sexiest man in America."[25]

So, spurred on by Pepper, Democrats in both chambers (but particularly in the House) sought to expand on the Bowen-Reagan plan. But there was one major check on their zeal—the insistence by Reagan and deficit-wary Democrats that any new benefits be fully financed. As Robert Pear noted in the *New York Times*: "From the start, it was clear to virtually everyone that the new program would have to pay for itself and could not increase the federal budget deficit."[26]

In fact, not only did Democrats agree that the proposal should be deficit neutral, but they also agreed that, like the President's plan, the costs of the new benefits should be borne exclusively by those who would benefit from them—current medicare beneficiaries.

Such a "user fee" was controversial for the Washington representatives of the major groups representing the interests of elderly Americans. In particular, these organizations included the influential AARP; the labor-backed National Council of Senior Citizens (NCSC); Villers Advocacy Associates (a lobby for low-income elderly people since renamed Families USA); and the National Committee to Preserve Social Security and Medicare, headed by James Roosevelt, son of FDR. Indeed, early on all the leading interest groups came out in opposition to what the Roosevelt group (as it was commonly called) dubbed "seniors-only" financing. "We are not convinced that the modest benefit improvements in the Stark-Gradison plan [which expanded on the Administration proposal; see below] justify the adoption of such a radical change in medicare's existing financing mechanism," AARP President John Denning testified at a March 1987 hearing of the Ways and Means Subcommittee on Health.[27]

But AARP, NCSC, and Villers (although not the Roosevelt group) soon realized that if medicare beneficiaries did not pay the costs, there would be no bill. Instead, they sought to make the benefits worth the added costs. Without saying so explicitly, the groups hinted early in the deliberations that adding an outpatient prescription drug benefit might make their members more willing to pay additional medicare premiums. As Villers Executive Director Ron Pollack testified at that same March 1987 hearing of the Ways and Means Subcommittee on Health: "I don't think there is any question—if we could do something on prescription drugs, I think that there would be significant enthusiasm on the part of the senior population, and I think that should be a very high priority."[28]

House Action

Equally as important as deciding that the cost of the new benefits would be borne by those who stood to benefit was negotiating how to spread that cost most fairly.

The first major proposal to reinvent the Bowen plan came in the form of a bill proposed jointly by Reps. Pete Stark (D.-Calif.) and Bill Gradison (R.-Ohio), the chairman and ranking Republican, respectively, of the House Ways and Means Subcommittee on Health. At first glance Stark and Gradison seemed an unlikely team. Stark was a self-made millionaire, liberal, and eccentric—during the Vietnam War he erected an eight-foot-high peace sign atop his bank in conservative Walnut Creek.[29] He was known for having a quick temper and a smart mouth that frequently got him in trouble (such as when he called former HHS Secretary Louis Sullivan a "disgrace to his race"). Gradison, in contrast, was the polite and reserved former mayor of Cincinnati, an economic conservative and social moderate who as a legislator was as thoughtful as Stark was impulsive.

But personality and ideological differences aside, Stark and Gradison were both serious and highly intelligent legislators. They had forged a close bond working on some of the most arcane issues in medicare policy, including refining the complicated formulas by which hospitals, doctors, and other health care providers are reimbursed.

Thus, only months after the successful conclusion of a bipartisan tax-reform bill, it seemed only logical that Stark and Gradison would team up on a bipartisan catastrophic costs measure. Indeed, their solid team was an effective deterrent to the efforts of Pepper and other liberals to add unlimited new benefits to the proposal. Chided Stark at a Health Subcommittee hearing in March 1987: "When you get Mr. Gradison and me and Secretary Bowen and the President all together, you had better reserve one of those puppies, my friend, because you are never going to get a chance for a breeding like that again."[30]

The Stark-Gradison bill, unveiled in late February 1987, sought to expand the benefits in the Bowen plan somewhat. Specifically, it provided lower, inflation-adjusted cost-sharing and slightly longer nursing home coverage. It also sought to solve the problem of the Bowen plan's regressive financing with a novel approach. Although it did propose raising the flat part B premium, it sought a smaller increase (about $1.30 per month, compared with Bowen's $4.92).[31] To finance the remainder, the bill proposed taxing the actuarial value of the government-subsidized portion of medicare coverage (the 75 percent of part B financed by general revenues). By tying payment of the new benefits to income taxes, rich medicare recipients would by definition be required to pay more than those of more modest means. According to Stark and Gradison's estimates, in 1988 Americans in the 15 percent tax bracket would have paid an additional $265 in income taxes, while those in the 28 percent bracket would have seen their tax liability increase by approximately $495. But, most importantly, most medicare beneficiaries—65 percent—would not have paid any additional tax because their incomes were too low.[32]

The political plus of this approach was that most medicare beneficiaries would get new benefits without paying much for them. What would come back to haunt Congress later was that well-off elderly Americans would foot the entire bill for their poorer brethren—something many of them would not appreciate.

As it turned out, the concept of taxing the actuarial value of medicare was politically a nonstarter. Organized labor fought it for fear of setting a precedent that could lead to the taxation of fringe benefits in general. Thus, when the bill reached the full Ways and Means Committee in May, the taxing proposal was replaced by the financing that would ultimately be adopted, although in somewhat modified form. Originally devised in the Senate Finance Committee, it was officially called a "supplemental premium," a surtax that would be collected along with income taxes for the estimated 40 percent of medicare part A beneficiaries with taxable incomes over $15,000. Gradison preferred to call it "a mandatory user's fee."[33] Opponents simply called it by another accurate name: a new tax.

But while Ways and Means was holding the line, the other committee with jurisdiction over the medicare program, Energy and Commerce, was pushing the edge of the envelope. When it came to medicare, the two committees had always behaved somewhat like sibling rivals: they often disagreed about the means to an end, but when they did finally marshall their resources, they generally held off all other challenges. The complicated jurisdictional lines also added to the general confusion surrounding medicare. Ways and Means had sole jurisdiction over part A (because it was funded by a payroll tax), the two panels shared jurisdiction over the voluntary part B, and Energy and Commerce had sole jurisdiction over the joint federal-state medicaid program for poor people. The original Stark-Gradison proposal was actually introduced as two separate bills (HR 1290 and HR 1291) to prevent Energy and Commerce from gaining oversight of part A.

Superficially, the leaders of the Energy and Commerce health subcommittee appeared similar to those heading Ways and Means: a California liberal Democrat and a midwestern Republican moderate. But Health and Environment Subcommittee Chairman Henry A. Waxman (D.-Calif.) and Edward R. Madigan (R.-Ill.) fostered a much different dynamic than did Stark and Gradison. Waxman was then the House's consummate liberal health expert. His tack was to try to bridge the gap between Pepper's desire to expand medicare as much as possible and Stark's wish to produce a bill that President Reagan would sign. Indeed, Waxman publicly sided with Pepper more than with Stark—and while others lauded the administration for getting the ball rolling, Waxman made clear that its proposal was insufficient. "With its limited gesture of assistance, the administration has come upon a car wreck and only changed the tire," Waxman said that March.[34]

With a more liberal membership, not to mention a committee chairman (Rep. John D. Dingell [D-Mich.]) with whom he tended to see eye to eye on health issues, Waxman was not only freer to seek more expansions than Stark, he had a virtual obligation to do so.

Waxman's first addition, made during subcommittee consideration, was an outpatient prescription drug benefit. Although adding such coverage to medicare had been a longtime goal for Waxman, this particular inclusion came with not only the blessing but also the urging of House Speaker Jim Wright, in an effort to pacify the powerful Claude Pepper. During the week of May 4, Democrats from the Ways and Means, Energy and Commerce, and Aging Committees met, and Wright reportedly emphasized that "adding a drug benefit would help put a Democratic stamp" on what had begun as a Republican initiative.[35]

Waxman also added to the bill another provision he had been seeking for many years—an increase in the amount of income a person living at home could keep when medicaid was paying for the nursing home care of his or her spouse. Congress had been inundated with examples of "spousal impoverishment" resulting from medicaid requirements that nearly all of a couple's income be devoted to nursing home care even if one spouse was still living in the couple's home.

But the rest of the bells and whistles added to the bill came not from Waxman but from other members of his subcommittee. They included provisions to add a "respite care" benefit to provide relief to those who care for sick and elderly loved ones at home (added by Doug Walgren [D-Pa.]); provide limited coverage for preventive screenings for breast and colorectal cancer (added by Cardiss Collins [D-Ill.]); add coverage for influenza vaccines (added by James H. Scheuer [D-N.Y.]); and expand medicare coverage for outpatient mental health services (added by Gerry Sikorski [D-Minn.]).

The expansion of benefits raised objections from panel Republicans, including ranking member Madigan, who otherwise supported the proposal. "This exercise is supposed to be to protect against catastrophes, not to add new benefits to medicare," Madigan complained at the subcommittee markup.[36]

But the add-on machine was in full swing. At Speaker Wright's "suggestion," the Ways and Means Committee voted to add a prescription drug benefit to its bill too, albeit one slightly less generous than what Waxman had included in the Energy and Commerce version. The Reagan administration cried foul. In a June 15 veto threat letter to the committee chairmen, HHS Secretary Bowen warned that such additional benefits, would "result in program cost increases that quickly outpace the bill's financing, greatly jeopardizing the stability of the program's design."[37]

But Democrats decided the administration was bluffing about a potential veto of its top domestic initiative. Besides, the leadership had to deal with a still unsatisfied Claude Pepper. Even with the drug benefit added, Pepper complained that the bill did not go far enough. "I believe it would be a tragedy to accept minor reform at a time when the country is overwhelmingly supportive of meaningful change," he said.[38]

By early July leaders had successfully brokered a deal between the Ways and Means and Energy and Commerce versions of the bill. The revisions trimmed back the extra benefits added by the latter committee somewhat (the preventive benefits were dropped and the respite care provision cut by one-third). But Pepper was threatening to scuttle the entire package by proposing to add an amendment to the bill that would provide "long-term home care" benefits to any American who needed it. Unlike the rest of the bill, Pepper's provision would have been funded exclusively by working Americans, by eliminating the cap on income subject to the medicare portion of the social security tax.

Pepper's threat was no idle one—few doubted that the chairman of the Rules Committee could easily muster enough votes in his own panel for the amendment to be offered during floor consideration. But bringing the amendment up would have put Democrats in an impossible position: risking the wrath of elderly Americans for voting against a fully financed long-term care provision, or facing a certain veto by voting for it.[39] Once again Speaker Wright came to the rescue. Over a private lunch, he persuaded Pepper to withhold the amendment, with the promise of a floor vote on it on another bill at a later date.[40]

With Pepper pacified, at least for the moment, the House easily passed the catastrophic coverage bill on July 22 by a vote of 302 to 127. But there was much ill ease even among the bill's supporters, some of it presaging the fights to come. Said Rep. Brian J. Donnelly (D.-Mass.), a Ways and Means health subcommittee member who helped write the bill but would later successfully fight for its repeal: "It's not too hard to imagine that in 5 years, senior citizens will be paying $50 a month for all the benefits in this bill. They can't afford it, we can't afford it, but it is a future Congress that will have to pay the price."[41]

Senate Action

The dynamic that drove the catastrophic costs legislation in the Senate was considerably different from the one that moved the bill through the House. In the end, however, both chambers wound up in nearly the same place.

The major difference was the role of the Finance Committee. Unlike in the House, where jurisdiction over medicare and medicaid is shared, in the Senate, Finance has sole jurisdiction over both programs. In 1987 the Finance Committee also included Democrats who were in many cases more conservative than the panel's Republicans. At the May 1987 Finance markup of the bill, new committee Chairman Lloyd Bentsen (D.-Texas) and Health Subcommittee Chairman George Mitchell (D.-Maine) found themselves fending off just the sort of add-ons eagerly added to the bill in the House. But in this case, it was Republicans, including former Aging Committee Chairman John Heinz (Pa.), former Health Subcommittee Chairman Dave Durenberger (Minn.), and John S. Chafee (R.I.), who sought to do the adding.[42]

In keeping with the more conservative approach, especially Bentsen's, the bill approved unanimously by the Finance Committee in May was not as generous as the House bill. In particular, it did not originally include a prescription drug benefit. Mitchell did promise to work with Heinz on developing such a plan, a task that would take the rest of the summer.

But it was not just its lack of a drug benefit that put the Finance Committee bill at odds with the Senate as a whole, and this became clear as the leadership tried to move the bill to the floor. In fact, the full Senate would not finish work on its version until October 27.

Although it was not the only reason for the delay, the continuing controversy over the proposed prescription drug benefit was a primary factor. Some of the time was taken up by the process of devising the plan, but the prescription drug industry used the delay to try to scuttle the proposal.

At first glance, the drug industry's opposition to adding coverage to medicare seemed a classic case of looking a gift horse in the mouth. Surely major third-party payment for the very consumers who were the heaviest users of their products would give these manufacturers a financial windfall, much as doctors had profited greatly from the creation of medicare in 1965. But the drug industry, led by the its trade group, the Pharmaceutical Manufacturers Association (PMA), knew that although medicare had generated a lot of business for hospitals and physicians, it had also resulted in significant federal oversight of fees. Noted Phillip Longman in *The New Republic*, the PMA opposed the prescription drug provision in catastrophic coverage "out of the reasonable fear that if the government were paying for all these drugs it might want to have some say over how much they cost."[43]

This was a chance the PMA's member groups clearly did not want to take. During the 1987 summer recess, the PMA spent an estimated $3 million on a grass-roots campaign. Campaign materials included sample mailgrams to be sent to senators and President Reagan that were distributed, to state and local officials who dealt with aging issues, and to other key individuals.[44]

Another problem that became apparent during the delay between committee and Senate floor action was the potential for duplication of benefits for those who had supplemental medicare coverage paid for in full or part by former employers. Michigan, the home state of Finance Committee Democrat Donald W. Riegle, Jr., had a large number of former auto workers with generous retiree health benefits. Riegle wanted to amend the bill to prevent anyone from being forced to pay twice for the same benefits. His amendment would require employers who offered such plans to either substitute new benefits or provide cash refunds equal to the actuarial value of the duplicated benefits.[45]

Federal retirees faced a slightly different but no less thorny problem. Because federal pensions were fully taxable whereas social security was partially tax-free, basing the amount of any supplemental premium on taxable income was problematic. Two retirees (one federal and the other private sector) could have the exact same income, but because of the tax status of their pensions, the federal retiree could be assessed a much larger supplemental premium. That particular problem became the province of yet another Finance Democrat, David Pryor, who also chaired the Governmental Affairs subcommittee that oversaw the federal civil service.

The time and trouble ultimately paid off for the bipartisan team in the Senate. On October 27, Heinz announced that with some small changes, Bentsen and the White House had agreed to support both the underlying catastrophic costs bill and the prescription drug program. Not only did the Senate adopt the drug amendment by an overwhelming vote of 88 to 9 (the bill ultimately passed 86 to 11), but members also added a string of inclusions that had the effect of making the Senate bill more like its counterpart that had passed the House. For example, Barbara A. Mikulski (D.-Md.), successfully pushed for the inclusion of "spousal-impoverishment" provisions like the ones Waxman had added in the House, while Bob Graham (D.-Fla.) was able to increase the frequency of partial coverage of preventive health screening services and flu and pneumonia shots. The Senate also adopted language from Riegle and Pryor to address duplication of benefits. However, presaging the concerns with complexity that would erupt later, at one point Pryor himself was unable to explain his addition, finally referring a reporter to a member of his staff.[46]

House-Senate Conference

Despite the broad support for the catastrophic bill both on the Hill and in public opinion polls, Congress did not even begin negotiations to write a final bill until early 1988. First the three committees involved—House Ways and Means, House Energy and Commerce, and Senate Finance—were tied up resolving the year-end deficit reduction bill. Then negotiations were further delayed by the desire to complete work on a major trade measure that also involved many of the same players.

Indeed, some thought the catastrophic bill conference might be adversely affected by some of the ill will surrounding the last days of the budget fight in late December 1987. As they had with their version of the catastrophic coverage bill, Senate conferees had cut a deal with the White House involving deeper cuts to medicare and less new spending for medicaid. That enraged House health negotiators, prompting Stark to call the upper chamber "an elitist group of millionaires" he would not want his mother to vote for.[47]

Although the House and Senate catastrophic coverage bills appeared nearly identical on the surface, they had major structural differences. An important one was whether to have only one or several "caps" on out-of-pocket spending. The Senate bill was designed with but a single threshold, $2,030 in 1989, after which medicare would pay for all covered services. The House bill, by contrast, included three separate thresholds, one for hospital care (the $580 "first-day" deductible), one for covered nursing home care ($175), and a third for all part B expenses ($1,043). (From the outset, prescription drug coverage proposed in both houses was to have a separate deductible.) The House's substantive argument was that more beneficiaries who were not hospitalized in a particular year would trip the lower part B cap than the combined single cap. But far more important was the jurisdictional issue between the Ways and Means and Energy and Commerce Committees. Ways and Means members and staff were adamant about keeping the hospital (part A) and part B caps separate. They thus hoped to prevent Energy and Commerce from wedging its way into oversight over the hospital portion of medicare that was solely within the jurisdictional province of the tax-writing panel.

A second consideration was how to split the costs between the "flat" premium all beneficiaries would pay and the "supplemental" premium that would only be assessed on wealthier beneficiaries. The House version raised 80 percent of its funds through the supplemental premium. Although that minimized the flat premium increase, thus protecting very poor Americans, it required those of middle income to pay considerably more than under the Senate version, which split the flat and supplemental premium 45 to 55. For example, a single beneficiary with an income of $15,000 would have had to pay a surtax of approximately $210 under the House bill, but only $87 under the Senate version.

Another key question was how to index the proposed out-of-pocket cap. In the Senate bill, the number of beneficiaries projected to trip the expense threshold each year was held constant at about 4.6 percent. On the other hand, the House bill would have gradually increased the number of beneficiaries who would tangibly benefit, starting at about 10 percent. To make up for the increased outlays, it would also have increased the premiums.[48]

Though arcane, the indexing issue went to the heart of what the entire catastrophic coverage program meant. Was it intended—as many of its backers claimed—to be primarily an "assets protection" program, like fire insurance? If that was the case, then it did not really matter how many beneficiaries actually collected on their policies; the "benefit" was merely having the protection. "The ones who will benefit most are the ones who do not need this coverage," said Pete Stark in 1988. "The ones who will benefit most are those who know it is there if they need it."[49] That view also justified charging more affluent beneficiaries higher premiums, because they had more assets to protect. Or was the program supposed to help elderly Americans pay predictable medical expenses? In that case, those who paid premiums but reaped no tangible benefits would feel cheated. In fact, the authors of the final product never actually decided which of the two models should prevail. They bet instead that they could strike a balance that would provide tangible benefits to as many beneficiaries as possible without hitting anyone too hard—a bet they would ultimately lose.

A key mistake was overestimating the knowledge base of medicare beneficiaries, most of whom only knew that they liked the program and wanted no cuts in it. But a surprisingly high percentage of medicare recipients did not know what the program covered and therefore did not know what most insured people had that they lacked. For example, a 1984 Gallup poll conducted for AARP found that 79 percent of respondents believed (wrongly) that medicare paid for most long-term nursing home care.[50] Complicating that was President Reagan's broad but vague promise on his official endorsement of the Bowen plan in 1987. Reagan had stated that his bill would provide elderly Americans with "that last full measure of security," without actually defining what that was.

From the beginning, this lack of clarity was a source of concern for groups representing elderly people. In testimony before the Ways and Means Health Subcommittee in March 1987, AARP President John

Denning noted that, with an out-of-pocket cap only for medicare-covered services, "Beneficiaries may wrongly assume that their total out-of-pocket liability in a given year will not exceed the cap level. As they gradually come to realize that a full range of essential medical services and products do not even count toward the 'catastrophic' cap, they are apt to feel disappointed, if not duped."[51] National Council of Senior Citizens Executive Director William R. Hutton concurred, testifying at that same hearing: "The greatest financial fear of many older Americans is the spectre of nursing home care and the last full measure of security they can be given is protection from the costs of long-term care. The president's comments, I greatly fear, will only cause seniors to shift from one false hope of relying on the medicare program to answer these needs to another of relying on the catastrophic plan that the Administration has proposed."[52]

Still, Congress did little in the several months between Senate passage of the catastrophic coverage bill and final conference action to fill the public knowledge gap. Instead, members of Congress concentrated on negotiating with one another. They assumed they could rely on public support for their cause, while direct-mail lobbies were hard at work undercutting that support.

Leading the fray was the National Committee to Preserve Social Security and Medicare, the aforementioned Roosevelt group. Named by the *Washington Monthly* in 1988 as one of the nation's worst public-interest groups, the National Committee was much disliked in Congress for sending out millions of misleading direct mail letters intimating to senior citizens that unless they sent the organization money, Congress would cut back or eliminate social security or medicare benefits. Opposed from the outset to the "seniors only" financing of the catastrophic costs measure and its failure to deal substantively with the long-term care issue, in early 1988 the National Committee put its mailing machine into action. The organization urged its estimated 5 million members to tell their elected representatives to oppose the catastrophic costs bill and support the long-term care bill being pushed by Claude Pepper instead. The campaign was launched without the consent of Pepper, who had agreed to hold off on pushing his bill until completion of the catastrophic costs measure. "He sees the two bills as complementary," a member of his staff said.[53]

Still actively trying to shape public opinion was the Pharmaceutical Manufacturers Association. Having endorsed the Senate version of the drug benefit, the PMA launched its own direct-mail campaign to kill the version passed in the House, a version drug manufacturers feared was more likely to ultimately lead to price controls. Throughout the House-Senate subconference to iron out the drug portion of the bill, the amount of money at stake was obvious from the number of anxious lobbyists from drug companies and other pharmaceutical groups who paced outside the closed meetings.

During the negotiations, members of Congress who were actually writing the bill downplayed reports that mail was running against the measure. "A lot of the elderly complained about social security when it was passed. A lot complained about medicare when it was passed," said Mitchell in May 1988. "As the benefits become clear to people over time, I think the program will become widely accepted."[54]

With a little public prodding from Pepper, conferees finished work on the bill May 25. That day, at a remarkable public session, Bowen not only backed off from what had been unwavering administration opposition to the House's so-called respite care benefit but also endorsed the final bill. As with original passage of the bill, both the House and Senate approved the conference report by overwhelming majorities: 328–72 in the House and 86–11 in the Senate (in the latter chamber, the same margin by which the original bill had passed seven months earlier). President Reagan signed the bill into law in a Rose Garden ceremony July 1, making it Public Law 100-360.

But in addressing each other's concerns, conferees had also sown the seeds of the bill's ultimate demise. Out of fiscal caution, and primarily because of continuing controversy over cost estimates from the Congressional Budget Office (CBO) and the Reagan administration, conferees decided to phase the program in slowly but collect the money up front to create a "contingency reserve." The financing was to go into effect almost immediately and took two forms. The first was a flat premium increase of $4 per month, effective January 1, 1989. The second was the supplemental premium, which was to be assessed for the 1989 tax year. Initially it was set at $22.50 per $150 of income tax liability, with a maximum of $800, and was estimated to be required of the 40 percent of medicare beneficiaries who would owe $150 or more in income taxes.

But in 1989, the only major benefit that would be available was the unlimited hospital coverage, which was projected to aid only an estimated 3.8 percent of medicare beneficiaries. Thus, by front-loading the financing, conferees ensured that all beneficiaries would pay more, but less than 4 percent would feel the effects of the new and improved coverage.[55] That potential problem did not go unnoticed by the conferees. "It's an election year, and there's a growing concern about asking people to pay right away for benefits they're only going to get in the future," said conferee Rep. Ron Wyden (D.-Ore.), referring to a discussion about how quickly to phase in the drug coverage.[56]

While they were collecting premiums up front in the name of fiscal responsibility, however, conferees also leaned toward the House position of trying to ensure that, ultimately, a higher percentage of beneficiaries would "tangibly benefit." According to CBO, an estimated 7 percent of beneficiaries would trip the part B cap, set at $1,370 in 1990 in what would have been its first year; 16.8 percent of beneficiaries would satisfy the $600 deductible needed to trigger prescription drug coverage in 1991, the first year for that benefit. That, of course, drove premiums higher than those envisioned in the Senate bill. But negotiators did moderate the higher premiums somewhat by agreeing to hold constant the total percentage of beneficiaries who would trip the caps each year at about 7 percent, rather than the rising percentage envisioned in the House bill.[57]

In a final decision certain to cause ill will with opponents, conferees agreed to the House provision making the supplemental premium mandatory for those who qualified for part A benefits. Part B remained voluntary—the increase in the flat premium could be avoided simply by dropping part B. But few beneficiaries were expected to do that, because part B remained heavily subsidized by general revenues, and part B coverage was a prerequisite for most medigap insurance policies.

Ironically, though, the bill was still carefully and expressly designed to be a good value even for those beneficiaries who would have to pay the most. For example, the cap on the supplemental premium was specifically set so that even those paying the maximum would not have to pay more than the insurance value of the new benefits. In fact, CBO estimated that because of medicare's lower administrative costs (and no set-aside for profits) compared with private insurance, in 1990 the catastrophic coverage program would cost a beneficiary $19 per month less than a comparable private medigap policy. The final bill also included the little-mentioned breaks for federal retirees and those with employer-provided medigap or other supplemental coverage.[58]

The Backlash

The outcry over the new law began even before the ink was dry. Before the 100th Congress wrapped up in late October 1988, members had introduced a half-dozen bills—one with 50 cosponsors—to delay, alter, and even repeal the new program outright. Although the initial spate of bills came from Republicans concerned about the wealthier senior citizens who would be hit by the new surtax, liberals concerned about the medicare beneficiaries who would bear the entire cost of the new benefits weighed in early as well. For example, Rep. Barney Frank (D.-Mass.) announced in January 1989 that he would introduce a bill that would freeze the supplemental premium, which was to phase upward over five years as the new benefits became available; repeal the flat premium increase; and make up the difference by doubling the cigarette tax (then 16 cents per pack).[59]

Driving the new bills were complaints from senior citizens who inundated town hall meetings, flooded phone lines, and piled congressional offices knee-deep in protest letters. Some of the outrage was individually motivated, but much of it was the result of organized opposition. The National Committee to Preserve Social Security and Medicare, which opposed the financing from the outset, announced in January 1989 that it was mailing 3 million letters to its members urging them to tell their elected officials to reconsider the financing. The National Committee was joined in early 1989 by a 40-group coalition spearheaded by the National Association of Retired Federal Employees (NARFE) and the Retired Officers Association—two groups whose members actually *were* disadvantaged in disproportionate numbers by the law, because they already had most of the new benefits. Other groups that ultimately jumped on the bandwagon against the new law included the Conservative Caucus; the National Taxpayers Union; and a series of grass-roots groups, such as the Las Vegas-based Seniors Coalition Against the Catastrophic Act.

All, of course, asked for money to keep their campaigns going. "Help the Conservative Caucus repeal the unfair Catastrophic Coverage tax by sending in an emergency gift of $15, $25, $50, or $100 today. . . . The sooner [we] can raise a war chest to kill this unfair law, the sooner your tax bill will go down," proclaimed one mailing sent, of all people, to Mrs. Dan Rostenkowski. Defenders of the law alleged—but never conclusively proved—that drug companies either helped found or gave substantial support to some of these grass-roots groups.

During the early months of the backlash, the authors of the law and its major backers, including the new Bush administration and AARP, attributed most of the complaints to a lack of understanding. "Right now, what's getting out is the cost more than the benefits," said Rep. Wyden in December 1988. Down to the end of the fight, backers insisted that much of the protest was from people who in fact would not be nearly as adversely affected as they had been led to believe. "Next April 15, 94.4 percent of seniors will discover they're not paying anywhere near $800," predicted Sen. John D. Rockefeller IV (D.-W.Va.) in September 1989. "But what seniors believe now is what counts."[60]

The AARP leadership in Washington struggled to maintain support for the law. In January 1989, the group released results of a poll conducted by Hamilton, Frederick, and Schneiders: two-thirds of respondents age 65 and older supported the new law while only 21 percent opposed it. But as dissension grew, AARP faced a rebellion of its own. More and more local chapters were coming out against the bill—a movement not lost on members of Congress. "In 14 different meetings I've attended across the country, representatives of AARP have been there opposing this bill and protesting its enactment," noted Rep. Edward Madigan (R.-Ill.) one of the bill's original authors, in April 1989.

A key mistake made by supporters of the law in early 1989 was basing their arguments on the fact that only a small minority of beneficiaries would have to pay much of a surtax. As a result, they underestimated the more widespread perception that most senior citizens seemed to have, whether by simple misunderstanding or deliberate deception. "If it's a good law, it's going to affect a segment of our society adversely," said House Ways and Means Committee Chairman Dan Rostenkowski in June. "And if you're going to try to revise it to satisfy the demands of that small segment, then you're really not legislating. The case is closed. Let's go on to the next case."[61]

The law's backers had what looked to be a glimmer of hope in April, when the Joint Tax Committee and CBO discovered that the surtax rates had been set higher than needed to pay for the new benefits and maintain the legally required contingency and reserve margins. The estimated $5 billion the tax would bring resulted from an underestimate of the number of senior citizens who fell into the various tax brackets affected by the surtax and the amount they would have to pay. Finance

Committee Chairman Lloyd Bentsen (D.-Texas) immediately proposed lowering both the cap and the rate of the surtax in response to pressure building in the Senate, which on April 12 voted 97 to 2 to urge the committee to hold hearings on the new law.

But that faint hope was dashed in July, when a CBO reestimate of the drug benefit showed it would be much more expensive than originally anticipated and would consume the entire surplus. The news grew even worse in August, when it was discovered that what was viewed as a minor expansion of medicare's limited nursing home benefit (already in force in 1989) would in 1990 cost not $400 million originally projected, but perhaps as much as $2.4 billion. Ironically, the tremendous run-up in nursing home costs was probably only halfway the result of changes made in the catastrophic coverage law. Rather, estimators said, much was due to a 1988 change in regulations that made it easier for nursing homes to receive medicare reimbursement.[62]

As resentment grew, the revolt spread from conservative Republicans to liberal Democrats. In late May, what many saw as the turning point for the entire program may have come at a press conference held by three leading liberals: Democratic Senators Tom Harkin (Ia.) and Carl Levin (Mich.), and Rep. David Bonior (D.-Mich.). The trio, backed by labor and other groups, proposed keeping the new program's benefits in place. Instead, they sought to get rid of the surtax and finance the benefits by eliminating the "bubble" in the 1986 tax-reform bill that lowered the income tax rate for the wealthiest filers from 33 percent to 28 percent. "The problem is some of the seniors are subsidizing the rest," said Levin. "We've never had one part of a group pay a subsidy for another."[63]

That was not quite true: in both medicare and social security, wealthy beneficiaries subsidize those who are poor. But with catastrophic coverage, for the first time the subsidy was so obvious it could not be missed. This was probably the key complaint about the program—that the wealthiest beneficiaries were indeed paying more ito keep costs down for those less well-off. However, even those paying the most were still getting considerably more from medicare than they were putting in— $719 per year more, according to CBO estimates. That was a point many seemed to miss.

Still, the subsidy was a top source of outrage. Among those seeking to capitalize on it was the Golden Rule Insurance Company, a major seller of medigap coverage. "Seniors have income because they saved;

the savings generate income for them. The AARP tax is a *tax on thrift*," proclaimed one of several advertisements the company ran in the *Wall Street Journal*.

Although there had been a few early skirmishes in committees and on the Senate floor, the rising tide of resentment finally reached its peak in June. During consideration of a supplemental spending bill, Senate leaders (who supported the law) narrowly averted an up-or-down vote on an amendment by Republican Senators John McCain (Ariz.) and Orrin Hatch (Utah) to delay further implementation of the catastrophic coverage program for a year. Instead, after two days of tense debate, senators voted to order the Finance Committee to reexamine the law with an eye toward reducing the surtax and making the program voluntary. The amendment, prepared by Senate leaders George Mitchell (D.-Me.) and Bob Dole (R.-Kan.)—two Finance Committee members who helped write the measure—was crafted to avoid a direct vote on the underlying McCain amendment that everyone agreed would have passed. Indeed, the depth of dissatisfaction with the program had become such that Minority Leader Dole was practically reduced to begging his members for support. "We need to recognize that this is a Republican initiative that we are about to dismantle here," Dole said. "This is a Republican administration and the president has a right to expect some support from the Republican side of the aisle."[64]

But although the Bush administration remained on record in support of keeping the program unchanged, it was clear that its political operatives were getting worried about the political implications as well, and their lobbying on the measure was all but invisible. "The administration was not just useless, they were actually hurtful," observed one aide to a senior Finance member.[65]

Newly installed Majority Leader Mitchell also took another tack—questioning the motives of McCain, whose legislative interests had not previously been in the health care arena. McCain's principal argument was that senior citizens wanted long-term care, not the coverage provided in the catastrophic coverage program. "How in the world are we going to get a long-term health care plan when we have basically drained the resources dry of senior citizens in this country for catastrophic health care coverage?" McCain asked. That aroused the ire of Mitchell, who as chairman of the Health Subcommittee in the previous Congress had not only worked on the catastrophic coverage law but had also introduced a major long-term care bill. Noting that few of those complaining about the law's failure to deal with the issue of long-term care had previously expressed interest in the matter, Mitchell stated: "There are some who would look at that record and say that the concern for long-term care for the elderly goes only so far as is necessary to defeat the catastrophic program."[66]

Many of the complaints came from senior citizens who professed to have known nothing of the new law prior to its enactment. This is surprising, considering the widespread attention the law received in both the print and electronic media during its turbulent trip to passage, not to mention the attention devoted to it by newsletters of senior citizens organizations both for and against enactment. "From the very beginning there was limited news coverage on this bill and seniors were not informed of the contents of the bill, nor were they aware that a bill such as the Stark-Gradison bill was being debated by Congress," testified Peggy Hinchey of the Ann Arbor, Michigan, Senior Citizens' Guild at a hearing before the House Republican Study Group in April 1989. Yet a NEXIS search found that major dailies carried 658 separate stories about Congressional consideration of the medicare catastrophic law between January 1, 1987, and July 1, 1988, the day President Reagan signed the bill. The *New York Times* alone printed 121 stories during those 18 months, an average of more than one a week during the entire time the bill was under consideration.

Still, on June 1 Daniel L. Hawley, founder of the Seniors Coalition Against the Catastrophic Act, asserted to the Finance Committee that the law was "debated and voted on in haste with little or no study . . . to gain favor with the seniors." That was more than Finance Chairman Lloyd Bentsen could stand. After watching Hawley with an expression one committee aide described as the same one he wore in the now famous 1988 vice presidential debate just before he upbraided Dan Quayle for comparing himself to the late John F. Kennedy, Bentsen exploded. "This wasn't passed in the dark of night. It wasn't slipped through. I started hearings on this in 1984 because of my deep concerns with this issue. It's a sincere, conscientious effort, Mr. Hawley, on the part of every member of this committee to do what he thinks is right for America."[67]

Because House rules made it easier to keep unrelated or undesirable amendments off the floor, supporters in that chamber were better able to keep opponents at bay until late June. Then the Ways and Means Committee began consideration of the annual must-pass budget reconciliation bill—a measure to which changes to the catastrophic law would be considered germane. It was clear that the issue would be joined there, among other reasons, because the panel's ranking Republican, Bill Archer (Tex.), had introduced the first anticatastrophic bill back in 1988.

But for Ways and Means Committee members, realizing that they had to do something to address the complaints proved much easier than figuring out what to do. For three weeks they were trapped. Doing nothing was impossible politically. Repealing the program provided a serious budget problem. The premiums were already being collected, and eliminating the program would add as much as $6 billion to the federal deficit in fiscal 1990, according to the CBO.[68] Reducing the surtax would have assuaged the political problem. But the funds would have had to be made up either by making the program less progressive (which most Democrats opposed) or by pushing some costs onto working Americans (which Republicans opposed). Making the program truly voluntary, as many senior citizens advocated, would have been financially untenable. Only those most likely to need the benefits would opt in, leaving too small a pool over which to spread the costs.

The committee ultimately did approve a plan that made the program more regressive, reducing the surtax and enlarging the increase in the flat part B premium as well as increasing the deductible for the new prescription drug benefit. (The latter change would probably have had to be made anyway—drug prices and use had risen so fast that a July estimate found that under the original deductible, 26 to 27 percent of beneficiaries would have qualified for reimbursement, compared with the 16.8 percent originally envisioned.) Like the original bill passed in the Senate, the compromise also made the program voluntary, but only if beneficiaries also dropped their part B coverage. That did little to dampen the outrage. "Why should people have to give up part B in order to get out of paying for catastrophic coverage they never asked for?" asked Judy Park of the National Association of Retired Federal Employees.[69]

The annual August recess demonstrated how far gone the catastrophic coverage law was. Energy and Commerce Committee member Mike Synar (D.-Okla.) said his town meetings were so single-issue–oriented that his staff took to calling his travels "the catastrophic tour." In what came to be the most emblematic moment of the bill's entire history, an elderly woman draped herself across the hood of Dan

Rostenkowski's car when he tried to avoid an ambush of protesters during a visit to a Chicago senior citizen center.

By the time Congress returned, it had a new leader of the repeal movement in the House—Brian J. Donnelly (D.-Mass.), who as a conferee helped write the original bill. "If senior citizens really want the program to go away, then fine, we'll make it go away," Donnelly said.[70]

The House tried to do just that on October 4, when representatives voted 360–66 to repeal the program (and waive the budget act to prevent automatic cuts that would otherwise have been triggered by the addition to the deficit). The totals included votes for repeal from 151 Democrats and 44 Republicans who voted for the bill when it first passed in 1987 and again when the final version was approved in 1988.

Ironically, the Senate, where repeal-related action had been going on sporadically all year, voted three days later to retain a shell of the program, although the plan devised by John McCain would have jettisoned the much-despised surtax. By a convincing 26–73 vote, the senators defeated an effort to repeal the program outright.

It took six more weeks to resolve the matter. The House continued to insist on repealing the program, and the Senate stuck just as steadfastly to the McCain proposal. The Bush administration simply stepped back and waited, promising to sign whichever plan the Congress approved. Grumbled Representative Sander Levin (D.-Mich.) of the administration, "They haven't even been involved enough to be ambivalent."[71] In the end, the Senate caved in, very quietly, just before 2 A.M. on November 22. The final legislation (HR 3607; PL 101-234) left intact a series of medicaid expansions for both elderly people and poor pregnant women and children, as well as authority for the so-called "Pepper Commission," a bipartisan group that was to make recommendations concerning health reform and long-term care. But all the new medicare benefits were struck from the books—not, noted several members, likely to return soon. Noted coauthor Rep. Henry A. Waxman just after the House's first repeal vote in October: "This is a tremendous setback for the move to broaden benefits for the elderly. There's a very sour feeling among many [of us]."[72]

Implications for Health Reform

The rise and fall of the Medicare Catastrophic Coverage Act was in many ways a frighteningly accurate foreshadowing of the 1993–94 debate over health reform. To some extent, as is discussed below, the outcomes of both efforts reflected similar circumstances. But the demise of the catastrophic coverage law also directly contributed to the failure of the broader health reform effort.

For starters, Congress's foremost health experts became gun-shy. For the dozen or so members of the House and Senate who wrote the catastrophic coverage law, to say the repeal experience was unpleasant is a gross understatement. Over the course of a year they saw their constituents, their colleagues, and interest groups that had professed strong support for the program turn on them one by one, accusing them of being inept at best and venal at worst. And by and large, these survivors of the catastrophic debacle were still at the helm of health policymaking in 1993. As of April 1994, Democratic Reps. Dan Rostenkowski, Pete Stark, John Dingell, and Henry Waxman remained the full committee and subcommittee chairmen with the most influence over the ultimate shape of a health reform bill in the House. (Rostenkowski's May 1994 indictment on corruption charges forced him to step aside, but throughout the deliberations he remained a voting member of the committee he had formerly chaired.)

On the other side of the Capitol, catastrophic coverage veterans George Mitchell, Jay Rockefeller, Bob Dole, Bob Packwood, Dave Durenberger, and John Chafee were the principal players in the ultimately unsuccessful Senate quest for a bipartisan health reform bill. House bill coauthor Bill Gradison, while no longer in Congress, remained an important player in health policy as president of the Health Insurance Association of America.

The reluctance these legislators felt was understandable. After all, health reform was catastrophic coverage writ large—a bill that would affect virtually every American, some in ways they would not like. Indeed, in a speech at Harvard on April 22, 1994, Ways and Means Chairman Rostenkowski recounted (not without some pain on his face) how it had felt to have angry senior citizens mobbing his car. He warned that he did not plan to proceed on health reform without significant public support.

But if those who led the fight on catastrophic coverage were reticent, their colleagues were downright phobic. Repeatedly during the health reform debate in 1993 and 1994, members of the House and Senate urged colleagues not to repeat the mistakes of the catastrophic coverage battle. Exactly what those mistakes were, however, varied with who was doing the warning. It can never be proved, but surely fear of an even more catastrophic political misstep on health reform acted as a brake on broader reform efforts.

At the same time, some of these factors that contributed to the downfall of catastrophic coverage will have to be overcome if Congress is ever to successfully reshape the nation's health care system. These political facts of life include seven key points:

1. *It is hard to explain and sell changes to people who do not understand the underlying system being changed.*

As polls demonstrated repeatedly, most medicare recipients did not know that the program left them vulnerable to financial ruin were they to contract a serious illness. Little wonder people failed to give Congress credit for fixing something few realized was broken. And the public was not alone in not understanding medicare. Said Stark during the catastrophic debate, "I don't think there are 300 [of 435] members of the House who could tell you extemporaneously what medicare benefits are."[73]

The lack of information on the part of both the public and Congress was a key factor in the repeal effort. For every Rockefeller or Stark on the Hill who could stand up in a meeting and rebut misinterpretations and false accusations about what the catastrophic coverage law would and would not do, there were dozens like Rep. Connie Morella (R.-Md.) whose town meetings were mobbed with angry federal retirees yet who could not begin to explain the various provisions intended to help ease their constituents' burden.

Acceptance of the catastrophic coverage law was also hindered by the lack of understanding senior citizens have about the way medicare is financed. The law was expressly designed so that even those few individuals who would pay the maximum would still receive a government subsidy for their benefits, albeit a reduced one. But many senior citizens continued to think either that they were currently paying the full costs of their coverage (through premiums and payroll taxes during working years) or else that they were entitled to the subsidies they were receiving in perpetuity. This culture of entitlementalization not only makes it difficult to address health policy issues, but it also makes it increasingly hard to address the deficit, which complicates social policymaking in general.

2. *A complex system will inevitably require complex changes.*

Of course this is not true on its face; Congress theoretically can repeal complex programs and replace them with simpler ones. But Congress has long tended to build on what already exists, not only with popular programs like medicare and social security, but even with less popular ones like welfare. Legislation—particularly social legislation—is almost always evolutionary rather than revolutionary. In that context, changes will be difficult to explain, particularly when people do not understand what it is that is being changed.

3. *Complexity is the friend of demagogues.*

The catastrophic coverage experience showed that tackling an inherently complex issue without adequate public education leaves huge opportunities for those who would mislead, whether intentionally or not. The central irony of the catastrophic coverage law is that for all but a very small minority of beneficiaries—the estimated 3.3 million who had supplemental coverage fully financed by someone else—the law was unarguably a good deal. Yet it was clear that either most elderly Americans were not complaining or, more likely, many of those who were simply were misinformed about how much they would ultimately have to pay. Said AARP's John Rother, "The most prevalent misconception about the bill is that everyone was going to pay the $800. I can't tell you how many calls I've gotten from people who said 'I live on my Social Security and a small pension, and I can't afford $800.' "[74]

This is an area in which the media has even more responsibility than Congress. Yet too often, reporters seem to write about the politics rather than the policy of an issue, primarily because they understand the former better than the latter and are afraid to make mistakes.

On the other hand, Congressional and organizational backers of the catastrophic coverage law failed to make their case to the public: for most, the new law was a better deal than private medigap insurance, if only because the government can provide the benefits at a lower cost.

4. *Rules for budget neutrality require strategies that result in redistribution. That creates losers, and losers are more motivated to complain.*

In the era of the deficit, legislating has become a zero-sum game. The only way to give to some people is to take from others. In the case of catastrophic coverage, however, Congress miscalculated—the redistribution was more radical than the benefits it was financing. Noted health policy analyst Marilyn Moon, "Certainly the final package did not represent as dramatic a change on the benefits side as did the financing mechanism intended to pay for the legislation."[75]

It is axiomatic in politics that those who are or stand to be hurt are much more vocal than those who will benefit. But the need for redistribution will make the losers more apparent and will guarantee an increase in the volume of complaints. In the case of catastrophic coverage, the new benefits did not make enough people happy to counteract the volume of complaints.

One strategy that does not work is to play semantic games, such as trying to pretend the surtax was not a tax. "This semantic obfuscation backfired," noted Moon. "Calling this tax a 'supplemental premium' seemed disingenuous. The backlash by [senior citizens] stemmed both from the size of the premium and the feeling that the elderly had been deceived."[76]

5. *When it comes to health, the only accurate estimate is that estimates will be inaccurate.*

The catastrophic coverage experience not only deepened public mistrust of Congress (and encouraged members of Congress to mistrust each other), it also led members of Congress to mistrust interest groups as well as estimators throughout the government. Without cost estimates that continually escalated, the catastrophic coverage law's backers might have been able to withstand the public assault. Without interest groups that did 180-degree turns under an onslaught from their own memberships, Congress might have been able to find a financially acceptable way to deal with the new cost estimates. Indeed, partly as a result of this legislative debacle, it appears that no one trusts anyone's numbers on anything when it comes to health care issues. But given how notoriously difficult it is to estimate costs for health care (because, unlike tax bills, buying decisions are based on emotions as much as cost), waiting for trustworthy numbers will almost by definition mean not doing anything.

6. *The fact that the repeal effort was driven primarily by those outside the committees of jurisdiction helped hasten the breakdown of the seniority, committee, and party norms that have traditionally helped Congress function.*

The catastrophic coverage experience significantly undermined the credibility of Congress's health policy leaders with the rest of the membership. Rank-and-file members trusted those like Stark, Waxman,

Mitchell, and Dole when they were told that senior citizens would support the catastrophic coverage law. When that support evaporated, those on the Hill lost a measure of trust. It is these sorts of battles that rapidly turned the Democrat-led Congress into an institution of 535 freelancers, incapable of accomplishing much of anything—and probably contributed to the Republican takeover in 1994.

7. *Congress is not out of touch; in fact, the opposite is true.*

Rather than demonstrating how out of touch Congress is with its constituents, the catastrophic experience actually showed how hypersensitive representatives and Senators are to constituent complaints. Indeed, had Congress weathered the storm of public opprobrium until April 15, 1990, when several million angry senior citizens would have discovered they did not owe anywhere near as much as they had been led to believe, the entire storm might well have blown over. No major piece of legislation, no matter how worthwhile or necessary, will ever enjoy universal support. Unless Congress learns to differentiate legitimate public opinion from interest group–induced whining, it may never pass controversial legislation again.

Chapter 7

Congress and Health Care Reform 1993–94

Julie Rovner

THE FAILURE TO reshape the nation's health system in 1993 and 1994 will most likely be remembered through the prism of Bill Clinton's presidency. But the battle was at least as much about Congress and how it deals with profound, large, and divisive issues.

The very public failure to enact even minimal changes to the health care system overshadowed the fact that the 103d Congress came closer to a major overhaul of the nation's health care system than any of the several Congresses that had tried before. Major attempts to pass legislation to ensure universal health insurance in the 1930s, the 1940s, and the 1970s never either saw a bill reported from any House committee nor floor debate in either chamber. In 1994 four major committees approved broad bills, three of which would have guaranteed coverage for every American. The Senate never reached resolution of the bill Majority Leader George Mitchell brought to the floor and voted only on the most tangential of issues, but for twelve days it did debate national health insurance.

And though the president and Congress played the leads in the drama, many of the featured players proved just as important to the outcome. A key role was played by the vast array of interest groups. They almost unanimously began the fight strongly in support of reform, only to ultimately either back away or devote their energies to killing off a particular piece of a plan under consideration. Many of these groups (including ones representing business, labor, the medical community, and the insurance industry) ultimately decried Congress's inability to pass a bill. But to a large extent it was their own fault. Each interest wanted only to cut off one of the patient's fingers, but each went after a different finger, and the cumulative effect was that the patient bled to death.

Another important factor was the growing partisanship in Washington. During the previous twelve years of divided government, with Republicans in control of the White House and Democrats of at least one house of Congress, each side had had a stake in compromising to get things done—enacting legislation for which they could later take credit at the polls. But with both the White House and Congress under Democratic leadership, Republicans could and did adopt a scorched-earth policy, refusing to participate in helping the opposition fulfill any of its campaign promises. Early in the debate the desire to stick it to the Democrats was tempered by Republican fears of retribution at the polls should they be perceived as blocking something the public strongly supported. But as public opinion turned against health reform, Republicans became bolder in their attempts to block passage of any bill, culminating in a barely disguised filibuster on the Senate floor. Republicans routinely denied having such a strategy for blocking any bill. Occasionally, however, it would slip into public view—such as during a particularly nasty fight on the House floor over the crime bill in August 1994, when a member of the House Republican leadership, Representative Dick Armey of Texas, told Democrats, "Your president is just not that important to us."[1]

That partisanship was both inflamed and tempered by the peculiar politics of health reform. It was inflamed by the fact that health reform is a uniquely partisan issue—universal coverage and cost containment go to the heart of questions of how involved government should be in the private lives of Americans. But at the same time, both parties suffered from major rifts within their own ranks. Democrats were divided among centrists who wanted to guarantee coverage for all by building on the existing system, liberals who favored a fully government-run "single-payer" system, and conservatives who wanted only minor changes based on free-market principles. Republicans were likewise divided between centrists who thought the system needed a major overhaul and conservatives who sought only minor fixes and wanted to minimize government involvement.

Congress was also still suffering the aftershocks from its last attempt to produce major changes to the health system—the 1988 Medicare Catastrophic Coverage Act. The bill, which added substantially to coverage under the federal program for elderly and disabled Americans, was to be financed completely by medicare beneficiaries themselves. But after elderly people revolted, Congress was forced to repeal the measure in 1989 before it ever had a chance to fully take effect. As a result, many members had lost trust in the bipartisan leaders on health policy in the House and Senate, most of whom remained in charge at the start of the 1993–94 battle.

Adding to the confusion and public doubt in an era of tremendous mistrust of anything devised inside the Capital Beltway was a fundamental inability to explain clearly what the various plans would cost and who would pay. Indeed, if the media is the fourth branch of government, the 1993–94 fight over health reform saw coronation of a fifth: the number crunchers. In a town where both parties were pledged to deficit reduction, producing a plan whose numbers "added up" was the ultimate goal. But just as anyone with a printing press or video camera could be called a media outlet, it seemed anyone with a computer and a set of assumptions could produce cost estimates. In the end it seemed no one believed anyone else's numbers. This played a not insignificant part in the transformation of public opinion from strongly supportive of to strongly opposed to major change.

Each of these factors could be dealt with separately; indeed, each could be its own book. But this case study instead examines the debate chronologically. As Doris Kearns Goodwin notes in the preface to *No Ordinary Time*, her biography of Franklin and Eleanor Roosevelt during World War II: "A president does not deal with issues topically. He deals with events and problems as they arise. By following the sequence of events ourselves, it is easier to see the connections."[2]

Prologue

By early 1992, health care reform seemed inevitable.

Just about everyone agreed that two key problems plagued the system. First, health care was too expensive, and costs were growing too fast. The $820 billion Americans spent on health care in 1992 was nearly double what they spent only seven years earlier.[3] At the same time, too many people lacked health insurance. Estimates varied, but most analysts put the number of uninsured Americans at between 30 and 35 million.

It was not so much that the public demanded change as it was the institutional players in the health care system. Business groups were brought to the table by the spiraling cost of purchasing health insurance for their employees. One study by the benefits consulting firm Foster

Higgins & Co. found that U.S. companies were spending as much as one-fourth of net earnings on employee health costs. Organized labor, a longtime backer of national health insurance, redoubled its efforts, because businesses were trying to pass the costs onto workers more and more, in the form of lower wages or higher cost-sharing for health care. The nation's governors were also up in arms over the spiraling cost of medicaid, the joint federal-state health program for poor Americans. Between 1980 and 1990, medicaid's share of state budgets had grown from 9 percent to 14 percent.[4]

But it was not just the purchasers of health care who were clamoring for reform. For the first time, major segments of the health care industry itself were ready for big changes. Doctors were brought to the table by increasing threats on their autonomy. They complained of what was termed the "hassle factor," massive paperwork and second-guessing imposed by insurance companies, who no longer paid every bill routinely. As the number of uninsured people grew, hospital budgets were increasingly strained as facilities cared for patients who could not pay, and by resistance those who could pay (through their insurance companies) felt toward absorbing the growing costs of that uncompensated care. Even health insurance companies were seeking changes. Many found themselves unable to compete effectively with firms that sought to exclude those with preexisting conditions and insure only the young and healthy and those least likely to use health care.

But complaints from interested parties were not enough to put health care reform on the political agenda. What Congress needed to make such reform an imperative was demand from the voting public, which is exactly what it got in November 1991. The special Senate election to fill the unexpired term of the late John Heinz (R.-Pa.) was not expected to be much of a race. The popular two-term former governor Dick Thornburgh, who stepped down as President Bush's attorney general to run, was expected to thrash 65-year-old political neophyte Harris Wofford, who was appointed by incumbent Democratic Governor Robert P. Casey after Heinz's death that April.

But Wofford (under the tutelage of campaign adviser James Carville, who would go on to offer similar advice to presidential candidate Bill Clinton) found a hot-button issue to exploit the worries of the recession-weary middle class—health care. "If criminals have the right to a lawyer, I think working Americans should have a right to a doctor," Wofford pronounced in his most famous television ad.[5]

Wofford's upset victory lit a fire under Democrats in Congress, who had already been preparing for another push on overhauling health care. But it had an even greater impact on Republicans. In the Senate, Republicans under the leadership of Rhode Island's John S. Chafee rushed to present a modest health care overhaul bill that about twenty legislators had been toiling on in private for more than a year. Even President Bush—whose chief of staff, John Sununu, had once suggested Congress should simply pass its annual appropriations bills and go home—rushed to devise a health plan of his own.

Not surprisingly, health care was a major feature of the 1992 campaign for the Democratic presidential nomination. But Bill Clinton was hardly the candidate most associated with health care. Nebraska Senator Bob Kerrey took that title, running a virtually single-issue campaign with a health plan so complicated even health reporters could not understand it. Former senator Paul Tsongas also emphasized the issue and became the first to call for "managed competition." This was an arcane, market-based plan devised by a group of academics and health industry executives who called themselves the Jackson Hole Group, after the location of their meetings in Wyoming. Former California governor Jerry Brown occupied the liberal end of the spectrum, advocating a single-payer system similar to Canada's under which the government would replace private health insurance companies.

It was no accident that candidate Bill Clinton's first health proposal bore a striking resemblance to the play-or-pay proposals that at the time had the most support among congressional Democrats. Under such a system, employers would have been required either to provide workers and their dependents with health insurance coverage or else pay a tax to the government, which would provide the coverage itself. But by mid-year, play-or-pay plans had been discredited by studies that showed most employers would end up "paying" instead of "playing," and that the proposal was really not much more than a back-door entry into a fully government-controlled health system. Thus, after Clinton had wrapped up the nomination, the candidate who wanted to please everyone adopted the ultimate compromise. At the suggestion of Princeton sociology professor Paul Starr, who was working on his campaign staff, Clinton adopted a proposal that sought to marry the market-based managed competition framework for providing coverage to all (the Tsongas approach)—including a requirement that employers cover their workers—with a more regulatory proposal for controlling costs.[6]

The president-to-be officially unveiled the proposal in a September 24 address given at the New Jersey headquarters of Merck, the nation's largest pharmaceutical company. In the speech he described his proposal: "Personal choice, private care, private insurance, private management, but a national system to put a lid on costs, to require insurance reforms, to facilitate partnerships between business, government, and health care providers."[7]

Development of the Clinton Plan

By the time President Clinton took office in January 1993, the cost and coverage problems in the health care system had only worsened. Health spending was now consuming one of every seven dollars spent. The number of uninsured Americans was still rising, reaching an estimated 38.5 million in 1992, with an estimated 100,000 more Americans losing coverage each month. The bills continued to wreak havoc with the federal budget. Noted the president in his first major address to Congress on February 17: "Unless we change the present pattern, 50 percent of the growth in the deficit between now and the year 2000 will be in health care costs. By the year 2000 almost 20 percent of our income will be in health care. Our families will never be secure, our businesses will never be strong, and our government will never again be fully solvent until we tackle the health care crisis. We must do it this year."[8]

President Clinton wasted no time getting down to business on health care reform. On January 25, on only his third business day in office, he announced the formation of a task force on national health reform whose mission would be to "build on the work of the campaign and the transition, listen to all parties, and prepare health care reform legislation to be submitted to Congress within 100 days of our taking office." The task force membership would consist of leading cabinet officials and other top appointees and would be headed by First Lady Hillary Rodham Clinton. "I am grateful that Hillary has agreed to chair this task force and not only because it means she'll be sharing some of the heat I expect to generate," the new president joked.[9] Unfortunately for the president, that was probably the last joke anyone within the administration would make about the health task force.

Ira Magaziner, an old friend of the president and a fellow former Rhodes scholar, was put in charge of staff on the task force. Magaziner was a millionaire business consultant who knew a lot about organizing but precious little about politics or the ways of Washington. To staff the task force, Magaziner assembled nearly five hundred people. They would come to be known derisively as "worker bees" and included experts from elsewhere in the federal bureaucracy; staffers from Capitol Hill; and economists, physicians, ethicists, and lawyers from the private sector.

Magaziner set up a process that was cumbersome, to say the least. As the *Washington Post* put it: "Task force members were divided into 34 groups and their work had to pass the oral exams of seven 'tollgates'— an exercise Magaziner imported from his consulting life. He once wrote Hillary Clinton outlining the 1,100 decisions that would have to be made."[10]

While the worker bees toiled away, the early buzz on the plan was all favorable. In February, a policy committee of the Business Roundtable, a group of two hundred chief executive officers of major U.S. corporations, endorsed Clinton's "managed competition" concept. Five days later, the AFL-CIO executive council announced that organized labor would be willing to support a broad-based consumption tax to pay for national health care reform. In March, the influential U.S. Chamber of Commerce endorsed managed competition as well.[11]

The public was on board, too. A March 1993 Harris Poll found broad support for most elements of the emerging Clinton health care plan. These included 82 percent support for requiring employers to offer health coverage to their workers, 78 percent support for limiting annual increases in insurance premiums, and 76 percent support for emergency, short-term price controls on prices charged by hospitals, doctors, and drug companies. A whopping 86 percent even said they supported the cornerstone of the little understood managed competition, the purchasing cooperatives that would bargain for lower insurance rates.[12]

But though the public remained enthusiastic about prospects for large-scale health care reform, there was precious little preparation for the inevitable costs to come. Noted Representative Sander Levin in April: "I'm afraid that the public thinks that everybody will have what they have now, and they won't have to pay any new taxes. Those mathematics don't work out."[13] The new administration was also painfully naive in continuing to insist that it could push major initiatives on health and the budget through Congress before the end of the year.

Indeed, the process was hardly going as smoothly as some of the press coverage may have indicated. A key misstep was the decision by

White House media officials to keep the names of the task force staff secret. Aides insisted that the decision was strictly pragmatic—if these people were to devise a plan in one hundred days to totally reshape one-seventh of the nation's economy, they hardly had time to field interview requests from reporters. But the secrecy raised suspicions even among those groups inclined to support the president's plan. Noted David Vladeck, head of Public Citizen's litigation group, "The administration is making a political mistake to shroud this in a cloak of secrecy. I know that some special interests have had access and others have not. There will be a political price to pay for that."[14]

Opponents of the plan immediately jumped on the secrecy issue. In early February, Representative William F. Clinger, Jr. (R.-Pa.) asked the General Accounting Office to review whether Hillary Rodham Clinton's inclusion on the task force triggered the Federal Advisory Committee Act, which required public meetings of task forces that include persons who are not officially federal employees.[15] Three groups adamantly opposed to most of the Democratic plans for health reform (led by the Association of American Physicians and Surgeons, which opposed all third-party payment for health services, including medicare) went even further by filing suit in federal court. They won an early round. On March 10, federal District Court Judge Royce Lamberth ruled that the task force's official meetings must be open to the public, although the working groups could continue to meet in private.

Another problem stemming from the secret deliberations was the continual stream of leaks to a press corps growing day by day and starved for information. In an interview in March 1993, task force press officer Bob Boorstin explained the source of most of the leaks: "The interest groups come in, and they say to Ira or to [his deputy] Judy Feder or to Mrs. Clinton or to someone else, 'well, this is what we want.' And then the member of the task force . . . says to them, 'well, here are the six options we're considering.' Then the interest group leaves and it calls a reporter and says 'you won't believe what they're considering. They're considering'—and then they pick the one option out of the six that is the most extreme; the one they hate the most, because they want it floated in the press so that it can be knocked down."[16]

It was not only the secrecy of the process, however, that began to sow seeds of discontent among concerned players, but also the rhetoric of the first couple themselves. In an attempt to gain public support, they often took to bashing the health care establishment, particularly insurance and drug companies. "The pharmaceutical industry is spending $1 billion more each year on advertising and lobbying than it does on developing new and better drugs," the president said at a February 12 visit to a Northern Virginia health clinic. "Meanwhile its profits are rising at four times the rate of the average Fortune 500 company. Compared to other countries, our prices are shocking."[17]

The task force process also proved problematic on Capitol Hill. Despite inclusion of key Hill staff members in task force working groups, many members not only felt left out of the process but also worried that the White House was trying to do *their* job. Complained Representative Pete Stark (D.-Calif.), chairman of the House Ways and Means Subcommittee on Health: "If [President Clinton] comes out with a completed bill and if he makes his first statement saying that he's drafted the bill in complete detail, he has all the revenue estimates, and he hopes this bill gets through the House in 30 days, then I think he is drawing a line in the sand that could cause problems."[18]

The administration, however, particularly the first lady, went to great lengths to keep Congress informed of its developing plan through frequent briefings. With the public so strongly on board the health reform bandwagon, Republicans by and large remained mild in their criticisms. Said Senator Phil Gramm following a meeting with Hillary Rodham Clinton on April 30, "I think this is a major problem. I think it's something we've got to deal with. I hope we can deal with it on a bipartisan basis."[19]

Indeed, many Republicans were not in the least offended by being excluded from the president's policy development process. Said Senator John S. Chafee, head of the Senate Republican Task Force on Health, "I personally don't want to be involved in the administration's process. I think it makes more sense for the administration to come up with what it believes is the right way to proceed, having put a lot of time and thought into it, and on our side the Republican senators would do likewise, come up with what we think is best . . . and then we can sit down and negotiate."[20]

In the end, a variety of factors (including the sheer complexity of the task, Magaziner's desire to produce a plan with every *i* dotted and *t* crossed, and the prolonged absence of the first lady, who left to be with her dying father in Little Rock) led to the task force's inability to meet the president's order to complete work within one hundred days. By early June, the plan was approaching completion, but President Clinton was ultimately forced to recognize a fundamental reality of his office—the president cannot take on too many big things at once. With the battle over the budget reaching a crescendo, advisers warned the Clintons that Congress and the public would be distracted by the unveiling of the health care bill. Ultimately the administration opted to shelve health care reform until the budget battle was completed, which would not happen until August. It had become clear that health care reform would not be enacted in 1993.

Unveiling the Plan

The bruising budget battle, in which not a single Republican in either the House or the Senate ended up voting for the plan, had a not insignificant impact on the administration's developing strategy for pressing the issue of health care reform. As *Congressional Quarterly* put it: "The most obvious lesson from the deficit-reduction war was the depth of congressional antagonism to taxes. In response, administration officials now say that the only outright tax [to be included in the health plan] will be on cigarettes. The rest of the money will be raised from employers, who will be asked to pay 80 percent of their workers' health insurance premiums, and from employees, who will pay the balance."[21]

But although the delay gave the administration time to gear up for its sales pitch for the health plan, it also gave opponents time to build their case. Among the first out of the box was the National Federation of Independent Business (NFIB), Washington's leading small-business lobby. If Bill Clinton "focused like a laser beam" on the economy, as he promised on the campaign trail, then the NFIB focused like a laser beam on defeating the central element of the Clinton health plan—the employer mandate that would require NFIB members to provide and pay for the lion's share of health insurance for their workers. In May the NFIB released a study claiming that the proposal on which the Clinton plan was based could put 18.2 million jobs "at risk."[22] This study was the first of many that claimed the employer mandate would put millions of Americans out of work and many small firms out of business.

The official launch of the Clinton health care reform plan came in the president's September 22 address to a joint session of Congress, although early drafts of the proposal had been leaked to the press two weeks before. However, despite leaks, doubts about the numbers, and a teleprompter glitch that early in the speech left the president staring at the text of the budget address he had delivered in February, Clinton still managed to make a masterful pitch: "This health care system of ours is badly broken, and it is time to fix it. . . . The proposal that I describe tonight borrows many of the principles and ideas that have been embraced in plans introduced by both Republicans and Democrats in this Congress. For the first time in this century, leaders of both political parties have joined together around the principle of providing universal, comprehensive health care. It is a magic moment, and we must seize it."[23]

Befitting a proposal that sought to reshape one-seventh of the nation's economy without raising substantial new taxes or scrapping the current system, the Clinton plan was both complex and lengthy—the first version delivered to Congress was 1,342 pages long.

Actually, for all the work done on it and layers of detail added to it, the proposal's core was not that different from the plan Clinton had outlined in his Merck speech during the presidential campaign a year earlier. It sought to build on the existing health care system by requiring employers to provide most workers and their families with health insurance and to pay most of the costs. In an attempt to cushion the blow, the plan offered generous subsidies to small businesses and those with low-wage–earning employees, as well as payments to families and individuals with low incomes to help pay their portion of premiums and other out-of-pocket costs. Overall spending would be controlled primarily through competition, but also by fallback limits on the amount premiums could increase each year. Such premium caps were a clever device that allowed the Clinton administration to claim (correctly) that it was not imposing price controls on medical services. But caps would have forced just such eventualities—or else outright rationing—on the insurance companies themselves.

At the heart of the proposal were regional "health alliances" that would pool premiums from businesses and individuals and negotiate with insurance companies. These alliances were what architects of managed competition originally called "health insurance purchasing cooperatives." (That terminology was dropped, one administration official told reporters at a briefing, because it sounded too communistic.) New name or no, the alliances quickly became the butt of jokes. For example, in a cartoon in the *New Yorker*, titled "Beltway Car Pool," three children—one a toddler in a car seat—are sitting in the back of a car. One is explaining to the other two: "Under the proposal, regional 'health alliances'—essentially, giant insurance-buying pools—would collect money from employers and individuals and in return offer them a variety of competing health plans. A national health board would control the alliances' budgets and prevent them from raising insurance premiums over a certain amount. Cool!"[24]

In fact, given the issue's complexity, it was a testament to Clinton's rhetorical skill that the first public opinion polls were so positive. A *Newsweek* poll conducted in the two days following the president's speech found that 79 percent of those polled thought the nation's health system needed either fundamental changes or a complete restructuring. Fifty-five percent thought the Clinton plan would be good for the country, compared with only 27 percent who thought it would be bad.[25]

But the storm clouds were already forming, particularly regarding whether the plan's numbers added up. The source of much internecine warfare within the administration, the numbers ultimately released to the press were at least publicly supported by all the president's key economic and health aides. The total cost of the plan over five years, explained Leon Panetta, then director of the Office of Management and Budget, would be $331 billion. Those funds would provide subsidies (the administration called them "discounts") to help cushion the impact of the employer mandate on small businesses and those with low-wage employees, help poor Americans pay their portion of the cost-sharing requirements, provide a full tax deduction for health insurance for self-employed workers, and finance new prescription drug and long-term care benefits for medicare beneficiaries. Panetta insisted that the entire amount could be financed by raising the cigarette tax by 75 cents per pack (bringing the total tax to just under $1); assessing a 1 percent tax on the largest corporations (those with more than 5,000 employees) that opted not to join the alliances; increasing tax revenues from lowered health care costs; cutting $124 billion and $65 billion, respectively, in medicare and medicaid; and cutting $40 billion in other federal health programs. Indeed, the Clinton administration insisted that not only would it have a $45 billion security cushion in case the subsidies cost more than anticipated, but the revenues raised would also leave $58 billion for deficit reduction.[26]

Not surprisingly, many found those numbers less than credible. As Tom Scully, who helped develop President Bush's health plan, noted: "The fundamental problem is you are going to cover 35 million new people. Currently, those people are roughly getting half the health care in the uncompensated system that they would get if they had insurance, so you're doubling their level of coverage, and that's got to come from someplace."[27]

Even some of the plan's supposed supporters were publicly skeptical. In a comment that would be badly misinterpreted, Senate Finance Committee Chairman Daniel Patrick Moynihan (D.-N.Y.) said on a Sunday-morning talk show that the administration was engaging in "fantasy" if it thought Congress would be willing to cut $124 billion from medicare.

Autumn 1993: Handing the Ball Off to Congress

Congress was certainly not just sitting around waiting for the administration to send its health bill up to the Hill. By the time legislators left for their August recess in 1993, more than twenty bills to reshape the health care system had already been introduced.[28] Most of those measures were from Republicans; Democrats had been asked by their leaders to hold back their bills until President Clinton had unveiled his own.

But not everyone heeded that request. Most notably, a bloc of nearly one hundred House Democrats had signed onto a single-payer bill, HR 1200, introduced in March by Representative Jim McDermott (D.-Wash.), one of two physicians in the House and a member of the Ways and Means Health Subcommittee. The bill (a companion to one introduced in the Senate by Minnesota Democrat Paul Wellstone, though with far fewer cosponsors) was simple compared with the Clinton plan. It would have eliminated the role of insurance companies in health care and made the federal government pay all the nation's health bills. Critics called it socialized medicine, but in fact it would have more closely resembled medicare than the government-run British health system. Doctors and hospitals would have continued to operate privately, and patients would have continued to choose where to get treatment and from whom. But the government would have paid all the bills—and controlled the costs.

The very simplicity of the single-payer plan made it stand out and gave it significant popularity. In most polls, the single-payer plan was the fairly consistent preference of about one-third of the public. But in the antigovernment mood pervading the country up to and after the 1992 elections, the Clinton administration never seriously considered going the single-payer route. Nevertheless, particularly in the House, the single-payer proposal had broad enough support that its backers had to be considered seriously.

On the other end of the Democratic spectrum was a slightly smaller but still sizable bloc that first introduced the managed competition concept in Congress in April 1992. Led by Representatives Jim Cooper (D.-Tenn.) and Mike Andrews (D.-Texas), members of the Energy and Commerce and Ways and Means Health Subcommittees, respectively, the Conservative Democratic Forum sought a purer and less regulatory system than President Clinton had devised. Specifically, the new version of the plan, introduced in October 1993, lacked the premium limits of the Clinton plan and (even more significantly) had no employer mandate. As a result, the bill did not pledge to cover every American, as did the Clinton bill or the single-payer plan. That was the source of much angst for the administration and backers of so-called universal coverage.

The 1993 version of what became known as the Cooper-Grandy bill (HR 3222) was the first major health bill to enjoy significant Republican support (twenty-two of its original fifty cosponsors were members of the then minority party).[29] Among its leading backers were moderate Representative Fred Grandy of Iowa (like Andrews, a member of the Ways and Means Health Subcommittee) and Senator Dave Durenberger of Minnesota, longtime ranking Republican (and from 1981 to 1986, chairman) of the Senate Finance Committee's Health Subcommittee.

At least nominally, House and Senate Republicans seemed more united than the Democrats. In the Senate, longtime health care leader (and Finance Committee member) John Chafee convinced twenty-three of forty-four of Republican senators (including Minority Leader Bob Dole of Kansas) to sign onto a unique bill that sought to guarantee universal coverage without either an employer mandate or government takeover of insurance companies. Instead, the bill pursued a third course, requiring individuals to purchase their own coverage and providing subsidies for those with low incomes. The plan included no spending controls or new taxes and derived almost all of its funding from reductions in medicare and medicaid.

The House Republican bill, introduced by Minority Leader Robert Michel (R.-Ill.), was considerably less sweeping but garnered even broader support, with 106 of 175 Republicans signing on.[30] It did not even aspire to universal coverage. Instead, it sought to make insurance more accessible by encouraging creation of purchasing groups and outlawing some of the insurance industry's practices, such as barring coverage for those with preexisting conditions and canceling coverage for people who get sick. (With some variation, such "insurance reforms" were common to all the bills.) The Michel bill also proposed tax-preferred "medisave" accounts, which would allow people to accumulate funds to pay most routine medical expenses, thus enabling them to carry only catastrophic insurance coverage. Such accounts had been longtime favorites of conservatives, because they would give consumers more control over health spending and provide personal incentives to limit such spending. Liberals argued that the medisave accounts could do more harm than good by discouraging preventive care (which would be out-of-pocket expenses) and drawing the healthiest people out of the regular health insurance pool, thereby leaving only the sick behind and driving insurance costs up.

Into this tangled web of interests strode what administration officials hoped would be its best weapon, Hillary Rodham Clinton. From September 28 to September 30, the first lady testified before members of each of the five major committees that handle health care in Congress (House Ways and Means, Energy and Commerce, and Education and Labor; and Senate Finance, and Labor and Human Resources) and answered their questions.

Even her critics admitted that Mrs. Clinton's appearances before the committees were a triumph. Speaking mostly without notes, Mrs. Clinton presented the plan clearly and concisely, seldom having to ask aides for help with the many and varied questions members threw out at her. She even gave as good as she got. During one exchange Representative Dick Armey (R.-Texas), a combative conservative who would lead the opposition to the Clinton plan, promised to make the debate "as exciting as possible." The first lady, remembering that Armey had earlier compared the Clinton health plan's alleged killing off of jobs to the actions of an infamous Michigan doctor who had assisted terminally ill patients commit suicide, replied, "I'm sure you will ... you and Dr. Kevorkian."[31]

But even Hillary Rodham Clinton could not answer everyone's questions. On October 14, in an ominous foreshadowing of the debate to come, a "Citizens' Jury" organized by a Minnesota think tank voted 24–0 that the system needed changing, but 19–5 that the Clinton plan was *not* the best way to do it.

The Citizens' Jury—twenty-four Americans selected to represent a cross-section of the public on criteria such as age, race, gender, geography, income, and political preference—spent five days in Washington undergoing a total immersion in the substance and politics of health care reform. Along the way they were briefed by some of the nation's leading health policy experts as well as three U.S. senators. But in the end, though members of the Citizens' Jury were convinced that the system needed to be changed, they had no idea what form that change should take. "We couldn't believe how complex this issue is," said the Jury's spokesman, Gregg Madden, a sales representative from New Hampshire.[32]

The jurors were hardly the only Americans confused about health care reform. Despite the education efforts of the media and the first family, a survey sponsored by the Kaiser Family Foundation and the Harvard School of Public Health conducted from September 30 to October 5 (a week *after* the president pitched the plan to Congress and the country and the first lady made her triumphant tour of Capitol Hill) found the public seriously lacked an understanding of even the rudimentary issues involved. For example, 68 percent of those polled had either never heard the term "managed care" (the system of integrating financing and delivery of health care on which the Clinton plan and many other proposals pinned their cost-control hopes) or could not define it. Just under 80 percent had never heard of or could not define "managed competition." Even some of the basics had yet to sink in. Despite the president's brandishing of a red, white, and blue "health security card" during his speech that would guarantee every American continuing coverage no matter what, 48 percent of those polled thought that under the Clinton plan workers who quit or lost their jobs might also lose their insurance. More than 40 percent did not know the plan would pay for preventive health services, another oft-repeated theme. But at the same time, 51 percent of respondents mistakenly thought the plan would cover nursing home care.[33]

"It's sort of embarrassing," admitted Robert J. Blendon, one of the survey's sponsors and a public opinion expert at the Harvard School of Public Health. "People say they're reading newspapers furiously and watching television, and then they can't answer any of the questions."[34]

But while the public was trying to figure things out, the Clinton administration was still putting the finishing touches on its voluminous plan. It ultimately took more than a month to deliver the plan in completed form to Congress, which the White House managed to do on October 27. It would be nearly another month (November 20) before the bill would be formally introduced.

Part of the delay was the effort by Democratic leaders in the House and Senate to sign up cosponsors. The Senate version of the bill, S 1757, was introduced by Senate Majority Leader George Mitchell with thirty cosponsors—twenty-nine Democrats and James M. Jeffords of Vermont, the only Republican in either chamber who would ultimately embrace the president's plan publicly. The House bill, HR 3600, was introduced by Majority Leader Dick Gephardt with ninety-nine cosponsors. House leaders were anxious to exceed the eighty-nine cosponsors who had signed onto McDermott's single-payer bill, HR 1200.[35]

But most of the delay was caused by internecine battles over committee jurisdiction. Which committees would ultimately be awarded referrals of the Clinton bill was important for reasons beyond the current fight. The precedent set by what was expected to be a rewrite of the entire health care system would have jurisdictional ramifications for years (perhaps decades) to come. Turf-conscious committee chairmen knew just how high those stakes were. "The discussions are interminable," a House leadership aide told *Congressional Quarterly* in October. "There are constant efforts by committee chairmen . . . to get as much of this bill as possible."[36] Indeed, the chairmen of the three primary House committees with health jurisdiction—Ways and Means, Energy and Commerce, and Education and Labor—each sought control of the entire measure. Noted *Congressional Quarterly:* "Asked what portion Energy and Commerce would handle, Chairman John D. Dingell, D-Mich., responded, 'We have health'."[37]

But unsnarling the jurisdictional tangle turned out to be simpler in the House than in the Senate. That is ironic; jurisdiction is more important in the House, where committees have relatively more influence, because opportunities to alter bills during floor debate are considerably more limited. The House bill was ultimately referred in its entirety to the Ways and Means and Energy and Commerce committees, and nearly whole to the third major committee, Education and Labor. Smaller pieces were referred to seven other panels: Veterans' Affairs, Armed Services, Rules, Post Office and Civil Service, Judiciary, Natural Resources, and Government Operations.[38]

In the Senate, noted the Congressional Research Service, "Normally bills are referred . . . to one committee only, i.e., the panel with jurisdiction over the 'subject matter which predominates.' Multiple referrals are rare and are invariably accomplished by unanimous consent."[39] But given the acrimony surrounding referral of the Clinton health bill in the Senate, unanimous consent was not even a possibility.

The Senate combatants were Daniel Patrick Moynihan (D.-N.Y.), chairman of the Finance Committee, and Edward M. Kennedy (D.-Mass.), chairman of the Labor and Human Resources Committee. Unlike in the House, where the jurisdictions of Ways and Means and Energy and Commerce were fairly evenly divided, Finance had long been the primary health affairs committee in the Senate. It had jurisdiction over all of medicare, all of medicaid, and (obviously) all taxes. Labor and Human Resources, on the other hand, had jurisdiction over the Public Health Service (including the National Institutes of Health and the Centers for Disease Control) as well as employee benefits through the Fair Labor Standards Act. But each chairman's passion for health reform was inversely related to his committee's claim. Kennedy had pushed for national health insurance for nearly a generation. In 1971, he had chaired the Health Subcommittee of the then Senate Labor and Public Welfare Committee and sponsored the Health Security Act. (It was in response to this national health insurance proposal that President Richard Nixon developed his memorable plan that would have required employers to provide coverage for their employees.) More recently (in 1988, 1989, and 1992), Kennedy had pushed various bills that would have mandated health benefits through his committee.[40] In contrast, in his first term as Finance chairman, Moynihan had been cool on the subject of health reform throughout the Clinton administration. A welfare expert, he worked closely with then Governor Clinton on the 1988 welfare overhaul, the Family Support Act, and made no secret of the fact that he would rather his committee work on welfare than health. "We don't have a health crisis," Moynihan said in a Sunday morning talk show appearance that gave the Clinton administration fits. "We *do* have a welfare crisis."[41]

The referee of this fight was Majority Leader Mitchell, hardly a neutral observer. A member of the Finance Committee, Mitchell chaired the Health Subcommittee from 1987 until he was chosen as majority leader in 1989. Though he had not worked on the issue as long as Kennedy, Mitchell was no less devoted to the goal of reforming the nation's health care system. Nevertheless, Mitchell found himself in a nearly impossible position. Kennedy was clearly more devoted to the issue than Moynihan and his relatively liberal committee more inclined to report a bill closely resembling the Clinton plan. Yet the Finance Committee, with its more moderate bent and its close 11–9 split between Democrats and Republicans, was taken more seriously by other senators and was also the most likely venue for a compromise that could ultimately pass the Senate.

Before the matter was resolved, things got personal and ugly. Reported the *Los Angeles Times*: "At the final moment before the bill was formally introduced . . . Kennedy prevailed through his superior mastery of the complicated Senate rules, leading Moynihan to threaten to publicly denounce Kennedy and to label the Clinton health plan a huge tax increase in disguise. (Kennedy and Moynihan's staff members deny that such an episode occurred, but sources from the White House and Capitol Hill insist that it did.)"[42]

In the end, Mitchell caved in. On November 20, S 1757 (the Clinton bill) was introduced and placed on the Senate calendar without being referred to committee. On November 22, Moynihan and Kennedy each introduced a bill drafted so that it could be referred without question to its respective committee. That day Chafee also introduced his bill (S 1770) with nineteen cosponsors, four less than had embraced the measure when it was unveiled in September.[43]

The jurisdictional fight was an important one. But its most important contribution was to effectively cede the public stage to the opponents of health care reform, who took it over willingly and to great effect.

The Opposition Steps Up to the Plate

By far the highest-profile opponents of the Clinton plan were Harry and Louise, the two stars in a series of commercials for the Health Insurance Association of America (HIAA). The ads sought to raise concerns so-called average Americans allegedly had about what the Clinton health plan could mean. As *National Journal* described it: "In the first and most provocative ad, the couple worries that the government will limit their choice of health plans and implies that the new plans would be less comprehensive than their current one. 'They choose,' Harry intones. 'We lose,' Louise concludes."[44]

Ironically, the HIAA was an unlikely nemesis of the Clinton plan. The once-united health insurance industry had splintered in recent years, with some companies pursuing more aggressive involvement in managed care (with the five largest ultimately uniting as The Coalition for Managed Competition) and others splitting off for ideological reasons. By the end of 1993, the HIAA represented companies with only about one-third of the nation's 180 million health insurance policyholders.[45] Although many of its membership's very companies were on the line, the HIAA had in fact already endorsed substantial reforms, including the highly controversial concept of universal coverage provided through an employer mandate.[46] Finally, the HIAA had lured away Bill Gradison, the ranking Republican on the Ways and Means Subcommittee on Health, to head its effort. A moderate who for years had worked successfully with the unpredictable Pete Stark, Gradison was one of the most knowledgeable House members of either party regarding health issues and a strong supporter of many reforms. Stark said one reason Gradison left Congress to head the HIAA was the pressure Gradison had felt from more conservative House Republicans (particularly Minority Whip Newt Gingrich) to stop collaborating with Democrats on health issues.

But though the HIAA supported many of the changes in the Clinton plan, the questions about bureaucracy and choice raised by Harry and Louise (the actors' real first names) proved irresistible to the media, who were searching for a way to illustrate opposition to health care reform. In fact, although the HIAA would ultimately spend $15 million on the ad campaign,[47] the Harry and Louise ads were broadcast more often on newscasts, exemplifying critics of the plan, than they were in actual paid spots.

Another ostensible ally of reform was the American Medical Association. In depicting the medical establishment as the enemy of reform and the friend of the status quo, the Clinton administration had been relatively careful not to antagonize doctors. This was not only because they represented the one sector of the medical community that enjoyed widespread public respect, but also because the administration was well aware of the prominent role the AMA had played in killing earlier health care reform efforts.

Indeed, the AMA was almost single-handedly responsible for the defeat of many national health insurance proposals, starting with the one advanced by President Harry S. Truman in 1949. In 1971 the AMA was allied with conservative Republicans who were pushing a tax credit plan as an alternative not only to Ted Kennedy's national health insurance bill but also to President Nixon's employer mandate proposal. By the late 1970s, the AMA had backed down slightly yet remained opposed to any significant federal role in the nation's health care system.

The AMA's concerns and the way it expressed them have remained remarkably consistent over time. More than money, doctors wanted autonomy and stewardship over the health care system. In 1949 the AMA launched what two chroniclers of the group's history called "one of the first nationwide political-public relations campaigns in U.S. history."[48] According to the authors, two reporters from the *Chicago Sun Times*: "[The public relations firm] promoted an image to capture people's imagination: an 1891 painting by the British artist Sir Luke Fildes of an old-fashioned doctor watching over a sick child. They printed 65,000 copies of a poster of the painting—to be hung in physicians' offices—with the headline: KEEP POLITICS OUT OF THIS PICTURE! The poster went on to describe compulsory health insurance as 'political medicine' that would create inferior medicine, red tape, and a heavy tax burden, and would bring 'a politician between you and your doctor'."[49]

After losing its battle against the creation of medicare and medicaid, the AMA reloaded for its next battle in the Nixon administration: "The AMA denied the system faced a crisis. It called the U.S. system the best in the world and insisted that many of the health problems cited by studies and experts were more likely the result of societal factors and economics than the absence of medical treatment. The few gaps in the system could be fixed, the AMA said, warning that frustration with rising costs should not automatically lead to the scrapping of the existing system."[50]

A decade later, however, as eroding health insurance coverage threatened physicians' own pocketbooks, the huge ship that was the AMA began to change course. Pressed in part by more activist, less conservative younger doctors, in 1990 the AMA formally adopted a plan that would have required employers to provide coverage to their full-time workers—the very idea it had opposed when it had been proposed by Richard Nixon.[51] During the task force process in 1993, the AMA continually hammered at the administration for not having more doctors involved in the actual writing of the Clinton plan. Yet at the same time AMA leaders met repeatedly with ranking administration officials, and in 1993 Mrs. Clinton and Vice President Al Gore both addressed AMA meetings.

The AMA's wish to have it both ways was illustrated in a letter sent by the organization's leaders to its membership on September 24, two days after President Clinton unveiled his plan on national television.

"The American Medical Association supports health system reform," the letter began. But the fifteen-page document went on to describe the AMA's "serious reservations about the president's proposal because it would limit choices by patients and physicians, undermine the quality of medical services, and lead to federal control of medical education and the physician workforce."[52]

It was ultimately the AMA's governing body, the House of Delegates, that would force its leadership's hand. On December 7, 1993, delegates voted to withdraw the AMA's previous support of the employer mandate and to give all financing options for universal coverage equal weight.[53] The AMA's turnabout was a significant blow to the Clinton administration at a time when public opinion on the health reform issue should have been about to peak.

It turned out, however, that the AMA's vote was engineered at least in part by the NFIB. The NFIB was devoting nearly all its energies to stripping the employer mandate from the bill, and not all of its activities were going on inside the Beltway. *Washington Post* reporter Michael Weisskopf dubbed the tactic by which state NFIB directors urged state AMA delegations to support the move to overturn the AMA endorsement of employer mandates "cross-lobbying." Wrote Weisskopf: "For the NFIB, one of the greatest critics of the Clinton plan, the cross-lobbying helped deny the president an influential ally on employer mandates."[54]

It was not only those who would be immediately affected by a change in the health care system who were gearing up in late 1993. As the air of inevitability regarding major change began to wane, some Republicans began to question the wisdom of their willingness to go along with reform efforts. Leading the charge was Bill Kristol, who had served as Dan Quayle's vice presidential chief of staff and had since ensconced himself at a think tank called the Project for a Republican Future. In a series of memos distributed not only to Republicans but also to the media (most of which would be printed nearly in their entirety on the *Wall Street Journal's* editorial page), Kristol was one of the first to argue loudly that Republicans should not attempt to improve the Clinton plan, but rather to kill it:

Any Republican urge to negotiate a "least bad" compromise with the Democrats, and thereby gain momentary public credit for helping the president "do something" about health care, should also be resisted. Passage of the Clinton health care plan, in any form, would guarantee and likely make permanent an unprecedented federal intrusion into and disruption of the American economy—and the establishment of the largest federal entitlement program since Social Security. Its success would signal a rebirth of centralized welfare-state policy at the very moment we have begun rolling back that idea in other areas. And, not least, it would destroy the present breadth and quality of the American health care system, still the world's finest. On grounds of national policy alone, the plan should not be amended; it should be erased.[55]

With that first missive, Kristol began to play a role in the shifting of Republican rhetoric on the health care issue. "Even though the memo never used the phrase 'no crisis,' conservative columnist Robert D. Novak fairly summarized its contents that way and several Republican leaders were soon adopting that rhetoric," wrote James A. Barnes in the *National Journal*.[56]

It was not that the Clinton administration did not expect the onslaughts from both the health care industry and the Republicans. Nor was it that the administration lacked its own strategy to sell its plan. It was just that the strategy it had did not work very well. Back in the spring of 1993, the Democratic National Committee (DNC) provided $100,000 in seed money to set up the National Health Care Campaign, which was to act as bipartisan backer for health care reform and to raise private funds to counteract the anticipated negative advertising. But the campaign never shook off being labeled a front for the Clinton plan, and it was ultimately reincorporated into the DNC as a special project. In August the DNC hired former Ohio governor Richard F. Celeste to serve as the political point person for selling the Clinton plan. However, the DNC was both outspent and outmanned by various interest groups and struggled unsuccessfully to be heard above the din.

In the meantime, the White House suffered setbacks on other fronts. After spending considerable time and effort successfully steering the North American Free Trade Agreement through Congress, the administration had adopted a deeply defensive mode. The Whitewater investigation was reaching fever pitch; foreign crises were escalating in North Korea, Haiti, and Bosnia; and the president was facing a spate of bad publicity from the story of two former Arkansas state troopers who claimed they had arranged extramarital liaisons for Clinton while he was governor.

The Battle Engaged

By the end of January 1994, it was clear the campaign for health care reform needed a jump start. Since it was first released September 22, public support for the Clinton plan had dropped from 67 percent to 48 percent, according to the *Washington Post*-ABC News poll. The percentage of respondents who thought they would be better off under the Clinton plan dropped even more sharply—from 77 to 52 percent.[57]

Momentum for reform was also slowed by a piece of good news. In December it was reported that medical price increases were slowing down. Medical prices rose by just 5.5 percent for the twelve months ending November 1993. The last time health care costs had increased that little was in 1974 (5.3 percent), when medical care was subject to President Nixon's wage and price controls. Analysts differed on the causes of the slowdown. Some attributed it to lower inflation in general, some to changes the medical industry and big business were making on their own (particularly the move to managed care), and others to an artificial suppression of prices by segments of the medical industry that feared what Congress might be gearing up to do to them. Analysts with long memories pointed out that the last time medical spending slowed was during the Carter administration, while Congress was considering a bill to limit hospital spending. After the bill was killed, spending jumped once again.[58]

Whatever the causes, President Clinton responded to the lull by devoting a significant portion of his January 25 State of the Union address to health care. At one point he brandished a pen and made what analysts variously described as the boldest or most foolish threat of his presidency: "I want to make this very clear. . . . If you send me legislation that does not guarantee every American private health insurance that can never be taken away, you will force me to take this pen, veto that legislation, and we'll come right back here and start over again."[59] Congressional Republicans were more than ready to rise to the challenge. Replied Bob Dole in the official Republican response: "Our country has health care problems, but not a health care crisis. But we will have a crisis if we take the president's medicine—a massive overdose of government control."[60]

Indeed, Republicans were rapidly backing away from universal coverage, particularly the so-called individual mandate in the Chafee bill. Dole mentioned in several interviews early in 1994 that he could already picture the Democrats' 30-second ad on the subject: "The Republicans don't want your boss to pay for your health insurance; they want you to pay for it."

The weeks that followed brought only more bad news for the embattled Clinton health plan. On February 2, nearly a year to the day after giving the Clinton plan a major boost, the Business Roundtable dealt it a major blow by endorsing the rival Cooper proposal. As the *Washington Post* noted:

Big business had backed the administration in its budget fight with Congress on the strength of White House promises of additional cuts in domestic spending. But the cuts never came. Many now believed the health plan would become an open-ended entitlement that would raise taxes and the federal deficit. "The only things these guys in the White House understand is a sharp stick up the nose," one executive told another as the session broke up. And a sharp stick it was. The Roundtable voted 60 to 20 to support the Cooper plan. In subsequent weeks, two other major business organizations, the National Association of Manufacturers and the U.S. Chamber of Commerce, came out against the Clinton plan.[61]

The Chamber of Commerce rebuke was particularly painful for the Clinton administration, because the organization had circulated draft congressional testimony that endorsed the concept of an employer mandate. But when House Republicans heard of the testimony, they unleashed a furious lobbying effort that forced Chamber leaders to back down. As Representative John A. Boehner (R.-Ohio) told the *Post*: "When we saw the Washington staff selling out our members again so they could stand arm-in-arm with the Clinton White House we felt we had to stop it."[62]

An even bigger blow came on February 8, when CBO, after much delay, pronounced that in its opinion, the numbers in the Clinton plan did not add up after all. Over the first six years the plan not only would fail to reduce the deficit, but it would also add $74 billion to it. Even more damning, CBO opined that the mandatory employer contributions toward workers' health coverage should be treated as on-budget federal receipts or (as Republicans had been proclaiming all along) a tax.[63]

Ironically, despite the media coverage, most of the CBO report on the Clinton plan was positive. The agency found that the plan would likely cover everyone, as claimed, and that the premium caps and medicare cuts would reduce national health spending in the aggregate as well as the federal deficit after the year 2004. The report even defended the plan's length and breadth: "Some critics of the proposal maintain that it is too complex. A major reason for its complexity, however, is that the proposal outlines in legislation the steps that would actually have to be taken to accomplish its goals. No other proposal has come close to attempting this. Other health care proposals might appear equally complex if they provided the same level of detail as the Administration on the implementation requirements."[64]

There was some good news for the Clinton administration: Republicans in Congress remained as deadlocked as Democrats over how best to proceed. A two-day summit of House and Senate Republicans in Annapolis, Maryland, failed to produce either the set of agreements members of the minority party sought or a list of proposals a sufficient number of Republican senators would support to block Democratic action.[65]

Committee Action

By March 1994, committee action should have been well under way if Congress was to complete work on such a massive bill before adjourning for the year in early October. But members were reflecting the doubts of their constituents—they wanted to proceed but were uncertain about which way to go. One thing was clear: the attack ads against the Clinton plan were doing their job. A *Wall Street Journal*/NBC News poll released March 10 found 45 percent of respondents opposed to the Clinton plan, with 37 percent in favor. Yet those same respondents still wanted strong action. When the elements of the proposal were described without identifying it as the Clinton plan, 76 percent said it had "some" or "great" appeal.[66]

An early indicator of trouble brewing was the March 2 announcement that neither of the two health-related subcommittees of the pivotal House Energy and Commerce Committee would be marking up a health bill. "At this point, we agree that the best way to achieve the

President's health care reform goals is to move directly to consideration by the full committee," said the joint statement from Chairman John D. Dingell (D.-Mich.), Health and Environment Subcommittee Chairman Henry A. Waxman (D.-Calif.), and Cardiss Collins (D.-Ill.), chairwoman of the Subcommittee on Commerce, Consumer Protection, and Competitiveness.[67]

The admission of gridlock was particularly ominous for several reasons. Most important, Energy and Commerce was seen as the committee whose membership was most representative of the full House membership; whatever it produced was most likely to ultimately become law. Energy and Commerce was also a key power center for health policy—led by Dingell, whose commitment to the issue dated back to his father, who preceded him in Congress and who introduced one of the first national health insurance bills in the 1930s. Dingell had introduced such a bill on the first day of each Congress in which he had served, to honor his father's unfulfilled goal. Dingell's power over health care issues was virtually matched by that of Health Subcommittee Chairman Waxman, a leading liberal legislator whose list of legislative achievements in health policy over the previous decade and a half could fill a book. Waxman presided not only over the successful effort to preserve medicaid from the reductions sought by the Reagan administration and Republican Senate in the early 1980s, but he almost single-handedly managed to expand the program during times of great budget tensions in the latter half of that decade.

It was left to the House Ways and Means Health Subcommittee to lead off the formal legislative action, which it did on March 8. But the proposal offered by Subcommittee Chairman Stark bore little resemblance to the Clinton plan. After consulting with his panel's Democrats, Stark scrapped Clinton's mandatory purchasing alliances, the premium caps, and most of the new bureaucracy. Instead, he built his vision of universal coverage on an existing program for which his panel already had oversight—medicare. Under the Stark plan, employers with fewer than one hundred workers could either purchase private coverage for their workers or enroll them in a new medicare part C (the existing program for elderly and disabled Americans includes part A for hospital coverage and part B for physician and outpatient costs). Those without jobs would also be covered by the new program. Stark's bill sought to control spending using existing medicare methodologies for regulating hospital, doctor, and other charges. Said Stark at the opening of the markup, "The plan achieves the president's objective, but without disrupting the good relationships that most Americans have with their doctors and without creating any new bureaucracies."

Republicans wasted no time getting to the heart of the issue when the subcommittee opened the bill for amendment on March 15. "This is an amendment I would describe as technical in nature," deadpanned Fred Grandy (R.-Iowa). "It's to strike the employer mandate." Republicans argued that the mandate in any form was a radical change. Said ranking Republican Bill Thomas (R.-Calif.), "In no way can you say that government mandating the role of business to pay for a structure it does not control is building on the current system." But Democrats who favored the concept of universal coverage united in opposition. "This is a fundamental decision here," stated single-payer proponent Jim McDermott. "If we accept this amendment we are essentially saying there will not be universal coverage."[68]

The Democrats ultimately prevailed, defeating the Grandy amendment by a 6–5 margin. The seventh Democrat on the subcommittee, Mike Andrews of Texas (an architect of the Cooper bill, which lacked an employer mandate), voted—as expected—with the Republicans.

The remainder of the markup proved a small-scale version of the large-scale debate. Liberal Democrats, led by McDermott, wanted to beef up the spartan benefits package Stark wrote into his bill. But committee members ultimately resisted, because they could not agree on how to pay for enhanced benefits. One proposal that was rejected was an amendment by Andrews, a leading tobacco industry foe, to raise the cigarette tax to $2 per pack. Stark's bill included the same 75-cent tax increase recommended by Clinton. Later, however, the panel voted to increase the tax by $1.25 to help finance expanded subsidies for small businesses that would be affected by the employer mandate. On March 23 the panel became the first subcommittee to report a bill when it approved Stark's proposal by the same 6–5 vote by which it saved the employer mandate. Along the way, the subcommittee voted down McDermott's single-payer plan, the Cooper and Michel bills, and (when the Republicans insisted) the original version of the Clinton plan. All the panel Democrats voted "present" on the Clinton bill to protest the Republicans' tactics and to save the president the embarrassment of "no" votes.

The next panel to formally take up health care reform was the Education and Labor Subcommittee on Labor-Management Relations. In keeping with that committee's left-leaning reputation, the bill Subcommittee Chairman Pat Williams (D.-Mont.) placed before his members on April 21 was clearly intended to set the liberal boundary of what the full House could ultimately consider. The bill included a benefits package even more generous than the one included in the original Clinton plan, and it provided more in the way of subsidies for small businesses. Over the course of the markup (which would consume much of six weeks) the bill would become even more generous, ultimately adding another $55 billion to the Clinton plan's cost over five years, according to CBO estimates.[69]

After fending off dozens of Republican efforts to scale the measure back, the subcommittee ultimately approved it on a straight party-line vote of 17–10 on May 25. On June 9 the subcommittee also approved by voice vote a slightly modified version of Representative McDermott's single-payer plan. The bill, HR 3960, was sponsored by subcommittee member and single-payer supporter George Miller (D.-Calif.), who needed to rewrite it slightly to give the committee jurisdiction. Williams was candid about the quid pro quo involved. By giving single-payer forces (who represented a majority of Democrats on the full committee) a vote on their plan, he told *Congressional Quarterly*, "They . . . are then willing at this subcommittee and full committee level to also cast a vote in favor of my mark."[70]

Among the thorny issues addressed by the subcommittee chaired by Williams was abortion. The Clinton bill attempted to duck the issue by including coverage for abortion but not actually mentioning the word. Instead, the bill merely called for coverage of "pregnancy-related services." Abortion remained one of the most troublesome issues in the entire health care reform debate. On the one hand, most private plans already provided coverage for elective abortions, so a national plan excluding such coverage would mean taking a benefit away from many women. On the other hand, although Congress in recent years had relaxed its strong antiabortion voting patterns, using federal funds for the procedure was still a line even many supporters of a woman's right to choose were reluctant to cross. Yet because of the various subsidies involved in the various incarnations of the Clinton plan, including abortion as a covered service would clearly mean spending federal funds to provide it.

On May 12 the Education and Labor Subcommittee turned back two separate attempts to amend the bill's abortion coverage. The first would have excluded abortion from the standard benefits package but made it available as optional, supplemental coverage. The other would have allowed states to decide whether or not the procedure were offered. Both amendments would be presented in similar forms at all subsequent markups and would in nearly every instance be defeated. But on May 11 abortion opponents had prevailed at the Health Subcommittee markup of the House Veterans' Affairs Committee, which was considering how a new health plan would affect the VA health care system. At the behest of subcommittee member Representative Christopher H. Smith (R.-N.J.), chairman of the House Pro-Life Caucus, the subcommittee passed (by an 11–8 vote) an amendment to limit abortions at VA medical facilities to cases of rape, incest, or endangerment of the mother's life.[71]

Following the two successful subcommittee markups at Ways and Means and at Education and Labor, Clinton backers got another boost in May from a CBO report critical of the rival Cooper plan. CBO Director Robert Reischauer told the Senate Finance Committee on May 4 that the bill would not only leave millions of Americans uninsured, but its financing mechanism would also fall billions of dollars short of the amount needed to fund the subsidies promised to low-income families to help them pay for private health insurance.

But senators at the hearing seemed more concerned about how slow CBO was in estimating the effects of various plans than about its evaluations of any particular bill. Reischauer and his seventeen health policy analysts had been working nearly nonstop for months to produce its formal evaluations and cost estimates for the raft of major health bills. As markups got under way, committee chairmen had to wait for official CBO scoring of their various proposals and amendments before they could proceed. Republicans complained that CBO favored Democratic plans, while Democrats protested that CBO was hamstringing the entire process. At one point a frustrated Bill Bradley (D.-N.J.) pointed out that the Clinton administration had taken far less time to process its numbers than CBO had. "What do they have that you don't?" the senator asked Reischauer. "Hundreds of thousands of employees," Reischauer snapped.[72]

The CBO report on the Cooper bill also put another divisive issue in health reform back into play—whether or not the federal government should continue to exclude employer-provided health benefits from taxation. The money at stake was one of the largest pots available in the health care reform game. In 1994, according to CBO estimates, the federal treasury was forgoing $74 billion in revenues by allowing employers to deduct the cost of employee health insurance from business taxes, and a comparable amount by allowing recipients of coverage to exclude it from their own income taxes. The effect of the deduction and exclusion, health analysts pointed out, was inherently inflationary—employers were encouraged to offer richer and richer benefits plans and employees to seek them, because both enjoyed a tax advantage from more coverage. Several bills, including the Clinton plan, included some limit on the tax preference for health benefits; but the Cooper plan was the only one to use it as its primary financing source. Under that bill, employees would still be allowed to receive health benefits tax free, but employer deductions would be limited to the lowest cost health plan in the area. Policy considerations aside, as *Congressional Quarterly* pointed out, advocating taxation of health insurance was politically risky for both sides: "Any Democrat who pushes the idea invites attack from Republicans that it would be taxing the middle class. Any Republican who tries it can expect the Democrats to level accusations that it would take away workers' health benefits."[73]

In May Senator Ted Kennedy strode into this mess with *his* incarnation of the Clinton plan. Despite his national reputation as the Senate's leading liberal, since taking over the helm of the Senate Labor and Human Resources Committee in 1987, Kennedy had proven himself a pragmatic and effective legislator. On a long list of controversial bills that would become law (including child care, the Americans with Disabilities Act, and the Family and Medical Leave Act), Kennedy showed he knew how and when to compromise, and he had benefited from strategic alliances with committee Republicans. Indeed, it was Kennedy who in September 1993 announced support for the Clinton bill from the only Republican who would ultimately sign on, committee member James M. Jeffords.

Unlike many other chairmen, Kennedy enjoyed the luxury of a panel stacked with liberals—indeed, the committee's reputation was that it was so liberal Kennedy could pass national health insurance out of it if he wanted to. But he chose instead to try to fashion something else—not a bill that would pass his committee, but one that could pass the full Senate. Changes Kennedy made to the Clinton bill to win Republican support included making the hated health purchasing alliances voluntary, exempting the smallest businesses from the controversial employer mandate (with the requirement that they pay a 2 percent payroll tax instead), and retargeting the small business subsidies to make better use of funds available. In a trademark public relations move, Kennedy's bill would also have allowed anyone to join the huge health insurance program for federal workers, the Federal Employees Health Benefits Plan. That would have, in effect, allowed anyone the same coverage enjoyed by members of Congress.

But Kennedy's strategy for attracting Republicans to the health care reform bandwagon failed. Complained ranking Republican Nancy Landon Kassebaum of Kansas, "The heavy regulation in the president's bill has not been eased; it has simply been moved around."[74] At the end of the marathon markup on June 9, the panel had adopted dozens of Republican amendments. However, the only Republican who would join in the 11–6 vote to approve the measure was Jeffords, who was already a Clinton bill cosponsor, and even his "yes" vote was a reluctant one.

The Labor Committee markup may not have produced a bill with bipartisan backing, but it did produce by far the most thoughtful congressional debate on health issues in 1994. Members spiritedly debated such second-tier but critical matters as who should guarantee privacy of medical records, who should hold the balance of power between doctors and insurance companies, and whether Congress or an appointed board should determine which benefits would be covered in a standardized package. Indeed, many of the issues the panel tackled clearly illustrated why health care reform had long been so difficult for Congress.

On the other side of Capitol Hill, House committees were also beginning to make headway on the massive effort. In the shadow of an impending indictment, House Ways and Means Chairman Dan Rostenkowski (D.-Ill.) scrapped plans to totally rewrite the proposal produced by Pete Stark's Health Subcommittee, and on May 18 he formally began deliberations on the subcommittee-approved bill. With Republicans making it clear they had no intention of supporting any of the Democratic plans, Rostenkowski's goal was evident: to find twenty votes from among the committee's twenty-four Democrats to report a bill from the thirty-eight committee members and keep health care reform alive. It would not be easy. The Democrats included several conservatives with grave doubts about the Stark bill's highly regulatory framework and employer mandate, as well as liberals like McDermott who found the benefits package in the Stark bill too paltry. Tobacco state legislators like Representative L. F. Payne of Virginia had to look out for interests back home concerned about the economic consequences of a dramatic increase in the federal cigarette tax.

Many outside observers thought the May 31 indictment of Rostenkowski on corruption charges signaled the beginning of the end of health care reform, much as the Tidal Basin antics of former Ways and Means Chairman Wilbur Mills had scuttled the last major attempt at health care reform twenty years earlier. But those assessments turned out to be premature. Under House rules, Rostenkowski was permitted to remain on the committee but had to temporarily cede the chairmanship to the next most senior Democrat, Florida's Sam Gibbons. Known mostly for his work on trade, Gibbons was an irascible 74-year-old considered by most to be a legislative lightweight.

But Gibbons surprised everyone. By June 9 he was ready with revisions to the subcommittee-approved bill. These included more freedom for businesses to self-insure (an important issue for larger companies), larger subsidies for small businesses and the working poor, a smaller tobacco tax, and a larger market for private insurance companies. On June 10 CBO concluded that the revised plan would, in fact, be deficit neutral.

On June 14 Gibbons won his first and probably most important victory, when the panel defeated a Grandy attempt to strike the employer mandate by a 20–18 vote. Then, just as his fragile Democratic coalition seemed ready to splinter, Gibbons received some unexpected help from the Republican leadership. The June 16 *Washington Post* included Grandy's complaint that House Minority Whip Newt Gingrich had instructed Republicans on Ways and Means to defeat the Gibbons bill outright rather than try to work out a bipartisan compromise. That infuriated Grandy, the lead Republican sponsor of the bipartisan Cooper plan. "It's disappointing," Grandy told the *Post*. "We now have a leadership that preempts policy with politics." In response, the Democrats rallied around Gibbons.[75]

But if the Republicans were helping Gibbons, the president was not. Faced with the probability that the Senate would be unable to pass a bill with an employer mandate to ensure universal coverage, the White House began hinting that it might accept what came to be known as "triggers." With the debate already all but incomprehensible, the trigger discussions made semantics even worse. Essentially, triggers came in two forms, hard and soft. Under a hard trigger, if market changes did not achieve near-universal coverage by a certain date (95 percent was the figure most often discussed), then an employer mandate would automatically take effect. Under a soft trigger, if the coverage threshold was not reached, Congress would be required to come back and review the issue. In the end, the entire discussion of triggers proved fruitless— opponents of the mandate found a hard trigger not different enough, and supporters of universal coverage thought the soft trigger not strong enough.

The only immediate impact of the discussions (besides further confusing the public) was to undercut the Ways and Means deliberations. Reported *Congressional Quarterly*: "Some members said the events were eerily reminiscent of [the 1993] battle over the Btu tax, a levy Clinton proposed then dropped in negotiations with the Senate after House members already had taken the difficult political step of voting for it. 'As a member who voted for the Btu tax, I've got to say, what are they doing?' said one committee Democrat."[76]

The administration quickly got the message. On June 21, the president told the Business Roundtable that he would not give up on his goal of universal coverage. The following day, after a meeting with Senate leaders, Hillary Rodham Clinton was even more explicit, announcing that "a bill that does not result in universal coverage . . . will not be acceptable."[77] That helped break the deadlock at Ways and Means, which managed to report the Gibbons bill on a 20–18 vote on June 30. Among the Democrats voting "no" was liberal McDermott, who complained that to win a majority, Gibbons had made too many concessions to doctors, insurance companies, and other special interests. Mc-Dermott threatened to urge the ninety-one cosponsors of his single-payer bill to walk unless the House leadership brought a bill to the floor that had a more generous benefits package and stronger cost containment provisions.

McDermott and his fellow liberals were much happier with the bill the full Education and Labor Committee had quietly reported out on June 23. Although the least watched of the markups (several of which were going on simultaneously), Education and Labor was among the most prolific of the committees. All told, in eight days of markup the panel considered ninety-seven amendments and approved fifty-one. It was also by far the most partisan of all the committees. During opening statements on June 10, Randy Cunningham (R.-Calif.) called the plan before the panel (a slightly modified version of the one approved by Williams' subcommittee in May) "an ugly child" that "smells as bad as dog's breath."[78]

The final Education and Labor package, approved by a vote of 26–17 (with two Democrats joining all the Republicans in opposition), had indeed set the liberal boundary of the debate. The Clinton plan's already generous benefits package was expanded to include dental care for children and adults, more mental health care, and more preventive services. During the markup, members also added $3.6 billion for school-based health clinics and a $2.5 billion program to bring more health professionals to rural and underserved areas. Later on June 23, the committee voted 22–21 to "report to the floor without recommendation" Miller's single-payer bill, HR 3960. Even without the favorable recommendation, Committee Chairman William D. Ford (D.-Mich.) had trouble rounding up votes to guarantee the single-payer plan a floor vote in the House, which had been his end of the deal by which the panel's single-payer supporters voted out his Clinton-plan–like bill.[79]

Foreshadowing what was to come, the two most important committees had the most trouble producing health care reform legislation. Despite the best efforts of John Dingell (who was considered, along with Dan Rostenkowski, among the most powerful committee chairmen on Capitol Hill), the Energy and Commerce Committee proved unable to report a bill and Dingell failed to even convene a markup. In a June 28 letter to Speaker of the House Thomas Foley, Dingell announced that neither the proposals he had floated along with subcommittee chairs Waxman and Collins "nor any other suggested legislation enjoys the support of a majority of Committee Members." Dingell referred in the letter to "certain members" who "were preoccupied with statewide campaigns for other offices"—thinly disguised references to Jim Cooper, who was promoting his own managed competition bill in his race to serve out Vice President Al Gore's remaining Senate term; and Jim Slattery (D.-Kan.), who ran an unsuccessful primary race for governor. Cooper and Slattery were considered key to the committee's ability to report a bill. However, neither would budge on any sort of employer mandate, and Dingell would not yield in his desire to report a bill guaranteeing universal coverage or nothing at all. "I am not going to report out a bad bill," Dingell told the Associated Press. "Nor am I going to allow my committee to report out a bad bill."[80]

But in the equally riven Senate Finance Committee, Pat Moynihan had no such lofty goals. He was determined to report a bill from his committee, whether or not the bill guaranteed universal coverage. As befitted its reputation as the most powerful committee in Congress, all eyes had been focused on Finance for months. Among its eleven Democrats and nine Republicans were most of the key players in the Senate's health care debate: Majority Leader Mitchell and Minority Leader Dole; key Clinton plan backers Jay Rockefeller (D.-W.Va.) and Tom Daschle (D.-S.D.); and leading Republican moderate John Chafee; as well as the Senate sponsors of the rival Cooper bill, John Breaux (D.-La.) and Dave Durenberger (R.-Minn.).

For months legislators on the Hill had been meeting behind closed doors, leaving reporters and lobbyists to cool their heels. Democrats met with Democrats, and Republicans with Republicans; the full committee membership met, and other senators split off in smaller bipartisan groups. The situation ultimately became so confusing that members were backing away from their own proposals. "I thought it was a good idea at the time," Breaux said in June of one of the trigger proposals he had devised only weeks earlier. "I don't think so anymore." Among the most remarkable flip-flops was the one made by Senator Robert Packwood (R.-Ore.), the panel's ranking Republican. A longtime backer of employer mandates who had introduced bills calling for them as early as the 1970s, Packwood was suddenly an ardent opponent. "I'm not going to compel people who are so vehemently opposed to it to cover their employees," Packwood explained at a June 14 press conference.[81] Cynics suggested Packwood's conversion was less the result of a policy shift than of his desire to please Minority Leader Dole, who could help Packwood in an ongoing ethics investigation stemming from charges of sexual harassment filed against him in November 1992.[82]

To confuse matters even more, no one was quite sure what Chairman Moynihan wanted or expected. One day he was for universal coverage and an employer mandate; the next he was trotting Republicans over to the White House to prove that he could not get any bill with universal coverage through his committee.

The deadlock was finally broken in part by the calendar. The July 4 deadline for completion of committee action was the first "real" one, to the extent that it would leave barely enough time left to get a bill finished before the November election. Majority Leader Mitchell—who not only was retiring from the Senate at the end of the year but had also declined a Supreme Court appointment to try to see health care reform through to enactment—specifically promised to have a health care reform bill on the Senate floor in July. Implicitly, that was a threat to Moynihan: if he could not get a bill out of Finance, Mitchell would take the Labor Committee bill instead.

Moynihan's salvation turned out to be a group of six moderate Democrats and Republicans who devised a plan that purported to cover 93 percent of Americans by 2005 without either an employer mandate or explicit spending controls. These six legislators (Republicans Chafee, Durenberger, and John Danforth of Missouri, and Democrats Breaux, Kent Conrad of North Dakota, and David Boren of Oklahoma) called themselves the "rump group" and formed the core of what would come to be called the "mainstream" group.

Pressed by Mitchell, Moynihan finally called a public markup for the week of June 27. To prove his point to the Clinton administration, the "mark" he presented to the committee included a modified hard trigger that would have guaranteed near-universal coverage by automatically imposing an employer mandate if 96 percent of Americans did not obtain coverage by 2000. But the committee quickly changed that. On June 30, as Ways and Means was successfully voting out its plan, Finance became the first of the committees considering health care reform to explicitly vote down an employer mandate. Only six of the panel's eleven Democrats voted to keep Moynihan's multilayered hard trigger in the bill. It was ultimately replaced with a soft trigger requiring Congress to vote on the recommendations of a nonpartisan commission for expanding coverage if 95 percent of Americans had not obtained coverage by 2002.

But even that was not enough to produce a majority. In the end, on the morning of Friday, June 30 (a day before the July 4 recess was to begin), Moynihan incorporated into his bill the proposal produced by the bipartisan rump group a week earlier. Ironically, it was the rest of the Republicans who were most upset by the prospect of seeing the bill rammed through—not so much because they disagreed with what was in it, but because it threatened what had been a significant display of Republican unity. "I can't speak for three of my colleagues," said Dole, "but the rest of us believed we could craft something all of us could support." Backers of the proposal were furious at being accused of rushing things. "We've talked about health care enough to make us all sick," retorted Breaux. "I don't think if we stayed here another two months we would know any more than we do today."[83] After a rare Saturday session, the committee voted 11–8 to report the only committee bill among the four that did not guarantee universal coverage.

Although the measure appeared to be a major defeat for universal coverage backers, it actually hurt Republicans more. Only three days earlier, on June 29, Dole managed to unite forty of the Senate's forty-four Republicans behind a measure they hoped would counter charges that they were "gridlock guardians" in the event they successfully defeated the Democrats' plans. The proposal was very much one with a least common denominator. It sought to guarantee all Americans "access" to coverage by barring insurance companies from discriminating on the basis of health status, encouraging formation of purchasing groups, and providing subsidies to very poor Americans. It included no requirements for coverage, no new taxes, and no cost-containment measures. The four abstainers—the three Finance Committee moderates in the rump group, and Clinton plan cosponsor Jeffords—were significant, because Dole needed forty-one votes to guarantee blocking of any Democratic plan.

Leadership Attempts to Reconcile

The narrow, partisan margins by which health care reform bills moved out of committee made it clear to House and Senate leaders that combining the bills into one that could win a majority in either chamber would be an uphill battle.

Abortion was a good example of how difficult reconciliation of bills would be. Although three of the four committees voted to include abortion as a covered service (with the Finance bill allowing employers to decide whether or not it would be included in their plans), a significant bloc of members, particularly in the House, made it clear they could not support any bill that included federal funds for abortion. The arithmetic was stark. With no Republican support, Democrats in the House could lose no more than thirty-eight votes and still pass a bill. Thirty-five Democrats signed a letter to Speaker Foley in June vowing not to vote for any bill that included abortion coverage. Their case was buttressed in July when the National Conference of Catholic Bishops, a key backer of universal coverage, called on Congress to strip abortion coverage from its health care reform bills. But the other side fought back. The same day the Catholic bishops held their press conference in

Washington, two abortion rights advocates called a press conference to announce that sixty-eight Democrats had signed a letter pledging not to support any health care reform bill unless abortion *was* included.

For Democratic leaders in the House and Senate, as well as the Clinton administration, the hope in July was clearly that as the moment of decision approached, the public would finally become involved enough to push some legislators off the fence. The public did in fact become more energized, but not in the way universal coverage backers hoped.

On July 22, the first of a series of bus caravans dubbed the "Health Security Express" left Portland, Oregon, on its way to Washington, D.C. The caravan was underwritten by three organizations that had been working closely with the Clinton administration on health care reform, and supported by dozens of other health, labor, and religious groups. Backers hoped the buses carrying uninsured Americans and others victimized by the failures of the health care system could recreate the successful bus trips of candidate Clinton two years earlier and rally public support for universal coverage. But at many stops the caravan drew more protesters than supporters. Citizens for a Sound Economy, a conservative antitax group that opposed the Clinton plan, operated its own hotline. Organizers rounded up counterdemonstrators against what its flyers called "The Phony Express: Special interests get a free ride to Washington D.C. to demand a handout." Administration speakers along the route (including the president, first lady, and several members of the cabinet) were heckled and shouted down. In Kentucky, Hillary Rodham Clinton was burned in effigy by tobacco farmers protesting increases in cigarette taxes.

Indeed, the din on both sides was almost overpowering. A study released by the Center for Public Integrity found that interest groups had spent at least $100 million to affect the outcome of the debate. In Washington, supporters of universal coverage held a press conference almost daily in an attempt to rally their troops. In one of the more imaginative events, Senators Paul Simon (D.-Ill.) and Paul Wellstone (D.-Minn.) held a mock lottery to draw names of the five senators who would theoretically lose their health insurance if Congress passed a bill to guarantee coverage to only 95 percent of Americans. Among the names drawn was that of Finance Chairman Moynihan.

Although public opinion remained badly divided, Congressional leaders pushed on. On July 21 Clinton met with House and Senate

Democratic leaders, who emerged to announce what everyone already knew—significant changes would be needed to find a bill that could pass either chamber. Wrote *Congressional Quarterly:*

> Now, as leaders cobble together final legislation for floor action in August, they have to hope their message will prompt needed flexibility from all sides. To pass a bill, Clinton and Democratic leaders need conservatives to embrace universal coverage and liberals to accept that it will be years before all Americans have access to affordable insurance.[84]

The House bill was unveiled first on July 29. Majority Leader Dick Gephardt, after marathon talks with virtually every House Democrat, ultimately decided to gamble by basing his plan on the Ways and Means bill. It included the controversial medicare part C program for small businesses and unemployed Americans and an employer mandate requiring coverage of 80 percent of most premiums beginning in 1997 for large companies and in 1999 for smaller firms. It called for a 45-cent increase in the cigarette tax (thought to be the maximum tobacco state legislators could accept) and a 2 percent tax on insurance premiums to help pay for subsidies for small businesses.

Although Gephardt was unsure he could find the votes to pass his bill in the House, Mitchell knew he could not even attempt such a proposal in the Senate. Mitchell's bill, unveiled August 2, would "set us on the road to universal coverage," as the senator put it, by seeking to guarantee coverage to 95 percent of Americans by 2000. If that threshold was not reached, state-by-state employer mandates could take effect that would require only employers of twenty-five or more workers to pay only 50 percent of premiums for workers and their dependents. The 95 percent "is not universal coverage," Mitchell conceded. However, it was clearly as far as he could go without risking the votes of moderate Democrats he desperately needed.[85] He could also go no further to the right without risking the votes of Senate liberals. Indeed, even the president recognized Mitchell's dilemma. Although the bill clearly failed to meet his bottom-line demand for universal coverage, on August 3 President Clinton declared that it did. "I believe it does meet the objective that I set out in the State of the Union and I would sign it," he said of the Mitchell bill.[86]

But while Democrats dithered, the calendar was becoming increasingly important. Leaders of both houses vowed to keep Congress in session through the start of the planned August recess to complete floor consideration of the health care reform bills. But House members were loath to vote for Gephardt's plan until they were sure the Senate would not turn around and kill even Mitchell's watered-down mandate. Still, House leaders denied the waiting game, at least in public. "We cannot possibly conduct House business on the basis of the Senate schedule,"[87] insisted Speaker Foley at his daily news conference August 4. "The Senate cannot conduct Senate business on the basis of the Senate schedule." Ultimately, the schedule was set so that the Senate would begin first, on August 9, and the House would begin on August 15. House leaders hoped that by then they would know what the Senate would do on the pivotal mandate issue.

Floor Action

But the Democrats' carefully planned schedule failed to take into account two separate problems—Senate Republicans and CBO. Along with the crime bill, both would ultimately distract members and the public and ruin the Democrats' plans for the health care reform bill.

From the very start, the formal Senate debate did not go smoothly. Mitchell proposed a schedule that would give the opening debate a high profile while leaving members time to complete action on other matters before turning to health care full time. Under Mitchell's plan, senators would debate the health care reform bill for four hours each on the evenings of August 9 and 10 with opening statements, and then turn to the amendments on August 11.

That left Republicans with a public relations dilemma. On the one hand, they would not consent to a strategy designed to give Democrats an advantage in getting their bill passed. On the other hand, they were concerned about being seen as blocking such major legislation—which could sway public opinion toward the Mitchell bill or, even worse, help forge Democratic unity. What the Republicans ultimately settled on was a device that could best be called a stealth filibuster. Publicly they simply claimed they needed time to examine the lengthy Mitchell bill and its potential ramifications and to explain their position to the American people. "We're not going to be rushed," said Bob Dole on August 9. "This issue is too important."[88] But in strategy meetings another tactic became clear: to take up as much time as possible, and if the clock ran out, so be it.

The tentativeness of both sides reflected a painful reality—neither side was sure who would prevail in the key vote on the Mitchell mandate. "Nobody knows how many votes there are for anything," admitted Dave Durenberger on August 11.[89] Indeed, unlike most Senate debates, the one on health care reform began with members truly trying to persuade each other—and the public—to join their cause.

Democrats prevailed on their colleagues' sense of history. "Medicare was a defining test for a Congress a generation ago," said Kennedy on the floor. "Social security was a defining test in the years of the depression. This legislation is the defining test for Congress today."[90] They also highlighted a traditional Democratic goal—fairness. Argued Harris Wofford: "How dare members of Congress, who have their health insurance paid for by their employer—the U.S. taxpayers—say it is impossible to provide the same kind of security to the people who sent them here. Why should middle-class Americans, who work hard, pay their taxes, and send their kids to school, not have that kind of security, too? It is a matter of simple justice."[91]

Republicans, in turn, played their strongest card—distrust of government. "This issue is about the role of government in a free society," argued Phil Gramm. "When my momma gets sick, I want her to talk to a doctor and not some government bureaucrat." As a backup, they also exploited the public's fear of change. "Congress is rarely shy about tinkering with things it does not fully understand, and health care is no exception," warned Nancy Landon Kassebaum.[92]

But while the right and left were duking it out on the Senate floor, the senators whose votes were sought most anxiously by both sides were holed up in John Chafee's hideaway office in a humid corridor of the Capitol. The rump group of six Finance Committee moderates was rapidly expanding into a formal "mainstream coalition" encompassing as many as twenty senators from both parties, all eagerly seeking that elusive middle ground that could address the health care problems most agreed on.

In the meantime, things were bogging down in the House. On the morning of August 11, House leaders put the health care debate off indefinitely. The official reason was that CBO had not finished scoring the Gephardt bill and the three alternatives expected to be offered on the floor. But off the record, aides confirmed that Democrats simply did not have the votes to pass any bill. Leadership staff was also distracted by having to round up votes for an unexpectedly close vote on the crime bill (a vote Democrats initially lost later that day in one of the uglier floor debates in memory). Leaders ultimately prevailed on the crime bill nine days later. But with CBO still not finished with scoring the health care reform bill, the Senate in an apparent holding pattern, and the atmosphere poisonously partisan, the House gave up and sent its members home on a delayed August break. Assuming by that time the Senate would have had to decide on the matter one way or another, Majority Leader Richard Gephardt announced that the House would take up the health care reform bill as soon as it reconvened in September.

It took Senate Republicans more than a week to finish their lengthy opening statements; Mitchell ultimately had to threaten to keep the Senate in session around the clock to convince Republicans that it was time to begin voting on amendments. Still, the first amendments members considered were all minor—for example, one to speed up a requirement that insurance plans provide preventive care to women and children, and another to strike from the Mitchell bill a $10,000 fine on employers who offered plans that failed to conform to the standard package of benefits.

As the two sides in the debate continued to shadowbox, attention turned to the mainstream coalition meeting in Chafee's hideaway office. On Friday, August 19, the coalition announced its agreement. The plan was not dramatically different from the one offered to the Finance Committee. It proposed changing insurance laws to ensure access, authorizing purchasing cooperatives, and providing subsidies to poor Americans to help them purchase coverage. It included a soft trigger requiring Congress to consider recommendations of a special commission if market changes did not sufficiently increase coverage. At the insistence of several members, it also sought to guarantee roughly $50 billion in deficit reduction over five years. The subsidies would be financed through deep cuts in medicare and medicaid, an increase in the cigarette tax from 24 to 69 cents per pack, and a tax on high-cost insurance plans.

Although the mainstream proposal satisfied those in the ideological center, it seemed unable to pull votes from those at either pole in the debate. "I'd rather do nothing than something that's a step backwards," complained liberal Paul Wellstone. Conservatives were equally unimpressed. Phil Gramm called the compromise just another incarnation of the Mitchell bill and said Congress should "stop carrying around this corpse, changing its clothes and putting more powder on its face."[93]

In the meantime, Mitchell also had to contend with the crime bill, which consumed four precious days of floor time from August 22 to 26. At the end, he reached the same conclusion House leaders had—the senators were simply too tired and angry to continue to debate on health care reform. After the Senate approved the crime bill late on August 25, Mitchell sent members home until September 12. The following day, after a meeting with the president, Mitchell announced that when the Senate returned it would not have enough time to pass a comprehensive bill. He would therefore spend the recess trying to reach agreement with the mainstream coalition on incremental steps.

The End

When Congress returned in September, for a while it seemed that it might actually take up a health care bill. Not only were those in the mainstream group nearing completion of a final package, but several other proposals were also being floated about. A group of Senate liberals proposed a plan, Kidsfirst, that would have guaranteed health insurance coverage for children and pregnant women. Others proposed even smaller packages, including one offered by two former governors, Bob Graham (D.-Fla.) and Mark Hatfield (R.-Ore.), that would have allowed states to move forward with their own plans more easily.

But it was not to be. As talks dragged on between Mitchell and the mainstream group and among him and his liberals, it became increasingly clear that there were not sixty votes—the number needed to break a near-certain filibuster—for any proposal. Both House members and senators were restive and wanted to go home and campaign. The public, despite three weeks of Senate floor debate, remained as confused as ever. The *New York Times* published a poll on September 13 in which 57 percent of those polled said Congress should try for minor changes before the end of the session. However, 50 percent of those same respondents said the president should veto a bill that failed to cover everyone.[94]

By late September, even the most ardent advocates of health care reform knew it was too late. As Energy and Commerce Chairman Dingell wrote in a September 20 letter to the president: "It is time for us to accept the fact that the health insurance industry, an assortment of small and large freeloaders, ideologues and their allies in the Congress have succeeded in their goal: preserving a status quo in which they prosper while millions of Americans suffer and our economy and competitiveness are made vulnerable. . . . Mr. President, the imperatives for health reform remain. The country owes you and the first lady a debt for your leadership, but it is time to give health care reform a decent burial and provide for its rebirth."[95]

In fact, the coup de grâce had been delivered in a private White House meeting earlier that day. House and Senate Republican leaders had reportedly told the president that if either congressional chamber sought action on any health care reform bill, no matter how small, they would block action on the GATT trade treaty that the administration badly wanted. House Minority Whip Newt Gingrich said he was concerned that even a small bill might grow in a last-minute conference committee with universal coverage proponents like Senator Rockefeller and Representative Waxman present.[96]

It was outright blackmail, but it worked. Mitchell officially pulled the plug on Monday, September 26, but not before firing off a final partisan shot: "Even though Republicans are a minority in the Congress, in the Senate they're a minority with a veto. They have the ability to block legislation and they have done so on health care reform. Therefore, it is clear that health insurance reform cannot be enacted this year."

For their part, as a reflection of the change in public perception, Republicans seemed happy to take the blame. Said Dole in a press conference immediately following Mitchell's, "There was an overwhelming consensus on the part of the American people to put on the brakes, and my view is we saw democracy in action. That's what happened. That's the way it's supposed to work."[97]

Conclusions

So how did something that was considered inevitable fail to materialize? Democrats blamed interest groups for scaring the public; Republicans blamed Democrats for overreaching. But the real answer is certainly more complex.

A key problem is one that militates against Congress's ability to make difficult decisions on any number of issues, not only health care reform. The sad fact is that when it comes to health care, most Americans are spoiled. They want the best and most up-to-date care available, they do not want to have to wait for it, and they want someone else to pay the bill. Although the president and first lady hinted about sacrifices in their stump speeches, no politician from either party was ultimately willing to tell the public that controlling costs would inevitably mean providing less care, or at least slower advances in medical technology. Conversely, keeping America's health care system the best in the world will mean spending an ever-increasing percentage of the nation's wealth on health care (particularly as the population ages, because older people consume more medical care services). The Senate floor debate could be fairly summarized as the Democrats telling the public they could have health care nirvana, and the Republicans telling them they could not. In that context, the Republicans deserved to win.

A related problem is the oft-repeated charge that Congress is out of touch with the American public. What makes Congress so timid, however, is that it is too much in touch. As Michael Wines wrote in the *New York Times*: "Its principal problem is not that it listens too little, but that it listens—and is shouted at—too much. . . . Modern Washington is wired for quadrophonic sound and wide-screen video, lashed by fax, computer, 800 number, overnight poll, FedEx, grassroots mail, air shuttle and CNN to every citizen in every village on the continent and Hawaii, too. . . . The cumulative effect has been to turn a somewhat slow and contemplative system into something more like a 500-channel democracy, with the clicker grasped tightly in the hands of the electorate."[98]

Complicating matters is that despite all the education efforts, at the end of the debate Americans still did not understand their health care system, not to mention the various changes proposed. That makes it easy for those who would mislead the public, whether intentionally or otherwise. Take, for example, the arguments against a government takeover of the health care system. What most Americans did not realize is that the government was already the largest payer in the nation's health care system. In 1993 the federal government alone paid 31.7 percent of the nation's $884 billion health bill. Federal, state, and local governments together paid 43.9 percent of the nation's bill.

This particular battle, however, was at least partly lost not so much because of those who sought to defeat the Clinton plan, but because of the ineffectiveness of those who supported it. Despite all the publicity revolving around the HIAA's Harry and Louise, few members of Congress or the media (much less the public) realized that the organization actually supported an employer mandate, or that the NFIB supported most of the proposed insurance market reforms. With some sort of substantive reform seemingly inevitable, those who backed most of the plan thought it was safe to devote their energies to the small parts they did not like. That left little support for building a public groundswell.

Finally, as with the Medicare Catastrophic Coverage Act that preceded it, Congress needs to learn that legislating in a zero-sum environment, in which someone must pay for everything, creates losers as well as winners. Because losers are quicker to complain, some mechanism must be found to highlight benefits of legislation to society as a whole, or else Congress may never again be able to address the nation's most pressing issues.

Chapter 8

How a Bill Did Not
Become a Law

Allen Schick

HEALTH CARE REFORM failed in 1994 because it did not have
the votes—not in Congress and not in the country, not
when Bill Clinton announced his plan and not when the legislative
effort collapsed, not before Harry and Louise took to the airwaves and
certainly not afterward. No postmortems, what-ifs, or finger-pointing
can change the fact that the overhaul of the nation's health care system
lacked majority support with the American public and in Congress. For
a brief period in the afterglow of Clinton's masterful speech to Congress
in September 1993, it may have appeared that sweeping reform would
carry the day. But even then the votes were lacking. Less than 40 percent of all House Democrats cosponsored Clinton's bill when it was
formally introduced on November 20, 1993, and only four more signed
on as cosponsors during the ensuing bargaining and lobbying by the
White House. The number of Senate sponsors never reached one-third
of that chamber's membership. In both the House and the Senate the
roster of sponsors included some key Democrats (such as Representative Pete Stark, chairman of the Subcommittee on Health of the House
Committee on Ways and Means, and Senator Daniel Patrick Moynihan,
chairman of the Senate Finance Committee) who were openly skeptical
about Clinton's proposals.

The needed votes might have been forthcoming if the White House
had proceeded differently or if Congress were a different institution.
The number of what-ifs is extensive. What if Clinton had accepted
incremental reform at the start rather than at the very end; if he had sent
Congress an outline rather than an overdetailed plan; if he had introduced the legislation earlier and not squandered scarce congressional
time; if he had reached out more to Republicans and depended less on

Democrats; if he had proposed smaller subsidies and less redistribution; if the subsidies had been targeted more strategically to supporters of reform rather than being spent on some who opposed it anyway; if he had attacked drug and insurance companies less and had worked for support from doctors and other affected groups more; if he had steered clear of health alliances and other novel arrangements and relied on familiar institutions instead; if his plan had less regulation and more competition; if, rather than entrusting reform to a special task force, he had worked at the outset with congressional committees and leaders. . . .

Although there is no end to speculation about what might have been, no postmortem can ignore the critical role Congress played in determining health care reform's fate. If Congress had acted on health care reform in 1994 as it had when previous presidents had called for enactment of universal coverage, the outcome might have been the same, even if Clinton had acted differently. In fact, during the peak of euphoria in late 1993, some observers predicted that no significant legislation would make it through Congress and that the drive to universalize coverage would be foiled by institutional barriers, just as previous ones had been.[1]

Much has been written about what Congress did to Clinton's legislative ambitions. It may be more productive, however, to inquire into what health care reform says about Congress than about what Congress did to health care reform. Clinton's failure confirms much of the conventional understanding of how Congress operates and how its legislative division of labor with the White House works. It says that Congress is influenced by the president's agenda as well as by public opinion and interest groups. The president has a stronger role in setting the legislative agenda than in dictating legislative outcomes, and these outcomes do not stray much from public sentiment. Interest groups play a large role in shaping the fine print of legislation.

In terms of the internal operations of Congress, health care reform confirms the importance of committees in the legislative process and the enlarged scope of parties and their leaders in formulating substantive policy. It highlights differences between the House and Senate but gives support to convergence theories that the two bodies have become more alike. Rules and procedures matter, in both facilitating and blocking legislative action; legislative time is precious, not only in the end-of-session rush to adjournment but also during midsession, when momentum often flags. Finally, the story of health care reform reinforces the conventional wisdom that Congress is discomfited by blatantly redistributive measures, especially when the stakes are so high and affected interests so powerful and vigilant.

Anyone seeking to explain what happened inside Congress should first look outside, to the influence of the president, public opinion, and interest groups. In the next three sections I consider these external influences accordingly. The picture that emerges is of far-reaching presidential demands that were only superficially backed by an apprehensive public while being strongly challenged by important interests. After examining the outside influence, it is necessary to look inside Congress to examine how the president's demands and legislative alternatives were handled by the political parties, committees, and leaders, and how they were affected by House and Senate rules and procedures. Once the external and internal conditions are reviewed, the failure of health care reform does not appear to be surprising or anomalous.

The President's Agenda

As John Kingdon has demonstrated, the president has the dominant position in setting the Washington agenda.[2] Congress might have taken up some version of health care reform in 1993–94 if it had not been prodded by Bill Clinton, but the odds are that the legislation would have been narrower and much less redistributive. Congress took up comprehensive reform because the president demanded that it act. It struggled with the issue for so long in the face of strong opposition and a shortage of votes because Clinton made health care reform the defining issue of the 1994 session. The president did much more than put health care on the agenda; he established the presumption that no matter how difficult the task, significant reform would be enacted. Clinton made health care the test of Congress's performance and of his own as well. So effective was the president in setting the terms by which Congress would be measured that health care reform did not slip from the legislative calendar until months after it was doomed. Congressional Democrats and some Senate Republicans could not let go when the votes were not forthcoming because they assumed that something would be enacted.

In retrospect, health care reform was like most agenda items: it was only one of a number of things of concern to Americans. Its failure was hardly an issue in the 1994 congressional elections. The conclusion to be drawn is not that reform was unimportant or that Americans did not really care about it. But the issue's prominence was greatly inflated by the president's extraordinary capacity to decide what Congress pays attention to. Health care reform will reemerge, though not necessarily with the same sense of urgency that it commanded in 1994.

The president's command of the agenda is accompanied by weakness in his ability to control legislative outcomes. Congress sometimes does nothing in response to presidential demands; and even when it acts, it typically makes big changes in the legislation.[3] The president's weak say over outcomes is not a personal shortcoming—though it can be overcome by strong presidential leadership—but an inherent feature of American politics. It is etched in constitutional arrangements that separate the president from Congress and establish distinct spheres of influence for each. The political separation of the two branches is the normal condition of American national government. But the independence of Congress in formulating alternatives has been whetted by protracted conflict, a long spell of divided government, and the weakening of presidential leadership in the aftermath of Watergate and Vietnam.

At times Congress accedes to presidential demands with few changes, but these tend to follow elections in which the president successfully claims a mandate, such as the elections of Lyndon Johnson in 1964 and Ronald Reagan in 1980.[4] Bill Clinton's 43 percent share of the popular vote in 1992 did not give him a mandate, but he nevertheless acted as if he had one. After all, his party now controlled both the White House and Capitol Hill, and it wanted to demonstrate that years of gridlock and finger-pointing were over. Clinton got much of what he wanted during his inaugural year, including a deficit reduction package that was significantly altered by Congress but still met his basic demands.[5] Perhaps this and other successes emboldened Clinton to believe that he could dictate the details of health care legislation; the public record indicates, however, that the president knew he had a tough fight on his hands.[6]

Clinton's health care reform was not derailed by its myriad details, though opponents gleefully pointed to its sheer size as evidence of the heavy hand of government. The legislation was done in by a few salient features—principally universal coverage, employer mandates, health alliances, and explicit and implicit controls. Although the legislative package was put together by a special task force headed by Hillary

Rodham Clinton, its basic elements were decided during the 1992 presidential campaign. Many details (such as financing) were filled in by the task force, but some of the most troubling features were locked in by the president long before the task force was organized.

In submitting detailed legislation to Congress, Clinton knew that compromise would be necessary. But in his January 1994 State of the Union Address, he drew the line on what he would yield:

> I am open, as I have said repeatedly, to the best ideas of concerned Members of both parties. I have no special brief for any approach, even in our own bill, except this: If you send me legislation that does not guarantee every American private health insurance that can never be taken away, you will force me to take this pen, veto the legislation, and we'll come right back here and start all over again.[7]

The problem with this veto threat is that it crimped Congress's capacity to generate acceptable alternatives. Universal coverage was not just one of the elements in Clinton's mammoth bill, but the defining characteristic of his legislation, its organizing principle, and the objective that shaped so much else in his health reform. Universal coverage meant that reform would be costly and controversial and would entail extensive regulation and redistribution. Universal coverage meant that government would play a prominent role in the new health system: Costs would have to be controlled, taxes would have to be raised, the types of services covered would have to be detailed, and every American would have to register with a bureaucratic entity.

Clinton directed his veto threat at Congress, but its impact was felt by congressional Democrats. Whether he intended to or not, Clinton held his own party hostage to demands for universal coverage. Perhaps congressional Democrats would not have been able to devise a passable alternative even if the president's demands did not limit their freedom to maneuver. As it is, they never had a chance. Universal coverage became the yardstick against which all alternatives were measured. Congressional Democrats could revise the details, but they could not come up with passable alternatives that deviated from the president's basic principle.

As long as it was in effect, the veto threat ruled out incremental steps of the sort considered by a mainstream coalition of Democratic and Republican senators in the final weeks of the 1994 session. Throughout most of the year, the president continued to insist on guaranteed insurance for every American. He argued that anything less than full coverage would make matters worse by encouraging cost shifting and diluting the effectiveness of cost controls. Clinton retreated from insisting on universal coverage in mid-July, signaling that 95 percent would suffice. But within a day he was forced to backpedal by supporters who insisted that anything less than 100 percent coverage was not worth the effort.[8] In the end, the president and his dwindling band of reformers would have taken just about any deal they could get, but by then it was too late to put health legislation back on track.

The demand for universal coverage was not the only impediment to Congress's ability to formulate a passable alternative. The budget was another. As Joe White explains in chapter 3, rules in place since 1990 require that the projected cost of entitlement legislation be offset so that there is no net increase in the deficit.[9] This rule compelled the president to send Congress a bill detailed enough to enable the Congressional Budget Office to estimate its budgetary impact. Any serious alternative to the president's plan also had to be sufficiently detailed to permit congressional budget experts to score it. This budget rule prevented House and Senate committees from marking up incomplete bills that highlighted the additional benefits to be provided but left out details on how reforms would be financed. Spending increases proposed in the quest for votes had to be traded off against other provisions that either cut spending or raised revenues. Whatever its advantages in strengthening budget control, this arrangement disrupted the free flow of alternatives, which is how Congress typically deals with measures placed on its agenda by the president.

In his September 22, 1993, address to Congress, Clinton acknowledged that "a lot of people . . . say it would be an outright miracle if we passed health care reform. But . . . in a time of change you have to have miracles. And miracles do happen."[10] Because miracles were not forthcoming, what Clinton needed was an alternative that had majority support. Producing such alternatives is Congress's most important legislative function. The task may have been difficult under the best of circumstances, but Congress did not have a free hand. It was encumbered by Clinton's demands, budget enforcement rules, and a public that wanted government to reform health care but was wary of governmental intrusion.

(Mis)Reading Public Opinion

The president was not the only one who favored universal coverage. Most Americans did too, but they wanted it without strings attached, without government control, and without having to pay for it through higher taxes or lower benefits. Congress's inability to devise a passable alternative was partly because interpreting public opinion was so difficult. When health care reform topped the congressional agenda, public attitudes were easy to misread and difficult to apply. Hundreds of polls were taken, both before the president unveiled his plan and after. Some were sponsored by interest groups that wanted to claim public support for their position, but many were by news media and other organizations with no axe to grind.

On the brink of the health care battle in 1993, most Americans were satisfied with the quality and availability of health care, but a majority nevertheless thought that the system needed major overhaul.[11] The percentage who were satisfied had decreased over the years, whereas the proportion who said that major changes were needed had edged up.[12] Americans were concerned about the cost of health care, especially about their ability to pay the expenses of major illness. This was not a new worry. But it was aggravated by recession and a sense of economic insecurity in the early 1990s as well as by cutbacks in the benefits provided by many employers.[13] In some polls a solid majority agreed that the country faced a health care crisis, but in others the percentage in agreement was much lower.[14] In the early 1990s, as in decades past, most Americans believed that government should be responsible for assisting those unable to pay for medical care.[15]

This configuration of public opinion—satisfied but worried, in favor of big changes but divided on whether the system is in crisis, and expecting the government to help those in need—pointed in the direction of Clinton's demand for universal insurance. In fact, almost three-quarters of those polled shortly after Clinton's State of the Union Address agreed that the president should veto legislation that fails to guarantee universal coverage, even if it would improve the country's health care system.[16] The principle of universal coverage continued to garner strong support in later months, even when congressional and public support for the Clinton plan flagged. A March 1994 *New York Times* poll found that 82 percent said it was very important that every American receive health insurance that could never be lost or canceled for any reason. Four months later, those holding this view had barely slipped to 79 percent.[17]

Why couldn't Clinton and congressional Democrats convert the public's endorsement of universal coverage into support for any of the House and Senate measures that promised cradle-to-grave insurance? The reason is that universal health protection came with features that many Americans did not like or that made them apprehensive about what care would be available in the future. Among many who already had health coverage, comprehensive reform stirred anxiety that services would be restricted. Telling evidence about the extensiveness of these fears comes from a *Washington Post* poll (see table 8-1) conducted shortly after the president presented his plan to Congress. Although almost three-quarters of those polled felt that the president had not told the public everything they need to know and about half said they knew only a little about his proposal, a majority nevertheless agreed that it was better than the existing system. But fewer than 20 percent of those surveyed thought that the quality of care they received would be improved. The same percentage (73 percent) that believed the Clinton package would help those who lacked insurance feared that it would hurt small businesses.

Probing beneath surface support for Clinton's proposal, the poll uncovered widespread anxiety among respondents that reform would make matters worse for people such as themselves. Substantial majorities feared that the choice of doctors or hospitals would be curtailed, the cost of their medical care would rise, and some types of services would no longer be available. They also worried that taxes would go up, there would be widespread fraud and abuse, quality of care would decline, and large and inefficient bureaucracy would be created.

Blaming these negative ratings on attacks from insurers and other opponents of comprehensive health care reform is expedient. But there is a simpler explanation for why Americans wanted reform but were wary of the Clinton plan. In explaining the failure of reform, the most salient feature of health care in this country is not that approximately 15 percent of Americans lack insurance but that 85 percent have it. To enact reform, Clinton had to extend coverage to those who were uninsured while also doing good (or at least being perceived as doing no harm) to the great majority of Americans who already had satisfactory care. The White House strategy was to lard reform with subsidies and controls—the former to induce powerful constituencies to support his

TABLE 8-1. *Public Attitudes Toward the Clinton Health Reform Plan*
Percent

General Attitudes	
Approve the Clinton plan	51
Disapprove of the plan	39
Don't know	10
Clinton plan is:	
Better than the present system	59
Worse than the present system	31
Same	2
The quality of your health care will:	
Get better	19
Get worse	34
Stay the same	44
Tax increases to pay for Clinton's plan:	
Support	40
Oppose	57
Don't know	3

Big Concerns About the Clinton Plan	
Might not have good choice of doctors or hospitals	72
The cost of medical care will increase	70
Some expensive services will not be available to all who need them	69
Taxes will have to be increased	68
There will be a lot of fraud and abuse	67
The plan will cost too much	66
Employers would eliminate existing jobs	64
The quality of your medical care will decline	64
Plan would create a large, inefficient bureaucracy	59
People who need it most won't get adequate medical care	56
The plan will pay for legal abortions	43

Source: ABC News/*Washington Post* poll, conducted October 7–10, 1993.

proposal, the latter to ensure that benefits not be taken away and that costs not get out of hand. Clinton urged that subsidies be doled out to big and small businesses, to low-income people and to retired workers, to elderly people and to anyone in need of home care. But the more Clinton tried to attract votes by aiding those with insurance, the more he risked alienating them by making costly and redistributive proposals that relied on the heavy hand of government regulation and control. Most of the 1,342 pages in Clinton's bill addressed health care provided to those Americans who were already insured. But the more he reached out to help and reassure this majority, the more he awakened fears that reform would take away some of the benefits they already had.

Of course, strident and sometimes misleading attacks by insurers and other opponents did not help, but it would be a mistake to assume that they conned Americans into turning against legislation that most of them actually favored. The opponents read the public opinion polls, just as the White House did, and they skillfully and unfairly portrayed reforms in ways that reinforced the anxieties felt by many Americans.[18]

A national survey sponsored by the Robert Wood Johnson Foundation found that attitudes toward health reform were strongly affected by advertising campaigns. Respondents were more likely to support change after hearing proreform messages and less likely to after hearing antireform ones.[19] The airwaves were filled with many more messages opposing reform than supporting it, and the advertising campaigns did have some effect in inciting public opinion on the Clinton plan.

Between September 1993 and June 1994, disapproval ratings for the Clinton plan soared from 24 percent to 53 percent, a rise that precluded enactment of anything closely resembling the president's version of health care reform.[20] In fact, more Americans trusted Congress than the president to handle such reform.[21] Yet public opinion did not offer sufficiently clear guidance on what direction Congress should take. On the one hand, most Americans persisted in believing changes should be made; on the other, they did not want the way their health care was provided to change. As health care reform wound down, a slim majority thought that the president should compromise and accept 95 percent coverage, but six out of ten respondents believed that Congress should continue to debate the issue and act on it the next year.[22]

In the summer of 1994 no less than in the fall of 1993, Americans wanted health care costs controlled, but they did not want controls enacted; they wanted the government to help but not to be in charge; and they wanted more spent on health care but complained that spending already was too high. In short, they wanted more government benefits and less government.

Congressional Democrats responded to these mixed messages by doggedly searching for votes that were not to be found. They stripped away the bureaucratic alliances that Clinton had proposed, giving Americans more choices than most already had, weakening cost controls, trimming employer mandates, and making other concessions to small businesses. But it was to no avail. Congressional Democrats and mainstream Republicans could not cobble together a passable compromise that navigated the contradictions and ambivalence of American public opinion.

That Congress did nothing in 1994 was a suitable denouement to the health reform story. The confusion and fears encountered by pollsters stalemated a Congress already battered by low public esteem and partisan strife. Looking back at the mood in America, the surprising thing is that Congress stuck with the task for so long. Many Americans who only one year earlier had wanted Congress to act were relieved when it did not. Once health legislation died, it quickly faded from public view. Democrats who had threatened to use it against Republicans in the congressional elections talked of other things instead, and Republicans who had feared that the failure of reform might be used against them also focused their attention elsewhere.

Fractured Interests

If American public opinion was split on health reform, so too were the many interest groups that joined the fray. And just as the contradictions in public opinion impeded reform, so too did divisions among and within the major groups with a big stake in the issue. That some powerful organizations, such as the American Association of Retired Persons (AARP) campaigned for reform while others such as the National Federation of Independent Business (NFIB) pulled out all the stops in opposition was not enough to block enactment of significant legislation. Business groups have opposed some recent legislation that became law—the 1993 Family and Medical Leave Act is an example—and politicians are accustomed to dealing with conflicts among interest groups. The stakes were higher this time, the lobbying more extensive, the mobilization of resources virtually unprecedented, and the divisions deeper than in most other legislative conflicts. Politicians were hampered by budget rules that limited the concessions they could make to important groups and by conflicts between large sectors of American society and within major organizations.

The entire health care sector was a battlefield in 1993 and 1994. Conflict raged between groups representing elderly people and those speaking for American business, between big and small companies, between business group leaders who wanted to develop a cooperative relationship with the new Clinton administration and rank-and-file members who demanded a harder line, between big insurers who fought for the right to select the physicians who would practice in their managed care operations and medical groups that fought for opening such operations to all doctors, and between physician groups that favored major changes in the health care system and those that preferred incremental adjustments.

Health care reform fell victim to hyperpluralism in American politics.[23] This condition refers to the vast growth in the number of interest groups and especially in the trade associations and "Washington representatives" seeking to influence national policy. Growth has occurred through a fissionlike process in which specialized interests separate from broader groups. As the number of associations has multiplied, the capacity of a parent group to represent specialized interests or to speak for the entire interest sector diminishes. Fissures have opened up within broad-based groups that have become transformed into "federations" of constituencies that do not see eye to eye on many of the issues that originally united them. By the time the health reform debate opened, for example, the Chamber of Commerce no longer spoke for American business, and the American Medical Association (AMA) no longer spoke for American medicine.

Although hyperpluralism is not new, its impact on health reform was sharpened by the redistributive character of the legislation. Within each sector—business, hospitals, physicians, insurers, workers, and so on—some would have gained and others would have lost, and deals made to secure the support of some subgroups would have put others at a disadvantage. Big employers with an older work force and many retirees would have benefited directly from subsidies from early retirees and indirectly from the abatement in cost shifting. Employers with a younger or part-time work force might have lost out, especially those who did not already pay for employee health insurance.

In some circumstances the fracturing of interests can facilitate compromise and mobilization of support for controversial measures. When a sector such as business or medicine is splintered among many groups that share some interests but not others, skilled politicians can play off some groups against one another, rewarding those that cooperate and punishing those that do not. The cost of assembling a majority may be lower when concessions have to be offered to some affected groups but not to all. In health care reform, however, the comprehensive sweep of the legislation complicated the politics of providing exclusive benefits to a relatively narrow band of groups. The legislation significantly affected just about every interest with a stake in health care. This was not a narrow-gauge measure that benefited some while not affecting many others. It forced just about everyone to choose sides. The final lineup was heavily weighted against the Clinton plan as well as against others devised by Democratic leaders in Congress.

If all anyone knew about health care reform is that the Chamber of Commerce, the Business Roundtable, the insurance companies, the AMA, the NFIB, and others were aligned against it, he or she would wonder why Congress took so long to walk away from the problem. But this was only the final lineup. During the year that health legislation roiled Congress, repeated efforts were made to win over business and medical groups. They were the prize; and when they slipped from Clinton's grasp, any prospect of sweeping overhaul of the nation's health care system died.

Health reform became a contest in which politicians lobbied the lobbyists. Reverse lobbying was practiced by Democrats and Republicans as well as by affected groups. The White House and congressional Democrats lost the contest because they lobbied Washington elites while opponents worked at the grass roots. They wasted benefits on those who were opposed to reform no matter what inducements were offered.

Fragile Coalitions

Interest groups have adapted to hyperpluralism by forming ad hoc coalitions on particular issues. The logic of coalition building derives from escalation in the number of groups. In a political world populated by thousands of groups, each can command only a sliver of influence. But it can gain clout by temporarily allying itself with others who share some of the same views on certain issues. The best coalitions are those that bring together disparate groups with different constituencies that are often on opposite sides of a question.

It did not work out that way in the fight for health reform, but it was not for lack of trying. "This was supposed to be the year," journalist David Rogers wrote in the summer of 1994, "that a broad-based coalition of interests would finally push health care reform into law." However, by then health reform had turned "into a classic confrontation, with business and medical interests lined up against the Clinton administration and its allies in labor and lobbies for the elderly."[24] The prore-form bloc tried to get both business and medicine on its side but had to settle for neither. After months of external pressure and internal friction, the Chamber of Commerce, the Business Roundtable, the National Association of Manufacturers, and the AMA came out against efforts by Clinton and Democratic leaders in Congress to devise a comprehensive measure that met the president's bottom-line demands.

Attempts at coalition building had only limited success. The Health Care Reform Project brought together natural allies such as the AFL-CIO, the AARP, the Consumers Union, and the Children's Defense Fund, as did Healthright (an alliance that included the American Federation of Teachers, the National Council of Senior Citizens, and the National Association for Home Care). Neither of these coalitions broadened the base for health reform.

Several business-labor coalitions were forged, including the National Leadership Coalition for Health-Care Reform, which actively campaigned for cost containment and also supported universal coverage and employer mandates. The coalition included ninety manufacturers, grocery chains, unions, and associations in the health professions and named former presidents Ford and Carter as its honorary chairmen. Another group of big companies joined the Corporate Health Care Coalition, which signaled its willingness to accept an employer mandate.

The White House tried to put together a Four Horsemen alliance to include hospitals, physicians, labor, and elderly persons by offering inducements such as restoration of proposed medicare cuts that would have boosted payments to hospitals by an estimated $250 billion over ten years.[25] This coalition endorsed the principle of universal coverage. However, it was compelled to paper over disagreements as to how health reform should be financed by coming out in favor of "shared responsibility," which could mean anything from employer mandates to taxing Americans to pay for health care.

The effectiveness of these coalitions was undermined by the refusal of major business groups to join them. Individual companies joined the coalitions, but the national trade associations did not. The coalitions called attention to schisms in the ranks of business and to conflicts played out not only in congressional committees but also in the Chamber of Commerce, the Business Roundtable, and the AMA.

Coalition building is the work of Washington elites, principally the leaders of national trade associations who negotiate the terms of agreement. But as the health care debate unfolded, it was increasingly influenced by grass-roots sentiment. Business interests and organized medicine, among many others, were adamantly opposed to the Clinton plan and to all Democratic alternatives that prescribed employer mandates and a strong government role in health care. When national groups moved to embrace comprehensive reform, they were pulled back by dissension in their ranks. In July 1994, for example, the AMA joined AARP and the AFL-CIO in endorsing universal coverage and cost containment. Within weeks, however, the AMA retreated from this position and sided with those wary of the Clinton proposal.[26] It was forced to quit the coalition because of state medical associations and rank-and-file members who vehemently opposed the stand taken by the national organization. The Chamber of Commerce experienced similar pressure when its national leaders sought out the White House for an accommodation on health reform. When some state chambers and constituents protested, the national leadership changed its mind. Its president acknowledged that the organization could not defy a substantial minority of its members and "expect to survive."[27]

Lobbying the Lobbyists

Why did the White House—with its enormous ability to target benefits to those who would vote its way—fail? Why were more corporations, many of which would have been major beneficiaries of reform, not convinced of the enormous advantages that would have accrued to them? And why did more medical groups not realize that health care was already being reformed by HMOs and huge insurance firms, and that they might be able to get a better deal from government-mandated care than from powerful market forces beyond their control?

The answer has to do with the split between Washington elites and the rank and file, ineffective targeting of interest groups by reformers, and instinctive distrust of government control by business owners and medical practitioners.

The revolt of the rank and file was not always spontaneous. It was spurred by cross-lobbying (interest groups lobbying one another) and by reverse lobbying (politicians lobbying interest groups). Lobbying the lobbyists fanned local opposition, which compelled national leaders to abandon support of comprehensive reform.

Both the AMA and the Chamber of Commerce were subject to vigorous lobbying by the NFIB, a .600,000-member association of mostly small and medium-size firms, many of which steadfastly opposed employer mandates, universal coverage, and other Clinton proposals. The AMA and the Chamber of Commerce were also lobbied by the White House and members of Congress. But though the White House worked to bring national leaders into the proreform coalition, the NFIB lobbied at the grass roots to pressure national groups to leave it. The White House offered legislative inducements, such as subsidies to business and fewer restrictions on doctors; the NFIB argued that these legislative favors would open the door to more government control. The NFIB won this battle because the Chamber of Commerce and the AMA were vulnerable to pressure from their membership ranks. Both are confederations of strong state associations, and both face growing competition from specialized groups.

The White House scored a temporary victory in July 1994 when the AMA, the AARP, and the AFL-CIO cosponsored a newspaper ad that endorsed "universal coverage with a standard set of comprehensive health benefits for every American by building on our current employment-based system . . . with a required level of employer contributions."[28] Although AMA leaders insisted that the ad merely affirmed the association's support of universal coverage, the statement was seen by others as a clear endorsement of Clinton's plan. House Republicans, led by Representative Newt Gingrich, attacked AMA leaders in a letter to all 450 members of the association's House of Delegates: "We are dismayed by the actions of the leadership of the AMA . . . [which is] out of touch with rank and file physicians."[29]

Even before this tempest, the NFIB launched a vigorous lobbying campaign designed to drive a wedge between AMA leaders and rank-and-file members. NFIB lobbyists met with representatives of more than half a dozen state medical associations. They encouraged NFIB state affiliates to warn their AMA counterparts that if employers were required to pay for health insurance, they would pressure the government to limit medical fees. Forced to balance proreform sentiments of some state medical groups and the antireform threats from others, the AMA emphasized its efforts to expand the rights of doctors to participate in HMOs and other health plans. In the end, the AMA supported the incremental proposals of the mainstream coalition, but these all came to naught.

The most aggressive case of reverse lobbying involved the Chamber of Commerce. Early in the Clinton presidency, Chamber leaders decided that cooperating with the new administration would enable them to do a better job protecting business interests than would outright opposition. The Chamber of Commerce softened some long-held positions in expectation of concessions from the White House. In line with its accommodating stance, a Chamber spokesman testified in October 1993 that "employers should provide and help pay for insurance," but that their share should not exceed 50 percent (rather than the 80 percent recommended by Clinton). The Chamber's turnaround sparked Representative John A. Boehner (R.-Ohio) to enlist dozens of House Republicans in calling their local chambers and demanding that the national organization withdraw its endorsement of employer contributions.[30]

Under pressure from all sides, the Chamber of Commerce commissioned a poll that showed 70 percent of its members opposed requiring employers to pay part of the cost of health insurance for their employees. Summing up the poll results, Chamber President Richard Lesher retreated from his earlier interest in compromise. "No government takeover, no mandates, no hurry," he asserted.[31] After the poll, Representative Boehner and other House Republicans met with Chamber of Commerce officials to discuss health reform and other issues. "Things have changed substantially there," he said; "they've come a long way."[32]

Reverse lobbying made a big difference in health reform because those doing the lobbying were people the affected group had to come to for favors. "When they're pursuing you," an official of the Health Insurance Association of America commented, "you have to wonder what happens next time you're pursuing them. Obviously, we're going to need help from these people in the future. You hate to turn any of them down."[33] Reverse lobbying usually did not involve explicit threats, but in at least one instance it did. When a major telephone company came out in favor of Clinton-type reforms, some key House Republicans warned that the telecommunications legislation it sought might be imperiled.[34]

The White House also lobbied the lobbyists, but it wasted opportunities by selecting the wrong targets. Lobbying inevitably involves the targeting of appeals, threats, and inducements to those whose support is sought. The best targets are those whose support makes a difference and who can be persuaded to change their minds. If a position already is locked in or has no bearing on the outcome, choosing it as a target makes little difference.

From the outset, the White House knew that it needed active support of key business interests. Sweeping reform could not be enacted if business was united in opposition. The president's plan scattered its largess to all types of businesses, but its most favored beneficiaries would be small companies, especially those that already provided insurance to low-wage workers. Many such companies would have been better off with reform than without it. But small business groups had a knee-jerk opposition to mandates and other government controls, even if they would have reduced health care costs.

Whether knee-jerk or otherwise, small business opposition led by the NFIB was unshakable. At no point during the health reform debate did the NFIB waver from outright opposition to employer mandates. Its vehemence was not toned down by the promise of government subsidies. Small business did not trust government and did not believe its promises. They did not want government telling them how to run their businesses, and they were not going to be swayed by government handouts.[35]

But instead of writing off small business interests as a lost cause, the White House and congressional Democrats engaged in a "mad political scramble to mollify" small companies. The House Education and Labor Committee reported a bill that would have capped health care premiums at 2 percent of payroll for some small companies—barely half the 3.9 percent proposed by Clinton. Not to be outdone, the House Ways and Means Committee promised tax credits, while the Senate Labor and Human Resources Committee reported a bill that would have financed health care through a payroll tax graded to the size of each firm's work force.[36]

Showering small business with legislative favors did not lessen its opposition to reform. Instead, it drew criticism from big companies that had been among the most vigorous champions of reform. Some major employers feared that they would have to pick up the tab for subsidies provided to small firms; a few calculated that, because they would have to pay for the benefits promised small business, their health costs would be higher after reform than before. In the end, the mistargeting of incentives lost some big business support without winning anything from small business lobbies.

In Congress Disassembled

How does Congress make law when powerful groups are mobilized in opposition, public opinion is confused and divided, and the president has demanded legislation that cannot be enacted? Evidently Congress did not find a satisfactory resolution of this quandary in 1994, for it failed to enact health reform. But the external pressures on Congress do not entirely explain its inability to act. After all, Congress did grapple with health legislation for the better part of a year. But the way it did increased the difficulty of enacting comprehensive reform. If it had proceeded differently, Congress might have enacted substantial legislation despite the formidable impediments it faced.

The first thing to note about Congress's consideration of health reform is that it worked on this extraordinary measure through ordinary legislative procedures. Health care legislation was assigned to the committees of jurisdiction, just as any other measure would be, but with the exception that this package was referred to more committees than usual. This was also a measure in which party lines formed early and were rarely crossed. The most unusual feature was the substantive role played by Democratic party leaders throughout the process, but especially after committees had reported legislation.

Extraordinary measures may demand extraordinary procedures to become law. These can include ad hoc task forces in lieu of standing committees, special rules in the House to restrict floor amendments, time-limit agreements in the Senate, bipartisan consultation through summit meetings or other arrangements, and omnibus measures that package diverse provisions in a single bill. Extraordinary procedures have two seemingly opposite characteristics: they broaden the scope of the legislation and restrict the ability of the floor to change the measure. These opposite characteristics are reconciled by deals that secure floor support by expanding the package's scope. During the Reagan and Bush years, the deals almost always were bipartisan; but with the advent of the Clinton administration, dealmaking generally involved negotiations among Democrats, with Republicans excluded in the House and marginalized in the Senate.

Since 1980, reconciliation has been the most frequently used extraordinary procedure. It allows a broad swath of legislation to be combined in a single bill, while typically limiting the number of floor amendments considered in the House and the amount of time allocated the bill in the

Senate. Every reconciliation bill reported to the House or Senate since the procedure was first used in 1980 has passed.[37]

It was undoubtedly with this record in mind that Senate Majority Leader George Mitchell ventured to suggest in 1993 that health reform might be taken up as a reconciliation bill.[38] This trial balloon burst almost immediately, and for good reason. Despite its legislative breadth, reconciliation is a compressed process. The relatively short interval between issuance of instructions in a budget resolution and action on a reconciliation bill renders this process suitable for making targeted, budget-driven changes in programs. But it is unsuitable for major changes in substantive policy, and certainly so for a measure as far-reaching as health reform.

And so health reform proceeded in regular order, which is to say it did not get very far. There was no reconciliation-type mechanism for forcing action nor special arrangements for bridging differences between and within the parties or for melding the diverse bills produced by various committees into a passable measure. When the regular order no longer sufficed to move the legislation forward, the House and Senate resorted to ad hoc measures by party leaders. And when this no longer sufficed, the legislation died.

Parties in Conflict

From the outset, health reform was a polarizing issue, with most congressional Republicans on one side and the splintered Democrats on the other. Each party contributed to the cleavage—the Democrats spurred on by the political hubris that came with their control of both the executive and legislative branches, and the Republicans through a scorched-earth policy determined to give their adversaries no legislative victories. In the afterglow of their 1992 election triumph, the Democrats were confident they would end the interparty gridlock that had characterized the Reagan-Bush years and the intraparty squabbling that had marred the Carter presidency. The Democrats were in charge and they would govern—alone if necessary, with Republican votes if the other party cooperated. The prolonged, secretive work of the health reform task force drove home the message that this Democratic initiative would proceed without much consultation with the Republicans. The White House wanted Republican support but was not willing to give much to get it. When Senator James Jeffords (R.-Vt.) agreed to cosponsor the Clinton bill, the White House put him on display as evidence of bipartisanship at work. But no other Republican joined the cause, although some professed strong support for health reform in principle. At times there was talk of a deal with Senator John Chafee, leader of a small group of moderate Republicans. Whether Chafee never got the message or was not really interested in cooperating with Clinton, he and the White House went their separate ways.

Chafee was not a free man in dealing with the Democrats; he had to be attentive to what fellow Republicans (especially Senate Minority Leader Robert Dole) wanted. Most Republicans were concerned that the Democrats would not give much in return for their votes. They feared that if the Democrats made concessions to get the bill out of committee, they would take them back on the floor. If they had to woo some Republicans to pass the legislation in the House or Senate, perhaps the Democrats would then ignore them in conference, when opposition would be weakest. This fear of being used and then ignored contributed greatly to Republican reluctance.

This refusal to cooperate was buoyed by the rise of a more militant brand of opposition in the Republican party. The new obstructionists claimed that Republicans would perpetuate their minority status in Congress as long as they settled for a marginal role on legislation. Newt Gingrich (R.-Ga.) was the political leader of this wing of the party and William Kristol its intellectual strategist. When a few Republicans on the House Ways and Means Committee, such as Fred Grandy of Iowa, offered amendments that would improve the prospects of reporting health reform legislation, they were pulled back by Gingrich. The immediate result was to unify committee Democrats, who then reported the bill without any Republican support. Nevertheless, Gingrich succeeded in driving home the point that Republicans should accentuate, not fudge, their differences with Democrats.

Operating out of the Project for a Republican Future, Kristol faxed a flurry of memos to congressional Republicans and others warning against bipartisanship in health reform. The first of these memos, sent in December 1993, argued that the "urge to negotiate a 'least bad' compromise with the Democrats, and thereby gain momentary credit for helping the president 'do something' about health care should . . . be resisted. . . . On grounds of national policy alone the plan should not be amended; it should be erased. But the Clinton proposal is also a serious political threat to the Republican party. Republicans must therefore

clearly understand the political strategy implicit in the Clinton plan—
and then adopt an aggressive and uncompromising counterstrategy
designed to delegitimatize the proposal and defeat its partisan purpose."[39]

Gingrich, Kristol, and the approaching congressional elections hardened Republican resolve, and the president and his fellow Democrats
were foiled in their attempts to probe for areas of compromise. Senator
Robert Dole became an especially elusive player, publicly expressing
his willingness to cooperate but taking a hard line when the Democrats
sought cooperation. Looking back at the 1994 election results, the Republican strategy worked. It sharpened the policy differences between
the two parties, helped defeat health care reform, and led congressional
Republicans to their biggest electoral victory in more than forty years.

Party Drift

Health care reform was not an isolated case of interparty conflict. In
recent years, party-line voting, with the majority of Democrats on one
side of the question and the majority of Republicans on the other, has
become much more pronounced. Table 8-2, drawn from data compiled
by *Congressional Quarterly*, shows polarization of the two parties at a
postwar high in the early 1990s. From 1966 through 1984, party-line
voting never exceeded 50 percent in either the House or the Senate. But
since the mid 1980s, the parties have diverged on a rising percentage of
roll call votes. The Democrats and Republicans were split on two-thirds
of the roll calls in 1993. If House and Senate roll calls on routine or
noncontroversial matters for which party affiliation has no bearing
were removed from the calculation, party-line voting might exceed
80 percent.

I believe the increased polarization of the parties has been based on
two main factors. One pertains to the composition of the parties, the
other to their relationship. There are fewer southern conservatives who
are Democrats than once was the case, and there are more who are
Republicans. "The Democratic Party," political scientist David Rohde
notes, "has gotten a lot more internally homogeneous, and Democrats
and Republicans have gotten a lot more different."[40] The long stretch of
divided government contributed to polarization, unifying congressional Republicans behind their president, with the Democrats in opposition. Table 8-3 shows that the increase in party-line voting has been

TABLE 8-2. *Partisan Voting in Congress, 1954–94*[a]
Percent

Year	House	Senate	Year	House	Senate
1954	38	47	1974	29	44
1955	41	30	1975	48	48
1956	44	53	1976	36	37
1957	59	36	1977	42	42
1958	40	44	1978	33	45
1959	55	48	1979	47	47
1960	53	37	1980	38	46
1961	50	62	1981	37	48
1962	46	41	1982	36	43
1963	49	47	1983	56	44
1964	55	36	1984	47	40
1965	52	42	1985	61	50
1966	41	50	1986	57	52
1967	36	35	1987	64	41
1968	35	32	1988	47	42
1969	31	36	1989	55	35
1970	27	35	1990	49	54
1971	38	42	1991	55	49
1972	27	36	1992	64	53
1973	42	40	1993	65	67
			1994	62	52

Source: *Congressional Quarterly Almanac*, 1992, p. 26-B; and *Congressional Quarterly Weekly Report*, December 31, 1994, p. 3658.
a. Partisan voting is the percentage of roll call votes in which a majority of Democrats voted against a majority of Republicans.

accompanied by rising party loyalty scores among both Democrats and Republicans. On major issues it is no longer unusual to find almost all Democrats on one side and almost all Republicans on the other.[41]

Polarization has been much more marked in the House than in the Senate, but it has increased in both chambers. In the House, the length of Democratic control and that party's aggressive use of rules to regulate floor action widened the gulf between the two parties. It has been a long time since House Republicans and Democrats genuinely cooperated on legislation. But even in the Senate, where the opportunity to

TABLE 8-3. *Party Unity Scores, 1961–94*[a]
Percent

Year	Democrats	Republicans	Year	Democrats	Republicans
1961	71	72	1981	69	76
1962	69	68	1982	72	71
1963	71	72	1983	76	74
1964	67	69	1984	74	72
1965	69	70	1985	79	75
1966	61	67	1986	78	71
1967	66	71	1987	81	74
1968	57	63	1988	79	73
1969	62	62	1989	81	73
1970	57	59	1990	81	74
1971	62	66	1991	81	78
1972	57	64	1992	79	79
1973	68	68	1993	85	84
1974	63	62	1994	83	83
1975	69	70			
1976	65	66			
1977	67	70			
1978	64	67			
1979	69	72			
1980	68	70			

Source: *Congressional Quarterly Almanac*, 1993, p. 17-C; and *Congressional Quarterly Weekly Report*, December 31, 1994, p. 3659.

a. The party unity score is the percentage of partisan votes (in which a majority of Democrats opposed a majority of Republicans) in which members of Congress voted with a majority of their party. A separate party unity score is computed for each member of Congress and is then averaged for all Democrats and Republicans to yield the scores shown in this table.

filibuster and the use of time-limit agreements to schedule legislative business have encouraged Democrats and Republicans to cooperate, party-line behavior has become much more marked in recent years.

But even when they fight, Democrats and Republicans manage to legislate. Almost two-thirds of the important laws enacted between 1949 and 1994 passed the House with bipartisan majorities.[42] Counting those measures approved by voice vote, barely one-quarter of the bills occasioned party-line voting on final passage. (Final passage refers here to House or Senate approval of the measure, not adoption of the conference report.) Bipartisanship was even more widespread in the Senate, where 69 percent of the bills passed with a majority of both Democrats and Republicans voting in favor and another 15 percent were approved by voice vote.

In fact, during periods of divided government there has been more bipartisan support for significant legislation than when a single party controlled the White House and Capitol Hill. Between 1949 and 1994, in the twenty years that the House and the White House were governed by the same party, the House passed 56 percent of significant laws with bipartisan majorities (table 8-4). But during the twenty-six years of divided rule during that period, the House passed 72 percent of major laws with majority support from both parties. The same pattern appeared in the Senate (table 8-5). During the years that the same party controlled the Senate and the presidency, 61 percent of significant laws were passed with bipartisan majorities; during the years of divided government, bipartisanship averaged 78 percent.

Why was Congress more partisan when political power was unified than when it was divided? In answering this question, it should be kept in mind that the data pertain only to measures that made it into law; they do not deal with those (such as health care reform) that fell victim to partisan conflict. During periods of divided control, Democrats and Republicans had incentive to bargain on important legislation, because few significant measures could be enacted if they failed to compromise. On the other hand, the majority party had an incentive to go it alone when it controlled both houses of Congress and the executive branch.

A comparison of the first years of the Bush and Clinton presidencies is instructive on this point. The 1989–90 (101st) Congress was a period of divided government and intense conflict between the Bush White House and congressional Democrats. That Congress enacted five significant laws (so designated by Mayhew). Each passed the Senate with bipartisan support, four by lopsided margins. Four of the measures also garnered bipartisan support in the House. The only exception was the 1990 deficit reduction law, with most House Republicans voting against the agreement negotiated by George Bush.

Bipartisan enactment did not mean, however, a lack of partisan strife. When government was divided, the two parties learned how to legislate when they disagreed. With Republicans ensconced in the White House for all but four years from 1969 through 1992, and the Democrats

TABLE 8-4. *Party Line Voting in House on Significant Legislation During Periods of Divided and Unified Control*

Congress	Year	Unified control			Divided control		
		Bipartisan vote	Partisan vote	Voice vote	Bipartisan vote	Partisan vote	Voice vote
81st	1949	0	2	0			
	1950	5	1	0			
82d	1951	0	2	0			
	1952	1	0	0			
83d	1953	1	0	0			
	1954	5	1	2			
84th	1955				0	0	0
	1956				1	0	0
85th	1957				1	0	1
	1958				2	0	2
86th	1959				2	0	0
	1960				2	0	0
87th	1961	4	2	0			
	1962	3	2	0			
88th	1963	1	1	1			
	1964	3	2	0			
89th	1965	4	5	0			
	1966	4	2	0			
90th	1967	3	0	0			
	1968	5	0	0			
91st	1969				4	0	0
	1970				6	1	2
92d	1971				3	0	0
	1972				10	0	0
93d	1973				6	2	1
	1974				6	1	0
94th	1975				3	2	0
	1976				6	2	0
95th	1977	3	3	0			
	1978	2	1	0			
96th	1979	1	2	0			
	1980	6	0	1			
97th	1981				1	1	0
	1982				4	1	1
98th	1983				2	1	0
	1984				2	0	2
99th	1985				1	0	0
	1986				4	1	2

TABLE 8-4. *(continued)*

		Unified control			Divided control		
Congress	Year	Bipartisan vote	Partisan vote	Voice vote	Bipartisan vote	Partisan vote	Voice vote
100th	1987				2	3	0
	1988				2	3	0
101st	1989				2	0	0
	1990				2	1	0
102d	1991				2	2	0
	1992				4	0	0
103d	1993	0	6	0			
	1994	1	2	1			
Total		52	34	5	80	21	11
Percent		57	37	5	71	19	10

Source: (List of major legislation) Charles O. Jones, *The Presidency in a Separated System* (Brookings, 1994), pp. 129–45; Stephen Gettinger, "View from the Ivory Tower More Rosy Than Media's," *Congressional Quarterly Weekly Report*, October 8, 1994, vol. 52, no. 40, pp. 2850–53.

(Vote counts) *Congressional Quarterly Almanacs*, 1948–93 (Washington: CQ Press); *Congressional Quarterly Reports*, vol. 52, nos. 5, 6, 12, 16, 47.

in control of the House for this entire period and the Senate for all but six years of it, the two parties were impelled to compromise, even on matters on which they were deeply divided. Conflict was most intense and party lines most sharply drawn during the amendment stage. Afterward, interparty bargaining—sometimes between the White House and congressional leaders, sometimes within Congress—often produced a compromise and bipartisan support on final passage.

During the 1989–90 Congress, as in others, many of the important votes were not on final passage but on floor amendments. As may be expected, partisanship was much more evident at this stage. For example, the 89–11 Senate vote in favor of the 1990 Clean Air Act was preceded by twenty-five roll calls (most on substantive amendments, some on procedural matters). Thirteen of these were decided by a bipartisan majority and twelve divided Democrats and Republicans. The House also passed the Clean Air Act with overwhelming support from both parties, as indicated by the 401–21 vote. As is often the case, the House considered relatively few amendments. One was rejected,

TABLE 8-5. *Party Line Voting in Senate on Significant Legislation During Periods of Divided and Unified Control*

Congress	Year	Unified control			Divided control		
		Bipartisan vote	Partisan vote	Voice vote	Bipartisan vote	Partisan vote	Voice vote
81st	1949	3	0	0			
	1950	4	0	2			
82d	1951	2	0	0			
	1952	1	0	1			
83d	1953	0	0	1			
	1954	3	2	3			
84th	1955				0	0	0
	1956				0	0	1
85th	1957				1	0	1
	1958				3	0	1
86th	1959				2	0	0
	1960				2	0	0
87th	1961	2	3	1			
	1962	3	1	1			
88th	1963	2	0	2			
	1964	2	1	2			
89th	1965	5	4	0			
	1966	5	0	1			
90th	1967	1	0	2			
	1968	5	0	0			
91st	1969				3	1	1
	1970				9	0	0
92d	1971				3	0	0
	1972				11	0	0
93d	1973				8	1	0
	1974				5	1	1
94th	1975				1	3	1
	1976				7	1	0
95th	1977	4	2	0			
	1978	2	2	0			
96th	1979	2	1	0			
	1980	6	0	1			
97th	1981	2	0	0			
	1982	4	1	1			
98th	1983	3	0	0			
	1984	3	1	0			
99th	1985	1	1	0			
	1986	6	0	1			

TABLE 8-5. *(continued)*

		Unified control			Divided control		
Congress	Year	Bipartisan vote	Partisan vote	Voice vote	Bipartisan vote	Partisan vote	Voice vote
100th	1987				2	1	2
	1988				6	0	0
101st	1989				2	0	0
	1990				3	0	0
102d	1991				1	1	2
	1992				3	0	1
103d	1993	0	6	0			
	1994	2	1	1			
Total		73	26	20	72	9	11
Percent		61	22	17	78	10	12

Source: (List of major legislation) Charles O. Jones, *The Presidency in a Separated System* (Brookings, 1994), pp. 129–45; Stephen Gettinger, "View from the Ivory Tower More Rosy Than Media's," *Congressional Quarterly Weekly Report,* October 8, 1994, vol. 52, no. 40, pp. 2850–53.

(Vote counts) *Congressional Quarterly Almanacs,* 1948–93; *Congressional Quarterly Reports,* vol. 52, nos. 5, 6, 12, 16, 47.

three had near-unanimous support, and two split the parties. The conference on this bill entailed vigorous bargaining between Democrats and Republicans to resolve matters in dispute.

If this pattern had prevailed with health care reform, legislation would have been reported by committee, Democrats and Republicans would have fought over floor amendments, and sufficient compromise would have been reached in conference to permit bipartisan passage. Health care legislation did not play out that way, but not simply because Clinton ignored the Republicans and went it alone with Democrats. By the time health reform was on the congressional agenda, the parties had become so polarized that their differences could not be bridged by normal legislative interaction. Party behavior on legislation was markedly different during the 1993–94 (103d) Congress than it had been four years earlier. With the election of Bill Clinton, the Democrats controlled the government and Republicans were united in opposition. Party cohesion scores soared, and party lines were more staunchly defended than they had been during times of divided government.

Interparty conflict began in the early stages of legislative activity and continued through House and Senate passage. According to tables 8-4 and 8-5, seven of the ten significant measures enacted in 1993–94 passed the Senate on party line votes, and eight of the House votes on passage were along party lines. Final passage of important legislation drew more partisan votes in the 103d Congress than in any previous Congress since 1949.

The 103d Congress began with partisan fighting in January 1993 and ended almost two years later with partisan stalemate. House Democrats designated two polarizing measures as HR 1 (the Family and Medical Leave Act) and HR 2 (the Motor Voter Registration Act). An earlier version of HR 1 had been vetoed by George Bush during the previous Congress. Passing this bill entailed eight party-line votes in the House and nine in the Senate. The Democrats outvoted the Republicans on all these roll calls, averaging more than 90 percent cohesion in the House and 95 percent in the Senate. The Republicans were united in opposition, scoring better than 80 percent cohesion in each chamber. Party lines also held in voting on HR 2, the voter registration bill, with 98 percent of House and Senate Democrats supporting their party's position and 95 percent of the Republicans voting against it.

Polarization persisted through votes on crime legislation, education reform, establishment of the national service program, and the 1993 budget reconciliation act. Of major legislation, only GATT drew bipartisan support, as many Republicans backed Clinton's trade liberalization policies.

Republican opposition got a boost during Senate action on a stimulus appropriation bill Clinton sought early in the 1993 session. At the start of debate, Republicans had the modest objective of reducing the bill's scope and price tag; by the time they were done, Clinton had to settle for a much smaller package than the Republicans had been willing to give him at the outset.[43] During consideration of the measure, Senator Robert Byrd (D.-W.Va.), a master of Senate rules, employed some parliamentary tricks to deter the Republicans from offering floor amendments.[44] This tactic backfired, for it unified the Republicans and emboldened them to threaten a filibuster. All but two of the twenty Senate roll calls on this measure had the parties aligned on opposite sides. In fact, the Republicans were unanimously in opposition on sixteen of the votes. As Senate action stalled, Senator Chafee observed "a hardening in the attitude of Republican senators." They had discovered that despite their minority status and their own disagreements over policy, they could block the new president's priorities.[45]

Early in his term, Clinton was criticized for not reaching out to Republican moderates before legislative positions became polarized. His best efforts may have been futile, however, for his election had the effect of hardening Congress along party lines. Every Senate Republican voted against the budget resolution, which was considered shortly before Senate action on the stimulus appropriations bill. The Republicans also unanimously opposed the 1993 budget reconciliation bill. With several Democrats defecting from their party's position, it took a tiebreaking vote by Vice President Al Gore to pass the reconciliation bill. This scene was repeated six weeks later, when the Senate adopted the conference report on the reconciliation bill with another tiebreaking vote.

Legislative action in 1993 gave Clinton advance notice of party polarization and the difficulties he would face the next year with health care reform. Facing unified Republican opposition, the president was held hostage to fellow Democrats who could demand substantial concessions before supporting his legislation. In the case of the reconciliation bill, recalcitrant Democrats forced the president to substitute a narrower tax on gas in lieu of the broad energy tax he had initially proposed. In the case of health care, there were many more defectors, and their demands cut to the heart of his program. The price for winning back Democratic votes in Congress was not simply substituting one energy tax for another. It entailed surrendering the president's commitment to universal coverage financed by employer-paid premiums.

In sum, health care legislation was trapped between two powerful trends in party relations. One was rising polarization and conflict, the other the looming congressional elections—and the growing conviction among Republicans that the more stalwart they were in opposition, the better their performance at the polls. Perhaps Clinton could have fashioned a strategy that appealed more to congressional Republicans; but even his best efforts might not have changed the outcome. Health care reform headed the legislative agenda during a transitional period in American politics—the probable end of a long stretch of Democratic dominance and the possible onset of a new era of Republican hegemony. When the parties are reversing positions, the gulf between them tends to widen, making compromise more costly for those threatened with loss of majority status and less attractive for those on the brink of power.

Committee Breakdown

The polarization of Democrats and Republicans hindered House and Senate committees in performing one of their critical functions: producing passable legislation. The Democrats could not count on Republican help to get health reform out of committee, and they feared that defections in their own ranks might block their ability to report and pass the legislation. Faced with a shortage of votes, House and Senate Democratic leaders urged rank-and-file members to vote unpassable bills out of committee. In health care reform, committee action was seen as an obstacle to legislation, not as a means of perfecting the measure and assembling votes needed for passage. These legislative chores would be performed, the leaders promised, after the committees were done and not before.

This may not be the way the legislative process is supposed to work, but it is the way much controversial legislation enacted in recent years has made it into law. If the House or Senate had voted on health legislation, the battle cry undoubtedly would have been: pass the bill now, we will fix it in conference. This tactic heightened the fears of Republicans and recalcitrant Democrats that any significant concessions won in supplying the votes to get the bill out would be bartered away later. Some House Democrats were also concerned that some hard choices they made would be undone by later concessions needed to pass the bill in the Senate.

As things turned out, none of the five committees with general jurisdiction over health care reform produced passable legislation. The committee (Energy and Commerce) whose membership was most representative of the parent chamber had the greatest difficulty, and it did not report anything. The two committees whose Democratic membership was least representative (House Education and Labor and Senate Labor and Human Resources) had the easiest time producing legislation, but what they reported could not have garnered majority support on the floor.

The House Education and Labor Committee made no effort to formulate a bill that could pass. This committee's Democrats saw their role as staking out a position to the left of the president's, in the hope that what finally passed would be more to their liking. Their bill put other Democrats on notice: they should not take the liberal wing of the party for granted, and party leaders searching for votes should not settle for less than the president had requested. This committee's bill was not taken seriously by Majority Leader Richard Gephardt when he tried to cobble together a compromise.

Unlike Education and Labor, the Democrats on the Ways and Means Committee were interested in making law, not a political statement. In line with its long record of success on the floor, this committee wanted to produce passable legislation. At one time, Ways and Means dominated the House through closed rules that barred floor amendments and impelled members to accept legislation on its terms. It also helped that Ways and Means Democrats had the lead role in parceling out House committee assignments to party members. But that role and most closed rules were taken away twenty years ago. This left Ways and Means no choice but to prevail by marking up bills and building coalitions that anticipate the preferences of the House. The committee has been most successful in this when Democrats and Republicans have cooperated. This possibility was precluded, however, in the health care reform markup when Newt Gingrich deterred Fred Grandy from offering amendments that would have made the bill more palatable to fellow Republicans. The reported bill would surely have been more likely to pass in the House if some Republicans on Ways and Means had helped develop it. Gingrich's demarche unified Ways and Means Democrats, thereby making it easier for the committee to report a bill. But it also pulled the committee away from producing enactable legislation.

Shortly before markup, Sam Gibbons replaced Dan Rostenkowski as chairman of Ways and Means. Under the circumstances, Gibbons did a remarkable job coaxing most committee Democrats to set aside their differences and back a bill honoring Clinton's pledge of universal coverage through a new part C medicare program for uninsured Americans. Gibbons had his hands full assembling a bill that could get out of committee; he paid little attention to devising a measure that could make it through the House. *Congressional Quarterly* described the reported bill as "a patchwork measure that fully satisfied neither wing of" the Democratic party.[46]

There is a good possibility that if Rostenkowski had chaired the markup, he would have steered it in a different direction. The former Ways and Means chairman knew that health care reform needed cheerleaders from business if it were to pass. He offered concessions to the insurance industry in exchange for its promise to temporarily pull the

Harry and Louise ads. In more than a dozen years as chairman of Ways and Means, Rostenkowski had quashed efforts to use legislation to make political statements. He wanted bills that could pass, not ones that could only be reported. He almost certainly would not have used a new scheme such as part C medicare as the starting point for the committee bill, and he would have been willing to offer substantial compromises to get Republican votes. Perhaps it would have all come to naught; but Rostenkowski would not have willingly settled for a bill that had to be salvaged by Majority Leader Gephardt.

The third principal House panel was Energy and Commerce. This sprawling committee had aggressively aggrandized its jurisdiction over the previous two decades and had parlayed its role in medicaid and medicare legislation to become a key player in health policy. John Dingell, who chaired the committee with a strong hand, was an ardent supporter of universal coverage and had an extraordinary knack for getting his way on legislation. Dingell unabashedly used his power as chairman to cajole committee members into line. He was adept at bottling up the measures he did not want (as he did for years with clean air regulation) and at mustering a majority for the bills he wanted (as he did in 1990, when clean air legislation was finally enacted after years of delay).

Because Energy and Commerce better mirrored the ideological makeup of the House than did other committees, it became the battleground in the fight for health care reform. But Energy and Commerce was also the center of opposition to the Clinton plan within the Democratic party. Led by Jim Cooper of Tennessee, whose own health reform proposal had neither employer mandates nor universal coverage, the band of Energy and Commerce defectors denied Dingell the votes he needed to report a bill. Dingell wooed Jim Slattery of Kansas with favors for small business, but he was no match for the grass-roots lobbying organized by the NFIB.[47] Like Clinton, Dingell offered concessions to those whose support eluded him. In the end, Dingell did not even take health legislation to markup; he simply notified Democratic leaders that the committee was unable to act.

The situation was somewhat more promising in the Senate, because the two committees with general jurisdiction over health reform had (like the Senate itself) a history of bipartisan cooperation. The two committees—Labor and Human Resources, and Finance—differed in makeup and political orientation, but Democrats on each had reason to seek accommodations with Republicans. Finance's 11–9 Democratic majority meant that unless some Republican support was forthcoming, a single defection could block legislation. Democrats had a wider (10–7) margin on Labor and Human Resources; however, Chairman Ted Kennedy had developed a working relationship with committee Republicans that sheltered his bills against filibusters and presidential vetoes. Kennedy was especially skillful at trimming his legislative ambitions to dampen Republican opposition while still achieving his core objectives.

Intraparty cooperation diminished in both committees after the election of Bill Clinton. Finance's work on the 1993 reconciliation bill split committee members along party lines, while the activities of Labor and Human Resources that were at the forefront of Clinton priorities, such as the national service program and education reform, distanced Republicans from Democrats. These committees could not wall themselves off from the partisan drift that enveloped Congress in the 1990s.

But they tried. Labor and Human Resources was the first congressional committee to report health reform legislation. Markup began in a cooperative spirit, with members of both parties joining in a 17–0 vote that defined benefits to be covered by health insurance. "One small step for health care, one giant leap for bipartisanship," Kennedy boasted.[48] But the first step became the last as Democrats outvoted Republican efforts to delete employer mandates, cost controls, and other features of the Clinton plan. As much as Democrats on Labor and Human Resources wanted to bring their Republican colleagues on board, they were unwilling to make the fundamental compromises needed to bridge the gap between the two parties. They could not walk away from the liberal convictions that had guided the committee for decades and shaped its legislative output. When the markup ended, Senator Jeffords (the only Republican sponsor of the Clinton plan) was the only member of his party to vote for the bill reported by the committee. The committee's bill was not passable, and the Democrats knew it. "This isn't the end," Kennedy remarked when the bill was reported; "it's really the beginning."[49]

The situation in Finance was a mess. The committee had a chairman who did not think the high priority accorded health care was warranted and who was skeptical that the Clinton bill or anything like it could pass. However, he had difficulty crafting a version that could. Finance's bill was written in markup, largely through the work of a middle-of-the-road coalition of Democrats and Republicans. They abandoned universal coverage and employer mandates and sought to cap government health spending but not private costs. Dozens of bills were considered in markup, and many were adopted with the support of a centrist bloc of six Democrats and Republicans. At times the Finance Committee reverted to its habit of "Christmas treeing" the bill—for example, adding subsidies for low-income mothers and infants, a block grant for community and home assistance for people with disabilities, tax breaks for various groups, and other benefits. The committee's bipartisan majority sought a middle-of-the-road position, providing a "soft trigger" for future consideration of universal insurance if more than 5 percent of Americans lack coverage by 2002. One of the most contentious issues was whether large multistate companies should be subject to state regulation. On this and several other issues, Majority Leader George Mitchell sided with the position that he believed would facilitate reporting of a bill, even if it was contrary to his own view. For example, Mitchell initially voted to permit state regulation of health insurance provided by large companies, but he switched his vote after being informed it would jeopardize centrist Republican support for reporting the bill.

Unlike the four other committees with general jurisdiction over health reform, Finance did muster some Republican votes. Moreover, Finance was the only committee in which Republicans had a significant voice in shaping the reported bill. Minority Leader Robert Dole, also a member of the Finance Committee, played a game of cat and mouse with Democrats and moderate Republicans, hinting that he would support a bill that was to his liking but backing away when concessions were offered. In the end, Dole introduced his own bill, signaling that he would only accept reforms that were too limited to draw Democratic support.

If the measures reported by the other committees were not passable because they were too partisan, Finance's bill was tainted because it was not partisan enough. Not enough Republicans supported it to offset the possible loss of Democratic senators who wanted stronger assurance that health care coverage would be available to almost all Americans.

Leaders as Followers

With all the committees done, health care reform had too many conflicting bills for consensus but too few popular bills for passage. The task of forging a passable bill fell to House Majority Leader Gephardt and Senate Majority Leader Mitchell, veteran lawmakers with a long-standing interest in health reform and keen grasp of the issues. Each had license to craft a bill from scratch, but neither could ignore the president's preferences or what had already happened in committee. Both were beholden to the political arithmetic of health reform—the elusiveness of Republican votes and the threat of Democratic defections. When they started, neither had a majority in his own chamber; when they ended, neither did either.

What Gephardt and Mitchell did have was a mandate to lead and the wishful expectation that somehow all the difficulties of the previous year would be resolved through brilliant tactics. The followership role the leaders took was of their own choosing, for they had elected at the outset not to get involved. House Speaker Tom Foley had decided to allow normal legislative routines to run their course. There would be no ad hoc task forces that bypassed standing committees and enabled the leaders to take charge, nor would there be special referral arrangements to the committees of jurisdiction. Foley refused to adjudicate among rival committee claims for jurisdiction, and he did not pressure the committees to expedite their work. Following the regular procedures was in accord with Foley's personal tastes, but it may also have been influenced by his predecessor's unhappy experience as an activist speaker. Jim Wright, the previous speaker, did take an early and active interest in the substance of legislation and pushed committees to produce according to his agenda. Perhaps the most telling lesson for Foley was that when Wright was forced to resign amidst allegations of misconduct, few Democrats had rallied to his side. Committee barons wanted leaders to keep the House on schedule, not to meddle in their legislative business. Given the schisms within Democratic ranks on health care reform, it is understandable that the leadership was reluctant to get involved until it was evident that nothing could pass without its active intervention.

The majority leader of the Senate has fewer formal powers than the Speaker of the House but a more substantive role in legislation. George Mitchell's main powers included being given the floor ahead of others and negotiating time-limit agreements. The latter thrust him into the center of legislative activity, not only through scheduling the Senate's work but also in negotiating legislative compromises and dealing with senators on their floor amendments. Mitchell also was a legislator in his own right and actively participated in the Finance Committee's markup of health care reform. Reforming health care was his number one career objective, as evidenced by his rejection of the Supreme Court seat Bill Clinton had offered him. But though he was involved in health care reform from the outset, Mitchell did not want to alienate fellow Democrats by stealing a march on their committees.

Although the House and Senate have become more alike over the years, the great difference in their size pulls them in different directions. The House is a committee-centered body, the Senate more floor-centered. The basic role of the House majority leadership is to use its control of the special rules that determine floor procedure for particular measures to facilitate passage of legislation recommended by committees. In practice, this means enabling the majority to get its way on the floor by restricting amendments that would materially alter the measure reported by committee or weaken its chances of passing. With health care reform, it meant that Gephardt would have to base his proposal on what House committees had done and would have to have reasonable assurance of majority support before taking it to the floor.

Gephardt had two reported bills to choose from, but only the Ways and Means bill had a chance of getting majority support. The Gephardt plan retained the main features of the Ways and Means bill, including universal coverage, employer mandates (at the same 80 percent rate that Clinton had proposed), a new part C medicare for uninsured Americans, direct subsidies for low-income persons, tax subsidies for companies paying low wages, and a broad benefits package. Although it added some bells and whistles to attract liberal and conservative Democrats (such as a single-payer option for states and a slower phasing-in of universal insurance), Gephardt's plan was no more passable than the Ways and Means bill on which it was based. Short of the needed votes, Democratic leaders deferred House consideration until the Senate acted.

Mitchell's mode of operation was similar to Gephardt's. He consulted widely, but almost entirely among Democrats. Mitchell saw his role as nudging liberal and conservative Democrats toward a centrist position on which enough of them could agree to constitute a majority. Like Gephardt, he did not do much to attract Republicans, fearing that their votes could be gained only by risking Democratic support. Unlike Gephardt, Mitchell did not need a majority before taking the bill to the floor—he knew the bill would be amended by the Senate. For him, floor action was to be part of the process of assembling a majority.

Mitchell's starting point was the Finance Committee's bill. Along with Finance, Mitchell settled for 95 percent coverage rather than a universal plan, but he devised a stronger trigger if actual coverage were to fall short of this target by 2002. Mitchell's version of an employer mandate capped this share at 50 percent, with an exemption for the smallest firms. Moreover, the mandate would not be implemented before 2002, and then only if other methods of achieving 95 percent coverage were not available. Mitchell's plan also walked the line between liberal and conservative views on cost controls, taxes, subsidies, and other issues.

Mitchell did not have a passable bill when he took it to the floor. At this stage, Republicans had little incentive to cooperate, because they had hardly played any role in drafting the new measure. Some moderate Democrats also withheld their support; health care reform still had too many controls and costs to suit their tastes.

Though the Mitchell bill got further in the legislative process than any other, it died far short of enactment. When health care reform was officially pronounced dead in September 1994, a coalition of centrist Democrats and Republicans was still at work, hoping to breathe life into it by means of incremental changes. Theirs was the last act on health care reform in the 1993–94 Congress and might be the first in a future Congress.

What Congress Learned About Itself

In the course of their failure to reform health care, members of Congress learned much about health policy and politics. They also learned how their own institution operates and why lawmaking has become so difficult and contentious. Arguably, health care reform is a special case with few implications for the more ordinary work of Congress. Representative Jim McDermott (D.-Wash.), the leading congressional proponent of a single-payer system, explained one way health legislation is different: "Usually a committee works on a bill, and then committee members say to the rest of us, 'Trust me, this is a good bill,' and we vote for it. But it's very dicey to accept a 'trust me' on this bill. . . . It affects every person in every member's district."[50]

Yet extraordinary cases, such as health care reform, enhance under-standing of how Congress operates precisely because they are so spe-cial. They shed light on institutional characteristics that might go unno-ticed in ordinary circumstances. Just as the great success of tax reform in 1986 provided insight on the value of bipartisan cooperation, the failure of health care reform in 1994 emphasizes the legislative costs of partisan conflict, weak leadership, and other obstacles to enactment.

In the remainder of this chapter, I set forth a number of propositions drawn from the health care reform experience. The lessons pertain to familiar features of Capitol Hill: the president and his agenda, interest groups and their demands, parties and public opinion, committees and leaders, and budget rules and budget scarcity.

1. A weak president should not make strong demands.

From beginning to end, Bill Clinton was the dominant figure in the health care reform debate. He put health care at the top of the agenda, established universal coverage as the bottom-line objective, and de-terred key congressional Democrats from seeking incremental reforms that fell short of this goal. In making demands, Bill Clinton acted like a strong president who had the resources to get what he wanted. In fact, Clinton was only strong enough to block the alternatives he did not want. He was weak in Congress because he was weak in the country and in his own party.

Clinton's 43 percent plurality in the 1992 election was not a green light for far-reaching change. Nor was his persistently low standing in public opinion polls. His own party was deeply divided on health care, but he cast his lot with liberal Democrats who held him hostage to promises they could not keep. Deciding not to give liberals the single-payer plan they really pined for, Clinton could not easily retreat from his second-best commitment to universal coverage. This commitment emboldened liberal Democrats to insist on nothing less than com-prehensive reform, while moderates and conservatives in the party still believed that the president would settle for much less.

When a weak president makes strong demands on Congress, he is likely to end up with legislative inaction or stalemate. Of course, Con-gress does not have to follow the president's lead. But in the absence of consensus on an alternative, legislators will be stymied by the unpass-able demands made on them. In the case of health care reform, no leading Democrat was willing to publicly tell the president that what he wanted he could not have. Rostenkowski might have tried if he had not been bought low by his own problems; Moynihan tried but was labeled a bungler or spoiler by fellow Democrats who did not like his message. Some of the politicians and experts associated with the task force put together by Ira Magaziner and Hillary Rodham Clinton said so in private, but their qualms were brushed aside. Republicans said so all along, but Clinton did not trust them to negotiate in good faith on more modest reforms. In the end, presidential weakness spread to congressional Democrats who found themselves doubly blamed—for following an unpopular president's unenactable demands, and for not enacting health reform.

2. *Incremental demands are more passable than comprehensive demands.*
Throughout the debate, proponents of universal coverage (and much else packaged with it) insisted that anything less was not worth the effort. They gave Congress an all-or-nothing ultimatum, which was reformulated into an almost-all-or-nothing option at the end. (Predictably, Congress did nothing.) They also discouraged Congress from enacting incremental improvement by labeling piecemeal reform as a misguided effort that would make matters worse.

Reformers were beguiled by a political hypothesis that has come into vogue in recent years: All political reform is difficult, but incremental changes may be even more difficult to enact than far-reaching ones. When change is comprehensive (the argument runs), the losses are spread widely, and particular interests cannot make a strong case that they have been treated unfairly. Nothing as far-reaching as health care reform has been on the congressional agenda during the past half-century or even longer, so this hypothesis must make up in grit what it lacks in evidence.

I begin with a different premise—that Congress is discomfited by redistributive legislation and clumsy in parceling out losses. Of course, Congress does pass much redistributive legislation, but, as I have argued elsewhere, it does so under the guise of distributing benefits.[51] With health care reform, however, there was no place for Congress to hide. In demanding comprehensive reform, the president and his congressional allies would have upset so much that was familiar about American health care. Just about every American would have been affected, including the 200 million who already had insurance. One-seventh of the economy would have been rearranged, and providers would have found their financial and working conditions greatly altered. Tens of millions would have lost out in some way, and tens of millions more would have feared that something of great value to them—their medical care—would be withheld. The prospect of such disorienting change alarmed millions of Americans. Opponents exploited these anxieties by portraying Clinton's plan as one restricting access to health services.

Incremental health care reform would also be redistributive, but on a much more modest scale. If Congress were to mandate community rating or to ban exclusions for preexisting medical conditions, it would have boosted insurance costs for many young workers and lowered them for older or high-risk persons. Nevertheless, legislation along these lines would have met with relatively little opposition, because the reformed health care system would have been similar to the one familiar to most Americans.

These and other incremental changes might have boosted the insured population to more than 90 percent. Adding more than 15 million people to the insurance rolls would have been no small accomplishment, even if it would have left millions more without insurance. Would this change have been worth it? No, say the all-or-nothing reformers, who fear that as the pool of uninsured Americans shrinks, the odds that politicians would pay attention to them would diminish. My own view is that incremental improvements should be preferred when they are all that can be enacted. This was the path tax reform took in 1986. The pure, comprehensive reform devised by Treasury tax experts was initially compromised by the secretary of the Treasury, then by the president, and finally by Congress.[52] Without the compromise, it is doubtful that significant reform would have been enacted.

3. Leaders should lead, not just follow.

Health care reform was legislation that called for leadership from the start. Given the scope of the reform and the foreseeable impediments to enactment, Democratic leaders in the House and Senate should have intervened long before it became evident that the committees of jurisdiction could not do the job. Leaders could have steered legislative work by establishing a task force, negotiating with Democrats, developing a consensus in their own party, strictly controlling the referral of bills to committee, or doing what they tried to at the end—devise a passable bill. Each of these tactics would have had the task of assembling a majority for health reform. That majority might have been found among Democrats or together with Republicans, but it could not materialize on its own without strong central guidance.

The leadership role in health care reform has been characteristic of recent Democratic leaders (with the exception of Jim Wright). Committees have had their way on legislation, and leaders have become involved only to resolve conflicts, schedule floor action, or work out deals needed for final passage. This laid-back leadership style often suffices. However, it did not in health care reform nor in campaign finance and lobbying reform, two measures with high priority in the 1993–94 Congress that died in the end.

Early leadership intervention is incompatible with the strong role for committees in the legislative process. Congress cannot have it both ways: leaders who dictate or actively shape legislation, and committees that perform their historic role of refining legislation. To justify a special role for party leaders, extraordinary conditions must be found that give strong indications that committees will not be able to perform. At least four such conditions were present in health reform: 1) committees in conflict on jurisdictional claims affecting the entire measure; 2) deep fissures within Democratic ranks on health legislation; 3) the difficulty of passing legislation without negotiated support of some Republicans; and 4) the measure's vast scope and complexity. The fact that health care reform had high priority for the president should not impart a special role to the leaders unless there is reason early on to believe that committees will not get the job done.

In 1995 the new Republican leadership in the House took a much more active role in substantive legislation. A comparison with the deposed Democrats is not entirely fair; the Republicans are not encumbered by a president of their own party or by committee chairs with independent power bases. If the Republicans hold on to power for an extended period, they may experience the same weakening of party leadership the Democrats did.

4. The role of committees should be to produce passable legislation.

Health care reformers neither bypassed congressional committees nor took committee work seriously. This posture left the House and Senate bereft of legislation with a chance of passing. If party leaders think committees are an obstacle or just another stage in the process, they should work around them. But once committees are entrusted with the time-consuming task of formulating legislation—a task that in this case took more than half a year of scarce legislative time—their marching orders should be to look ahead to what awaits the bill on the floor and not just to form the minimum winning coalition needed to get the measure out of committee.

The Democrats were not wholly to blame for the committees' failure to formulate measures that could appeal to a majority of the House or Senate. The unwillingness of Republicans (except some on the Senate Finance Committee) to seek common ground in markup pushed committees bills to the left. If Republicans on the House Ways and Means Committee had come forward with centrist amendments, the committee might have reported a bill without the provisions for part C medicare that alarmed providers, insurers, and big and small business, among others. Of course, Republicans wanted the committees to produce unpassable bills, which is exactly what happened.

The committee bills were not harmless errors, because they were grist for the measures put together by the leadership. There would have been no part C medicare in the Gephardt bill if there was no such provision in the bill devised by Ways and Means. Moreover, the committee bills stimulated unrealistic expectations in the liberal wing of the Democratic Party on what might be won in health care reform.

5. *The more unified party is the stronger party.*

Health care reform went down to defeat because Republicans were more united against it than Democrats were for it. If the reverse had been the case, the legislation would have become law.

Health care reform is not the only instance in which Democrats fought one another. The party unity scores presented in table 8-3 convey a misleading impression of cohesion in the Democratic ranks. As they neared the end of forty years of domination, House Democrats were deeply split, as they had been throughout that period. More than sixty House Democrats had combined economic and social conservatism scores of twenty-five or lower in 1993; about the same number had combined scores above ninety.[53] Broad measures of Democratic voting behavior in Congress show less dissension than once was the case. In the 1960s, the spread in the conservative coalition scores of northern and southern Democrats was typically more than 50 percentage points; in recent years, it has been about 40 points.[54] But these averages reflect the fact that the South now has a contingent of liberal Democrats in the

House. Conservative Democrats are about as conservative as they once were. Though there are fewer of them, there are still enough to block liberal ventures such as health care reform.

Bill Clinton sought the middle ground on health care that would reconcile the disparate wings of the Democratic party, or so he had hoped. But he found that the principal liberal and conservative alternatives to his proposal were quite popular among congressional Democrats.[55] Party leaders were understandably reluctant to jump in when fellow Democrats were so divided. But this was arguably the very situation that demanded aggressive leadership.

Republicans proved that it is easier to be united in opposition than in support. Although there was substantial disagreement among them, they were nearly unanimous in their dislike of Clinton's bill and, as the debate progressed, increasingly united in their determination to deny the Democrats a legislative victory.

6. Major reform needs bipartisan support.

With each party going its own way, the Democrats tried to craft comprehensive reform with no Republican participation in the House and little in the Senate. Had they succeeded, health care reform would have squeaked through with a razor-thin margin, just as other partisan legislation has in recent years. Some Democrats, notably Pat Moynihan, suggested that a strategy focusing on a minimum winning coalition is inappropriate for such truly sweeping change. This strategy wrote off Republican support, either because it was not available or deemed not worth the price.

Moynihan was right. Comprehensive reform should be consensual, not only in Congress but across the country. What the Democrats saw as Republican obstruction was more than that, for it reflected the unease Americans felt about what reform had in store for them. Consensual reform would have required that Democrats trim their legislative objectives and Republicans abandon some long-held positions. But that is the way tax reform was enacted a decade ago, and it was the only way health care reform could win majority support in Congress.

Health care reform vexed Congress at the end of Democratic rule and on the brink of Republican control. But reform was not the cause of this changing of the guard; it was the victim.

If there are lessons to be drawn from this, they are most likely to be applied by congressional Republicans, who demonstrated at the start of the 1995 session that they had the leadership and the unity so lacking among Democrats in 1994. It remains to be seen whether Republicans use these political resources to confront the hard choices of health care reform. Doing nothing may be appropriate in the short run; but the longer Republicans are in charge, the more they will learn that the problems of health care will not be remedied by legislative stalemate and inaction.

Notes

Chapter One

1. A summary of the recommendations of the Renewing Congress Project and their impact on congressional reform is contained in Thomas E. Mann, "Renewing Congress: A Report from the Front Lines," in James A. Thurber and Roger H. Davidson, eds., *Remaking Congress* (Washington: CQ Press, 1995).

Chapter Two

1. My understanding of jurisdictional politics in Congress has benefited from conversations with Bill Brown, Charlie Johnson, Tom Duncan, Bob Dove, Paul Rundquist, Carol Hardy Vincent, and especially Walter Oleszek, as well as many other congressional staffers. Of course, the responsibility for any errors in this chapter is mine alone.

2. *Organization of the Congress*, H. Rept. 103-413, 103 Cong. 1 sess. (Government Printing Office, 1993), p. 154.

3. *Budget Process: Testimony of Hon. Charles W. Stenholm, Hon. Barbara Mikulski, Hon. William F. Clinger, Jr., Hon. Robert E. Wise, Jr., Hon. Jim Kolbe, Hon. Christopher Cox, and Hon. William Orton,* Hearing before the Joint Committee on the Organization of Congress, 103 Cong. 1 sess. (GPO, 1993), p. 21.

4. *Committee Structure*, Hearings before the Joint Committee on the Organization of Congress, 103 Cong. 1 sess. (GPO, 1993), pp. 613–15.

5. Steven S. Smith, *Call to Order: Floor Politics in the House and Senate* (Brookings, 1989). See especially chapters 2 and 5. See also Barbara Sinclair, *The Transformation of the U.S. Senate* (Johns Hopkins University Press, 1989); David W. Rohde, Norman J. Ornstein, and Robert L. Peabody, "Political Change and Legislative Norms in the U.S. Senate, 1957–1974," in Glenn R. Parker, ed., *Studies of Congress* (Washington: CQ Press, 1985), pp. 147–88.

6. More generally, the Republican committee assignment process has been reformed so that the Speaker of the House can control or influence the selection of most members of the party's Committee on Committees. Mary Jacoby, "Big States Big Losers in Gingrich's Plan for Committee on Committees," *Roll Call,* December 1, 1994, p. 3.

7. Guy Gugliotta, "In New House, Barons Yield to the Boss," *Washington Post*, December 1, 1994, p. A1.

8. House Republicans are also continuing their previous practice of using informal task forces to supplement or bypass standing committees on complex issues. Major Garrett, "GOP Drops Overhaul of House Committees," *Washington Times*, November 29, 1994, p. A4.

9. *Operations of the Congress: Testimony of House and Senate Leaders*, Hearing before the Joint Committee on the Organization of Congress, 103 Cong. 1 sess. (GPO, 1993), p. 19.

10. News conference with Rep. David Dreier regarding committee reform, December 2, 1994, U.S. Capitol Building. As a former vice chairman of the Joint Committee on the Organization of Congress and the current chairman of the Subcommittee on Rules and Organization of the House (Committee on Rules), Dreier is a leader for House Republicans on congressional reform issues.

11. "D.C., Marine, Post Office Committees on Chopping Block," *National Journal's Congress Daily*, November 15, 1994, p. 2.

12. Michael Weisskopf, "Industries Fight for Footing in New House," *Washington Post*, November 22, 1994, p. C1.

13. These reforms still constitute the most significant reform of the House committee system since 1946. Three standing committees were abolished and approximately 20 percent of the jurisdiction of Energy and Commerce was transferred to other panels.

14. For general treatments of committee jurisdictions and the bill referral process, see Charles Tiefer, *Congressional Practice and Procedure: A Reference, Research, and Legislative Guide* (New York: Greenwood Press, 1989), pp. 68–87; and Walter Oleszek, *Congressional Procedures and the Policy Process*, 3d ed. (Washington: CQ Press, 1989), pp. 85–89. More generally, I have benefited from numerous memoranda and issue briefs about jurisdictional issues prepared by Judy Schneider of the Congressional Research Service, U.S. Library of Congress.

15. Tiefer, *Congressional Practice and Procedure*; Oleszek, *Congressional Procedures and the Policy Process*. See also David King, "The Nature of Congressional Committee Jurisdictions," *American Political Science Review*, vol. 88 (March 1994), pp. 48–62.

16. Split referrals (different panels receiving different parts of a bill) are also permitted in the House. Although some portions of the Contract with America received split referrals, they are relatively rare.

17. "Ways and Means Likely to Keep Health Care Jurisdiction," *National Journal's Congress Daily*, November 18, 1994, p. 1.

18. The bill was S.2320, *Universal Health Care Act of 1992* (SCORPIO files, U.S. Library of Congress).

19. Oleszek, *Congressional Procedures and the Policy Process*, pp. 86–87.

20. *Committee Structure*, Hearings, p. 620.

21. The Indian Affairs and Veterans' Affairs Committees marked up narrower portions of the Clinton bill.

22. Appropriations bills were dropped from the sample. Because the data in Tables 2-2 and 2-3 were gathered before the end of the 103d Congress, the 102d

was the most recent Congress for which comprehensive referral information was available. A less systematic look at referral patterns during the 103d Congress suggests that health referrals did not change significantly relative to the 102d. The referral data were gathered through the efforts of Carol Hardy Vincent.

23. During the 103d Congress, a "single-payer" reform proposal introduced by Rep. Jim McDermott (H.R. 1200) was referred to five committees: Armed Services, Energy and Commerce, Post Office and Civil Service, Veterans' Affairs, and Ways and Means. A more conservative reform alternative introduced by Rep. Jim Cooper (H.R. 3222) was referred to four committees: Education and Labor, Energy and Commerce, Judiciary, and Ways and Means. Judy Schneider, "Referral of the Clinton Administration's Health Security Act and Other Health Care Reform Measures to Committees of the House and the Senate," Washington, Congressional Research Service, February 24, 1994.

24. Garry Young, "Committee Gatekeeping and Proposal Power Under Single and Multiple Referral," *Journal of Theoretical Politics* (forthcoming). Young finds that multiply referred bills, controlling for other factors, are less likely to pass. See also Roger Davidson, Walter Oleszek, and Thomas Kephart, "One Bill, Many Committees: Multiple Referrals in the U.S. House of Representatives," *Legislative Studies Quarterly*, vol. 13 (February 1988), pp. 3–28. On the potential implications of jurisdictional fragmentation for policy coherence, see Thomas E. Mann and Norman J. Ornstein, *Renewing Congress: A Second Report* (American Enterprise Institute and Brookings, 1993), pp. 13–29. See also Roger Davidson, "Committee Politics in a Besieged Congress," paper delivered at the Conference on Congressional Change, Center for Congressional and Presidential Studies, The American University, October 8, 1994.

25. Six bills referred to the District of Columbia Committee and 28 bills referred to the Post Office and Civil Service Committee are included in the total for the Committee on Government Reform and Oversight, which received jurisdictions over issues previously considered by the first two panels. Two health-related bills were referred to the Merchant Marine Committee during the 102d Congress and are included in the totals for the panels receiving jurisdiction—one went to Resources, the other to Transportation and Infrastructure.

26. A somewhat different ordering is presented in Frank R. Baumgartner and others, "Committee Jurisdictions in Congress, 1980–1991," paper presented at the annual meeting of the American Political Science Association, September 1–4, 1994. This study relies on hearings as a measure of jurisdictional involvement in the health care arena. However, bill referrals—the data used here— clearly provide a more proximate indicator of legislative jurisdiction and involvement. If we rely on hearings, for example, the Select Committee on Aging was a major health panel during the 1980s. But the Aging Committee had no legislative jurisdiction and was abolished in 1993 because House members viewed it as unnecessary and wasteful. On the use of hearings as an indicator of legislative jurisdiction, see also King, "The Nature of Congressional Committee Jurisdictions," pp. 48–62; Bryan D. Jones, Frank R. Baumgartner, and Jeffrey C. Talbert, "The Destruction of Issue Monopolies in Congress," *American Political*

Science Review, vol. 87 (September 1993), pp. 657–71; John Hardin, "Congressional Activity on National Health Insurance Proposals: How Political Change Influences Legislative Organization," paper presented at the annual meeting of the Midwest Political Science Association, Chicago, April 14–16, 1994.

27. During the recent transition to Republican control, the Republican leadership considered stripping Ways and Means of its prerogatives over medicare benefits. But they discarded the proposal because it would have separated jurisdiction over medicare benefits from the financing mechanism (which, as dedicated revenue, would have remained with Ways and Means). Two decades earlier, Rep. Wilbur Mills, then chairman of Ways and Means, had used the same argument when the Bolling Committee considered a similar transfer. Mill's letter can be found in *Letters and Statements from Members, Groups, and Individuals Regarding the Work of the Select Committee on Committees*, Committee Print, House Select Committee on Committees, 93 Cong. 2 sess. (GPO, 1974), pp. 40–42.

28. King, "The Nature of Congressional Committee Jurisdictions," pp. 52–53.

29. On the distribution of jurisdiction over medicare, I have benefited from conversations with the House parliamentarians, as well as the work of a number of scholars at the Congressional Research Service, particularly Judy Schneider, Paul Rundquist, and Carol Hardy Vincent.

30. Steven S. Smith and Christopher J. Deering, *Committees in Congress*, 2d ed. (Washington: CQ Press, 1990).

31. Not-for-attribution interview conducted by the author with Senate staffer.

32. Judith H. Parris, "The Senate Reorganizes Its Committees, 1977," *Political Science Quarterly*, vol. 94 (Summer 1979), pp. 319–37.

33. *The Senate Committee System: Jurisdictions, Referrals, Numbers and Sizes, and Limitations on Membership*, Committee Print, Committee to Study the Senate Committee System, 94 Cong. 2 sess. (GPO, 1976), p. 16.

34. See testimony of Norman J. Ornstein and Thomas E. Mann, in *Committee Structure*, Hearings, pp. 495–96.

35. *Committee Structure*, Hearings, p. 733.

36. The Senate Judiciary Committee has been less active on health measures than its House counterpart, in part because the House Judiciary Committee often receives bills as part of a multiple referral. Health bills are seldom referred to more than one panel in the Senate.

37. For example, see Mann and Ornstein, *Renewing Congress*, pp. 13–31; Davidson, "Committee Politics in a Besieged Congress."

38. Smith and Deering, *Committees in Congress*. See also David E. Price, "Policy Making in Congressional Committees: The Impact of 'Environmental' Factors," *American Political Science Review*, vol. 72 (June 1978), pp. 548–74. On the importance of issue-specific variation for legislative participation, consult Richard L. Hall, "Participation and Purpose in Committee Decision Making," *American Political Science Review*, vol. 81 (March 1987), pp. 105–27.

39. Karen Tumulty and David Lauter, "Turf War Over Health Plan Smolders in Senate," *Los Angeles Times*, September 27, 1993, p. A5.

40. Alissa J. Rubin, "Members' Health Concerns Now Center on Turf Wars," *Congressional Quarterly Weekly Report*, October 9, 1993, p. 2735.

41. Glenn R. Simpson, "Dingell Warns a Joint Referral on Health 'Recipe for Disaster,'" *Roll Call*, October 14, 1993, p. 1.

42. Rubin, "Members' Health Concerns Now Center on Turf Wars," p. 2735.

43. Spencer Rich and Dana Priest, "Three House Panels Move to Assert Primacy Over Health Bill," *Washington Post*, October 24, 1993, p. A20.

44. Janet Hook, "Clinton Pushes Health Debate to Center Stage in Congress," *Congressional Quarterly Weekly Report*, September 18, 1993, p. 2457.

45. Spencer Rich, "Senate Chairmen in Tug of War Over Health Plan," *Washington Post*, November 24, 1993, p. A1.

46. Tumulty and Lauter, "Turf War Over Health Plan Smolders in Senate," p. A5.

47. Rich, "Senate Chairmen in Tug of War Over Health Plan," p. A1.

48. Richard E. Cohen, "Ready, Aim, Reform," *National Journal*, October 30, 1993, p. 2582.

49. Alissa J. Rubin, "Leaders Using Fervent Approach to Convert Wavering Members," *Congressional Quarterly Weekly Report*, July 30, 1994, p. 2144.

50. Alissa J. Rubin, "All Will Touch the Reform Bill, But Rules Panel Will Shape It," *Congressional Quarterly Weekly Report*, November 6, 1993, p. 3051.

51. Beth Donovan, "Senate Labor First Out of Gate with Approval of Overhaul Bill," *Congressional Quarterly Weekly Report*, June 11, 1994, p. 1522.

52. David S. Cloud, "Gibbons' Patched-Together Health Bill Now Faces Test on the Floor," *Congressional Quarterly Weekly Report*, July 2, 1994, p. 1793.

53. Beth Donovan, "A Disappointed Dingell," *Congressional Quarterly Weekly Report*, July 2, 1994, p. 1796.

54. Not-for-attribution interview conducted by author with House staffer.

55. "Healthcare Jurisdiction Plan Drafted," *National Journal's Congress Daily/A.M.*, July 22, 1994, p. 5.

56. On the advantages of multiple points of access within the congressional committee system for the consideration of comprehensive health care reform, consult Mark A. Peterson, "Congress in the 1990s: From Iron Triangles to Policy Networks," in James A. Morone and Gary S. Belkin, eds., *The Politics of Health Care Reform* (Duke University Press, 1994), pp. 103–47.

57. Chuck Alston, "Powerful Veterans' Groups at Political Crossroads," *Congressional Quarterly Weekly Report*, July 1, 1989, pp. 1602–03.

58. Ibid, p. 1603.

59. Smith and Deering, *Committees in Congress*, p. 79.

60. Letter from Robert L. Jones, Executive Director of AMVETS, from the files of the Joint Committee on the Organization of Congress, 103d Congress.

61. Letter from Roger A. Munson, National Commander of the American Legion, from the files of the Joint Committee on the Organization of Congress, 103d Congress.

62. Bill McAllister, "Program Continuity Pledged as 'Mr. Veteran' Steps Down," *Washington Post*, November 17, 1994, p. A21.

63. *Committee Structure*, Hearings, p. 559.

64. Some veterans groups, such as the American Legion, support proposals to open up VA hospitals to individuals with a connection to the military, such as Defense Department retirees. Some sharing of health care resources exists between the Veterans Administration and the Department of Defense. Kitty Dumas, "Aiming to Maximize Resources in the Era of Scarcity," *Congressional Quarterly Weekly Report*, June 13, 1992, p. 1708.

65. *H.R. 2824—Proposed Rural Health Care Pilot Program And Expanded Sharing of Federal Health Care Resources*, Hearing before the House Subcommittee on Hospitals and Health Care of the Committee on Veterans' Affairs, 102 Cong. 1 sess. (GPO, 1992), p. 5.

66. Ibid., testimony of James N. Magill, Director, National Legislative Service, Veterans of Foreign Wars, p. 19.

67. The Senate Veterans' Affairs Committee may be somewhat less responsive to veterans organizations under the chairmanship of Alan Simpson, who has described congressional relations with the veterans groups as "veteran-o-mania." Alston, "Powerful Veterans' Groups at Political Crossroads," p. 1602.

Chapter Three

1. Robert D. Reischauer, "The Congressional Budget Process," in Gregory B. Mills and John L. Palmer, eds., *Federal Budget Policy in the 1980s* (Washington: Urban Institute Press, 1984) pp. 385–413 (especially p. 406). The original conference paper was from September 1983.

2. Viveca Novak, "By the Numbers," *National Journal*, February 12, 1994, pp. 348–52; Steven Pearlstein and David S. Broder, "Clinton and the Analysts: A $133 Billion Difference of Opinion," *Washington Post*, February 9, 1994, p. A4; Hilary Stout and David Rogers, "CBO Disputes Cost Estimates in Health Plan," *Wall Street Journal*, February 9, 1994, p. A3.

3. Robert D. Reischauer, "Don't Let This Chance Go By," excerpts from his remarks, in *Washington Post*, February 11, 1994, p. A25.

4. Paul Starr, "Seductions of Sim: Policy as a Simulation Game," *The American Prospect*, no. 17 (Spring 1994), pp. 19–29 (especially 28–29).

5. The latter may be easily changed in the 1995 (fiscal 1996) resolution.

6. There are two numbering schemes because this provision was once in section 302 of the Budget Act. That section was moved to 602 because of the addition of some provisions in the 1990 legislation. These were supposed to be temporary, however, so some who were used to referring to a "302(a)" still do so rather than switch twice.

7. The permanent appropriation consists of the collections from the dedicated revenue source, the "HI" part of the social security payroll taxes.

8. The difference between formal annual appropriation and the reality of permanent entitlement is recognized by distinguishing "mandatory" appropriations such as those for medicaid from "discretionary" appropriations such as those for the National Institutes of Health (NIH).

9. For a more thorough discussion see Joseph White, "Presidential Power and the Budget," in Thomas D. Lynch, ed., *Federal Budget and Financial Management Reform* (New York: Quorum Books, 1991), pp. 1–29. On blame avoidance, see R. Kent Weaver, *Automatic Government: The Politics of Indexation* (Brookings, 1988).

10. This is usually issued in February or March, that is: Congress of the United States, Congressional Budget Office, *Reducing the Deficit: Spending and Revenue Options* (Government Printing Office, March 1994).

11. For an account of the measures and much of the politics, see David G. Smith, *Paying for Medicare: The Politics of Reform* (New York: Aldine de Gruyter, 1992); for more on the budgetary context, see Joseph White and Aaron Wildavsky, *The Deficit and the Public Interest: The Search for Responsible Budgeting in the 1980s* (University of California Press and The Russell Sage Foundation, 1989 and 1991).

12. Thus, in 1982 and 1984, Ways and Means and especially Finance helped set the targets; in 1983, when the budget resolution required savings that those committees did not advise, the committees ignored it.

13. The exception that proved the rule was within another bill with new, non–medicaid-related funding, the Medicare Catastrophic Coverage Act of 1988. For a summary see: Kaiser Commission on the Future of Medicaid, *The Medicaid Cost Explosion: Causes and Consequences* (Menlo Park, Calif.: Henry J. Kaiser Family Foundation, 1993), pp. 12–16.

14. Ibid., p. 14.

15. "Power" here should be understood to include not only a group's own resources but also the sympathy or opposition it meets with from others. The effect of that sympathy was shown nicely in the reaction of Rep. Marge Roukema (R.-N.J.) to the abortive summit deal of 1990. "If they're savaging medicare," she remarked, "it's going nowhere. Deficit reduction on the back of the elderly sick? This is madness." Quoted in White and Wildavsky, *The Deficit and the Public Interest*, p. 585.

16. Smith, *Paying for Medicare*, p. 232.

17. Ibid., p. 208. When presented with too weak a system in the last-gasp negotiations in 1989, Representative Stark therefore vetoed it. "As for the physicians," Smith reports, Stark "would get them through budget reconciliation and the update, just as before."

18. Ibid., pp. 127–65.

19. For a description of the importance of regulatory measures to the Clinton cost control scheme, see Joseph White, *Competing Solutions: American Health Care Proposals and International Experience* (Brookings, 1995), pp. 223–50.

20. It is also difficult to do anything about the tax deductibility of health insurance that is both fair and administratively viable; see the discussion in chapter 8 and the appendix of White, *Competing Solutions*.

21. Much of the discussion here is based on research compiled for Joseph White, *Treasured Authority: Appropriations Politics in Congress* (Brookings, forthcoming), for which special thanks are due to the Bradley Foundation for its support as well as to another that prefers not to be named.

22. Federal health-related spending also includes substantial expenses for federal employees and their dependents, including those in the military.

23. Many authorizations are enacted for single years and therefore are supposed to be reauthorized annually, but those reauthorizations often do not pass. Disagreement about issues such as school prayer and busing of children to schools, for example, made passing a Department of Justice reauthorization nearly impossible during the 1980s. The poor odds of success are worsened when, in the face of that difficulty, chamber leaders decide to give more promising legislation preference in allocating time for floor debate. Furthermore, all players know that, even though there are procedural objections to appropriating for unauthorized programs, those objections will be overcome for any established activity of the government. The fact of appropriation, once passed, continues the agency's activity. This reduces the need for reauthorization. A more extensive discussion of the authorization/appropriation relationship is presented in White, *Treasured Authority*.

24. A good example is financing of housing programs, which is discussed in White, *Treasured Authority*.

25. Some staff regret that they have few positive relationships with OMB, explaining that the appropriations staff and OMB examiners have very similar jobs and should be on the same side. But, the appropriators explain, OMB is too oriented toward reflecting officials' priorities rather than the law as it has been written by Congress and signed by the President. OMB also tends to make unrealistic proposals in order to claim the president has met his budget targets. Appropriators believe OMB does not have to be accurate but that both they and the agencies do, because appropriations are real money instead of proposals; that is, what the agency gets, not what OMB proposes, determines how the agency runs. Although the appropriators' perspectives are largely accurate, it should be noted that even if they were not, they would still control the committees' behavior!

26. White and Wildavsky, *The Deficit and the Public Interest*, pp. 290–91.

27. The literature on AIDS is voluminous and I cannot do justice to it here. For a stunning history of the early years of the AIDS epidemic, see Randy Shilts, *And the Band Played On: Politics, People, and the AIDS Epidemic* (Penguin Books, 1988); on the French experience with the blood supply, see Jane Kramer, "Letter from Europe: Bad Blood," *New Yorker* (October 11, 1993), pp. 74–95; for a synthetic consideration of AIDS policymaking in the context of other health hazard surprises, see Christopher H. Foreman, Jr., *Plagues, Products & Politics: Emergent Public Health Hazards and National Policymaking* (Brookings, 1994).

28. A brief summary of AIDS policymaking during the Reagan administration, beginning with the June 5, 1981, report, is in Richard Sorian, *The Bitter Pill: Tough Choices In America's Health Policy* (McGraw-Hill, 1988), pp. 203–37.

29. The subcommittee's full name is the Subcommittee on the Departments of Labor, Health and Human Services (HHS), and Education and Related Agencies. It is normally known as Labor/HHS. Labor/HHS has jurisdiction over the Public Health Service, including CDC and NIH. It also funds the medicaid program, though because that spending is considered mandatory, the subcom-

mittee pays little attention to its figures. *Congressional Quarterly Almanac* (Washington: CQ Press, 1982), p. 254.

30. *Congressional Record* (May 25, 1983), p. H3340, remarks of Rep. Green. Continuing Appropriations Resolutions (CRs) technically are vehicles to extend appropriations temporarily into a new fiscal year until new regular bills are enacted and signed. During the 1980s, however, more and more of the appropriations came to be enacted in full-year CRs, until all appropriations were enacted in CRs for FY87 and FY88. This form of enactment had little effect on Appropriations Committee action, but it did give Congress some bargaining advantages over the administration. See Joseph White, "A Crazy Way to Govern?", *Brookings Review*, vol. 6 (Summer 1988), pp. 28–35.

31. See the history of a $12 million addition to a supplemental appropriations bill in 1983. When Roybal proposed it in subcommittee, Natcher refused, but when the administration claimed it wanted the money by transfer, Natcher amended his own bill on the House floor. See *Congressional Record* (May 25, 1983), pp. H3336–44; *Congressional Quarterly Almanac 1983* (Washington: CQ Press, 1983), p. 511.

32. The story is in Shilts, *And the Band Played On*; see also *Congressional Record* (August 1, 1984), remarks of Rep. Weiss, pp. H8156–57; *Congressional Record* (September 25, 1984), pp. S11800–05, remarks of Senator Cranston and text of the memo. Some of the funding was put in a FY84 supplemental bill and some in the regular FY85 Labor/HHS text.

33. Thus in 1983, a point of order could have been raised against Natcher's floor amendment adding $12 million to the supplemental; nobody did so. See *Congressional Record* (May 25, 1983), p. H3343, remarks of Rep. Conte: "Everyone is a coauthor of this amendment because no one raised a point of order against it."

34. Thus even while offering an amendment calling for shutting down bathhouses, Rep. Robert Dornan (R.-Ca.) supported extra spending; see *Congressional Record* (October 2, 1985), p. H8030.

35. For a series of articles on the subject, see *Science*, vol. 237 (August 21, 1987), pp. 841–53.

36. *Congressional Quarterly Almanac* (Washington: CQ Press, 1987), p. 516.

37. *Congressional Quarterly Almanac* (Washington: CQ Press, 1987), pp. 404, 453–54 (quote p. 454). Earlier disputes included Rep. Dornan's bathhouse amendment in 1985. Occasionally a fight would occur in the entirely symbolic arena of the budget resolution, as when Senator Pete Wilson proposed switching funds from legislative postal funds to AIDS and Alzheimer's disease research in 1986. Because only appropriations spend money, this move was pure posturing. See *Congressional Quarterly Almanac* (Washington: CQ Press, 1986), p. 550.

38. *Congressional Quarterly Almanac* (Washington: CQ Press, 1988), pp. 706–13. That year President Reagan, in a valedictory, requested about as large an increase as Congress wished to provide. That year's almanac index has 40 separate AIDS categories.

39. This procedure first takes effect for FY96, for the budget round occurring within the executive branch at this writing. The director would now be ap-

pointed by the Secretary of HHS, not the director of NIH. The amount of budgetary power to be given to the director of OAR was quite controversial. The compromise was that funding would be allocated among institutes in accord with the plan, but institutes would make internal funding decisions. *Congressional Quarterly Almanac* (Washington: CQ Press, 1993), pp. 357–65; see also the Committee reports and the bill language (for example, Section 2353 (a) (6)).

40. The authorization proposed $880 million for FY94, and the Labor/HHS bill provided $579.4 million; *Congressional Quarterly Almanac* (Washington: CQ Press, 1993), p. 641.

41. See the conflict with Senator D'Amato reported in *Congressional Quarterly Almanac* (Washington: CQ Press, 1993), p. 637.

42. See the exchange between Rep. Natcher and Dr. Roper in House Committee on Appropriations, *Departments of Labor, Health and Human Services, Education, and Related Agencies Appropriations Hearings for Fiscal Year 1992*, 101 Cong. 2 sess. (GPO, 1992), pt. 3, pp. 330–31; for the record between Rep. Hoyer and Dr. Roper, see pp. 396–98.

43. Ibid, pp. 330–31, 395–96.

44. U.S. House, Committee on Appropriations, *Departments of Labor, Health and Human Services, and Education and Related Agencies Appropriations Hearings for 1991*, 101 Cong. 2 sess (GPO, 1992), pt. 4A, p. 45.

45. Ibid. See the exchanges between Rep. Pursell and Dr. Raub at p. 31, Rep. Conte and Dr. Broder at pp. 314–16, Rep. Natcher and Dr. Fauci at p. 1156, and Rep. Conte and Dr. Fauci at pp. 1160–61.

46. In addition to the previous citations, see the exchange between Rep. Myers and FDA Commissioner Dr. David Kessler in U.S. House of Representatives, Committee on Appropriations, *Agriculture, Rural Development, Food and Drug Administration, and Related Agencies Appropriations Hearings for 1993*, 102 Cong. 2 sess. (GPO, 1993), pt. 6, pp. 75–76.

47. Thus the new chairman of House Appropriations, Bob Livingston (R.-La.), retained much of the previous committee staff.

48. Many of the points in the following section are elaborated on and documented more thoroughly in White, *Competing Solutions*.

49. It is also the federal/state division for hospital care in Australia; see White, *Competing Solutions*.

50. That was the basic principle of S.1770, the "Chafee-Thomas" bill.

51. Both Chafee-Thomas and H.R. 3222, known as either "Cooper-Grandy" or "Cooper-Breaux," employed this approach. These were the two main "moderate" alternatives at the time the Clinton bill was introduced. Each bill also limited the tax deductibility of employer contributions for health benefits to a value that would depend on the standard benefit package. Each bill involved a tax hike for persons with greater benefits, and the size of the tax hike would be unknown until the commission made its proposal. Both bills would have had Congress vote on the commission proposal, but each was set up to prevent amendments and make disapproving the proposal very difficult.

52. The dynamic is hardly unique to health care; it was part of welfare reform design as well.

53. See Bill Clinton, "The Clinton Health Care Plan," *New England Journal of Medicine*, September 10, 1992, pp. 804–06; also see the text of candidate Clinton's address on health care at Merck Pharmaceuticals, Rahway, N.J., September 24, 1992 (transcript).

54. The relevant CBO reports are a June 1992 staff memorandum, "The Effects of Managed Care on Use and Costs of Health Services"; an August 1992 staff memorandum, "The Potential Impact of Certain Forms of Managed Care on Health Care Expenditures"; a May 1993 CBO Study, "Managed Competition and Its Potential to Reduce Health Spending"; a July 1993 CBO Paper, "Estimates of Health Care Proposals From the 102nd Congress"; a November 1993 Memorandum, "Behavioral Assumptions for Estimating the Effects of Health Care Proposals"; and a March 1994 Memorandum, "Effects of Managed Care: An Update." For examples of analyses by other scholars, see John F. Sheils, Lawrence S. Lewin, and Randall A. Haught, "Data Watch: Potential Public Expenditures under Managed Competition" as well as Verdon S. Staines, "Potential Impact of Managed Care on National Health Spending," *Health Affairs* (March 1993), vol. 12 supplement; see also Robert H. Miller and Harold S. Luft, "Managed Care: Past Evidence and Potential Trends," *Frontiers of Health Services Management*, vol. 9, no. 3 (Spring 1993), pp. 3–54.

55. David B. Kendall, "Health Care Price Controls: A Cure Worse Than the Disease" Progressive Policy Institute, Policy Briefing, June 9, 1994. PPI is the think tank arm of the DLC; Kendall was one of the staff who authored the Cooper-Grandy (or Cooper-Breaux) Managed Competition Act, H.R. 3222.

56. I mean to make no claim here as to whether President Clinton himself believed the claims for cost control from competition. Clearly some people in his administration did and some did not.

57. That benefit package, as noted above, was not specified in the bill, so CBO was being asked to make assumptions about what the bill's commission would decide.

58. Congressional Budget Office, "An Analysis of the Managed Competition Act," (April 1994), pp. 42–45.

59. See, for example, Congressional Budget Office, *Reducing the Deficit*.

60. I have no idea if the pattern described below was a strategy chosen by Dr. Reischauer, and I can imagine that it resulted from a series of choices in writing the report on the Clinton plan. But the approach followed logically from the constraints described above and the previous history of CBO. I can say that when I have described this pattern to a few CBO employees, no one has contradicted me publicly or privately.

61. The parallel between this summary and the contents of CBO's analysis can be easily seen by scanning the table of contents for Congressional Budget Office, *An Analysis of the Administration's Health Proposal* (February 1994).

62. CBO, *Analysis of the Administration's Health Proposal*, pp. 35–36.

63. CBO, *Analysis of the Administration's Health Proposal*, pp. 69–77.

64. CBO, *Analysis of the Administration's Health Proposal*, pp. 41–50.

65. Novak, "By the Numbers," p. 348.

66. Ibid., p. 349.

67. Stout and Rogers, "CBO Disputes Cost Estimates In Health Plan," p. A3; Steven Pearlstein and David S. Broder, "Clinton and the Analysts: A $133 Billion Difference of Opinion," *Washington Post* (February 9, 1994), p. A4.

68. David Rogers, "CBO Chief Is Doubtful of Cost Controls Under Conservative Health-Care Plans," *Wall Street Journal*, February 10, 1994, p. A6.

69. CBO could only advise on budgetary treatment; see "Analysis of the Administration's Health Proposal," p. 41. On reactions see Stout and Rogers, "CBO Disputes Cost Estimates," p. A3.

70. For a fuller critique see Joseph White, "When Should Health Care Be Included in Government Budgets? A Comparative Perspective," paper delivered at the 1994 Research Conference of the Association for Public Policy Analysis and Management, Chicago, October 29, 1994; for an example of CBO staff thinking, see Robin Seiler, "Applying Federal Budget Concepts to National Health Care Reform Proposals," from the same conference.

71. My thanks to Roy Meyers, formerly of CBO, for identifying this mindset in commenting on Robin Seiler's paper, cited above.

72. It depends, of course, on one's definition of weaknesses. CBO would not show that the administrative or financial aspects of the McDermott-Wellstone American Health Security Act of 1993 were inferior to the Clinton Health Security Act; however, that bill's explicit use of taxes and government insurance likely foreclosed it politically. For CBO's analysis, see its manuscript, "H.R. 1200, American Health Security Act of 1993," December 16, 1993.

73. Not out of obedience to political masters, but because whichever bill is most prominent is the one for which accurate budgetary analysis is most important, to prevent irresponsible legislation.

74. Rogers, "CBO Chief is Doubtful." The trouble was, no one else had ever met the kind of medical market Durenberger had in mind, either. The last time anyone had seriously proposed estimating the effects of budget policy on the grounds of a theory about behavior that had not been observed in practice was the supply side tax cut of 1981. As a matter of budget policy, whatever one may say about the economics, that was not an encouraging example.

75. Quoted in David Stockman, *The Triumph of Politics: How the Reagan Revolution Failed* (Harper & Row, 1986), p. 176.

76. This analysis ignores another level of controls, forced "sequesters," on two grounds. First, those particular rules, which suggest that paying for a tax cut with spending cuts would still force a sequester, can easily be changed within the FY96 Budget Resolution. Second, the incentive for a Democratic administration to cut spending further by initiating the sequester is rather hard to discern.

77. A balanced budget amendment might produce some further pressure for cuts. However, since the amendment was not in place at this writing and would not take effect even if ratified until 2002, it cannot be part of a report on the influence of current budget procedures. I will note only that during budget crunches higher levels of government tend to subject transfers to lower levels of government to disproportionate cuts. Programs such as medicaid and the various categorical grants for health services should be especially at risk if the amendment is ratified. But they already are.

Chapter Four

1. David G. Smith, *Paying For Medicare: The Politics of Reform* (Aldine de Gruyter, 1992), pp. 200–209.
2. Thomas R. Oliver, "Analysis, Advice, and Congressional Leadership: The Physician Payment Review Commission and the Politics of Medicare," *Journal of Health Politics, Policy and Law*, vol. 18 (Spring 1993), pp. 113–73; Smith, *Paying for Medicare*, pp. 167–173.
3. Physician Payment Review Commission, *Annual Report to Congress*, Washington, D.C., March 1, 1991, pp. 116–28.
4. Ibid., p. 128.
5. Physician Payment Review Commission, *Annual Report to Congress*, Washington, D.C., March 1, 1992, pp. xiv, 23–25.
6. Henry J. Aaron, *Politics and the Professors: The Great Society in Perspective* (Brookings, 1978), p. 9.
7. Lawrence D. Brown, "Knowledge and Power: Health Services Research as a Political Resource," in Eli Ginzerg, ed., *Health Services Research: Key to Health Policy* (Harvard University Press, 1991), p. 35.
8. Roger Benjamin, *The Limits of Politics: Collective Goods and Political Change in Postindustrial Societies* (University of Chicago Press, 1980).
9. Jeffrey C. Miller, "The Role of Information in Public Policy Making," *Health Policy on Target*, August 1, 1994, pp. 2, 7.
10. Geoffrey Vickers, *The Art of Judgment: A Study of Policy Making* (London: Chapman and Hall, 1965), p. 86.
11. David R. Mayhew, *Congress: The Electoral Connection* (Yale University Press, 1974), p. 5; R. Douglas Arnold, *The Logic of Congressional Action* (Yale University Press, 1990).
12. Arnold, *Logic of Congressional Action*.
13. Allen Schick, "Informed Legislation: Policy Research Versus Ordinary Knowledge," in William H. Robinson and Clay H. Wellborn, eds., *Knowledge, Power, and the Congress* (Washington: CQ Press, 1991), p. 101.
14. Schick, "Informed Legislation," p. 101; Charles E. Lindblom and David K. Cohen, *Usable Knowledge: Social Science and Social Problem Solving* (Yale University Press, 1979), p. 12.
15. The narrative of this example is derived from my personal involvement with the issue as a legislative assistant in the Senate.
16. David E. Price, "Comment," in William H. Robinson and Clay H. Wellborn, eds., *Knowledge, Power, and the Congress* (Washington: CQ Press, 1991), p. 127.
17. Smith, *Paying for Medicare*, pp. 101–105.
18. Oliver, "Analysis, Advice, and Congressional Leadership"; Smith, *Paying for Medicare*; I was also personally involved with the issue while working in the Senate.
19. Schick, "Informed Legislation," p. 100.
20. Richard Rose, *Lesson-Drawing in Public Policy: A Guide to Learning Across Time and Space* (Chatham, N.J.: Chatham House, 1993).

21. Karl R. Popper, *Objective Knowledge: An Evolutionary Approach* (Oxford University Press, 1972), p. 81; and David M. Ricci, *The Tragedy of Political Science: Politics, Scholarship, and Democracy* (Yale University Press, 1984), p. 116.

22. Brown, "Knowledge and Power," pp. 26–33.

23. Ibid., pp. 26, 28, 31.

24. Smith, *Paying for Medicare*, pp. 182–190.

25. John W. Kingdon, *Congressmen's Voting Decisions*, 3d ed. (University of Michigan Press, 1989), pp. 29–71.

26. Daniel Yankelovich, *Coming to Public Judgment: Making Democracy Work in a Complex World* (Syracuse University Press, 1991), p. 42.

27. Daniel Yankelovich, "What Polls Say—and What They Mean," *New York Times*, September 17, 1994, p. 23.

28. Cristine Russell, "How Much Do People Know about Health?" *Washington Post*, March 1, 1994, Health section, p. 6.

29. Darrell M. West and Diane J. Heith, "Harry and Louise Go to Washington: Political Advertising and Health Care Reform," paper prepared for the 1994 annual meeting of the American Political Science Association.

30. Mollyann Brodie and Robert J. Blendon, "The Public's Contribution to Congressional Gridlock on Health Care Reform," *Journal of Health Politics, Policy and Law*, vol. 20 (Summer 1995), pp. 403–10; Lawrence R. Jacobs and Robert Y. Shapiro, "Don't Blame the Public for Failed Health Care Reform," *Journal of Health Politics, Policy and Law*, vol. 20 (Summer 1995), pp. 411–24.

31. Arnold, *Logic of Congressional Action*, pp. 3–146.

32. Robert J. Blendon and John M. Benson, "Public Opinion Update on Health Care Reform #1, #2, and #3," reports prepared for the Health Subcommittee, U.S. House Committee on Ways and Means (Harvard Program on Public Opinion and Health Care, Harvard School of Public Health, November 19, 1993, December 9, 1993, and January 25, 1994).

33. An example is "Long Term Care in America: Public Attitudes and Possible Solutions," prepared for the American Association of Retired Persons by The Daniel Yankelovich Group, Inc., January 1990.

34. An example is "Public Attitudes on Health Care Reform: Summary," national public opinion survey conducted for the Employee Benefit Research Institute, EBRI Report Number G-43 (The Gallup Organization, Inc., April 1993)

35. West and Heath, "Harry and Louise Go to Washington."

36. "Trade-Offs & Choices: Health Policy Options for the 1990s," survey prepared for Metropolitan Life Insurance Company (New York: Louis Harris and Associates, Inc., 1990).

37. "An Analysis of the Jobs-at-Risk Associated With Mandated Employer Health Insurance," a report prepared for The Partnership on Health Care and Employment (Washington: Consad Research Corporation, 1990).

38. "Analysis of Hospital Expenditures and Revenues, 1979–1989," a study prepared for the Federation of American Health Systems (Washington, D.C., Lewin/ICF [division of Health & Sciences International], April 1991).

39. American Society of Internal Medicine, "The Hassle Factor: America's Health Care System Strangling in Red Tape" (Washington: ASIM, 1990).

40. Jack L. Walker, Jr., *Mobilizing Interest Groups in America: Patrons, Professions, and Social Movements* (University of Michigan Press, 1991).

41. Frank R. Baumgartner and Bryan D. Jones, *Agendas and Instability in American Politics* (University of Chicago Press, 1993), pp. 175–92.

42. Mark A. Peterson, "Political Influence in the 1990s: From Iron Triangles to Policy Networks," *Journal of Health Politics, Policy and Law*, vol. 18 (Summer 1993), pp. 395–438.

43. Joel D. Aberbach, Robert D. Putnam, and Bert A. Rockman, *Bureaucrats and Politicians in Western Democracies* (Harvard University Press, 1981).

44. Keith Krehbiel, *Information and Legislative Organization* (University of Michigan Press, 1991), pp. 60–66. Arnold, *Logic of Congressional Action*.

45. Krehbiel, *Information and Legislative Organization*, p. 62.

46. Bruce Cain, John Ferejohn, and Morris Fiorina, *The Personal Vote: Constituency Service and Electoral Independence* (Harvard University Press, 1987).

47. Norman J. Ornstein, Thomas E. Mann, and Michael J. Malbin, *Vital Statistics on Congress, 1987–88* (American Enterprise Institute, 1987), pp. 147–48.

48. Robert Pear, "With Long Hours and Little Fanfare, Staff Members Created a Health Bill," New York Times, August 6, 1994, p. 7.

49. Ibid.

50. Roger H. Davidson and Walter J. Oleszek, *Congress and Its Members*, 2d ed. (Washington: CQ Press, 1985), p. 256.

51. Allen Schick, *Congress and Money: Budgeting, Spending and Taxing* (Washington: Urban Institute, 1980).

52. Terry M. Moe, "The Politicized Presidency," in John E. Chubb and Paul E. Peterson, eds., *The New Directions in American Politics* (Brookings, 1985), pp. 235–271; Mark A. Peterson, "Health Policy Making in the Information Age: Is Congress Better Informed than the President?" paper prepared for the Conference on Governance in an Era of Skepticism: Administrators and Politicians, sponsored by the International Political Science Association Research Committee on the Structure and Organization of Government, Stockholm, Sweden, September 16–18, 1992; Schick, *Congress and Money*.

53. Steven Pearlstein and David S. Broder, "Clinton and the Analysts: A $133 Billion Difference of Opinion," *Washington Post*, February 9, 1994, p. A4.

54. Robert J. Samuelson, "CBO's Wishful Thinking," *Washington Post*, February 16, 1994, p. A19; Editorial, "Accounting for Health Care," *Washington Post*, February 9, 1994, p. A22.

55. Adam Clymer, Robert Pear, and Robin Toner, "For Health Care, Time Was a Killer," *New York Times*, August 29, 1994, pp. A8.

56. Robin Toner, "Budget Director, the Conscience of Congress, Turns Ideas Into Dollar Signs," *New York Times*, August 21, 1994, p. A32.

57. Smith, *Paying for Medicare*, pp. 54, 79.

58. Oliver, "Analysis, Advice, and Congressional Leadership"; Smith, *Paying for Medicare*, pp. 167–69.

59. Oliver, "Analysis, Advice, and Congressional Leadership," p. 145.

60. Smith, *Paying for Medicare*, p. 116.

61. Kevin Merida, "Hill Health Care Gets a Closer Look," *Washington Post*, March 21, 1994, p. A17; Robert Pear, "Health Care Debate to Shift to Federal Employees' Plan," *New York Times*, September 7, 1994, p. A1, A10.

62. Clymer, Pear, and Toner, "For Health Care, Time Was a Killer."

63. Alissa J. Rubin, "Clinton Task Force All Ears On the Subject of Overhaul," *Congressional Quarterly Weekly Report*, May 22, 1993, pp. 1293–95.

64. Oliver, "Analysis," p. 145.

65. Mark A. Peterson, "From Vested Oligarchy to Informed Entrepreneurship: New Opportunities for Health Care Reform in Congress," paper prepared for the 1994 annual meeting of the Midwest Political Science Association.

66. Moe, "The Politicized Presidency," pp. 235–271.

67. This issue is covered with respect to OTA in Bruce Bimber, "Institutions and Ideas: The Politics of Expertise in Congress," Ph.D. dissertation, Massachusetts Institute of Technology, 1992.

68. Oliver, "Analysis, Advice, and Congressional Leadership," p. 149.

69. Brown, "Knowledge and Power," pp. 40–41; Daniel M. Fox, "Health Policy and the Politics of Research in the United States," *Journal of Health Politics, Policy and Law*, vol. 15 (Fall 1990), pp. 481–500.

70. The answer is not always encouraging. See Thomas R. Wolanin, "Congress, Information and Policy Making for Post-Secondary Education: Don't Trouble Me with the Facts," *Policy Studies Journal* vol. 4 (Summer 1976), pp. 382–94.

71. Charles W. Anderson, "The Place of Principles in Policy Analysis," *American Political Science Review*, vol. 73 (September 1979), pp. 711–23; Carol H. Weiss, Ed., *Using Social Research in Public Policy Making* (Lexington, Mass.: Lexington Books, 1977); Carol H. Weiss, "Measuring the Use of Evaluation," in James A. Ciarlo, ed., *Utilizing Evaluation: Concepts and Measurement Techniques* (Beverly Hills, Calif.: Sage, 1981), pp. 17–33; Carol H. Weiss, "The Circuitry of Enlightenment," *Knowledge: Creation, Diffusion, Utilization*, vol. 8 (December 1986), pp. 274–281; Carol H. Weiss, "Congressional Committees as Users of Analysis," *Journal of Policy Analysis and Management*, vol. 8 (Summer 1989), pp. 411–431; Fox, "Health Policy and the Politics of Research," pp. 481–499; Rudolf Klein, " Research, Policy, and the National Health Service," *Journal of Health Politics, Policy and Law*, vol. 15 (Fall 1990), pp. 501–523; Jonathon Lomas, "Finding Audiences, Changing Beliefs: The Structure of Research Use in Canadian Health Policy," *Journal of Health Politics, Policy and Law*, vol. 15 (Fall 1990), pp. 525–542; Paul A. Sabatier, "Knowledge, Policy-Oriented Learning, and Policy Change: An Advocacy Coalition Framework," *Knowledge: Creation, Diffusion, Utilization*, vol. 8 (June 1987), pp. 649–692.

72. Weiss, *Using Social Research in Public Policy Making*, p. 17.

73. Aaron, *Politics and the Professors*, pp. 165–66.

74. Brown, "Knowledge and Power," p. 39.

75. William C. Hsiao, "Objective Research and Physician Payment: A Response from Harvard," *Health Affairs*, vol. 8 (Winter 1989), pp. 72–75; Klein, " Research, Policy, and the National Health Service," pp. 501–523.

76. Carol H. Weiss and Michael J. Bucuvalas, *Social Science Research and Decision-Making* (Columbia University Press, 1980), p. 172.

77. Robert Pear, "Report Criticizes the Objectivity of the Federal Watchdog Agency," *New York Times*, October 17, 1994, p. A1.

78. Oliver, "Analysis, Advice, and Congressional Leadership," p. 115.

79. Ibid., pp. 139, 145.

80. William G. Manning and others, "Health Insurance and the Demand for Medical Care: Evidence from a Randomized Experiment," *American Economic Review*, vol. 77 (June 1987), pp. 251–77; Morris L. Barer, Robert G. Evans, and G. L. Stoddart, *Controlling Health Care Costs by Direct Charges to Patients: Snare or Delusion?* Occasional Paper 10 (Toronto: Ontario Economic Council, 1979).

81. Paul C. Weiler, *Medical Malpractice on Trial* (Harvard University Press, 1991).

82. *Skinner v. Mid-America Pipeline Company*, 490 U.S. 212 (1989).

83. Julie Kosterlitz, "Radical Surgeons," *National Journal*, April 27, 1991, pp. 993–97.

84. E. E. Schattschneider, *The Semi-Sovereign People: A Realist's View of Democracy in America* (Holt, Rinehart and Winston, 1960); Kay Lehman Schlozman and John T. Tierney, *Organized Interests and American Democracy* (Harper & Row, 1986), pp. 58–87.

85. Peterson, "Political Influence in the 1990s"; Mark A. Peterson, "Institutional Change and the Health Politics of the 1990s," *American Behavioral Scientist*, vol. 36 (July 1993), pp. 782–801; Mark A. Peterson, "Health Care and the Hill: Why Is This Year Different from All Others?" *PS: Political Science & Politics*, vol. 27 (June 1994), pp. 202–207.

86. Theodore R. Marmor, "A Summer of Discontent: Press Coverage of Murder and Medical Care Reform," *Journal of Health Politics, Policy and Law*, vol. 20 (Summer 1995), pp. 495–501; Mark A. Peterson, "The Health Care Debate: All Heat and No Light," *Journal of Health Politics, Policy and Law*, vol. 20 (Summer 1995), pp. 425–30.

87. Kingdon, *Congressmen's Voting Decisions*, pp. 242–61.

88. Rudolf Klein, "Research, Policy, and the National Health Service," *Journal of Health Politics, Policy and Law*. vol. 15 (Fall 1990), pp. 501–23.

89. Peterson, "Health Care Debate"; Paul Starr, "What Happened to Health Care Reform?" *American Prospect*, no. 20 (Winter 1995), pp. 20–31; James Fallows, "A Triumph of Misinformation," *Atlantic Monthly*, January 1995, pp. 26–37.

90. Aaron, *Politics and the Professors*; Anthony Barker and B. Guy Peters, "Introduction: Science and Government," in Anthony Barker and B. Guy Peters, eds., *The Politics of Expert Advice: Creating, Using and Manipulating Scientific Knowledge for Public Policy* (University of Pittsburgh Press, 1993), pp. 1–16; Klein, "Research, Policy, and the National Health Service."

91. Toner, "Putting Prices on Congress's Ideas," p. 32.

92. Weiss and Bucuvalas, *Social Science Research and Decision-Making*, pp. 30, 170.

93. Robert J. Blendon and others, "How Much Does the Public Know About Health Reform?", *Journal of American Health Policy*, vol. 4 (January/February 1994),

pp. 26–31; Tom Hamburger, Ted Marmor, and Jon Meacham, "What the Death of Health Reform Teaches Us About the Press," *Washington Monthly*, vol. 26 (November 1994), pp. 35–45; Kathleen Hall Jamieson and Joseph Cappella, "Newspaper and Television Coverage of the Health Care Reform Debate, January 16–July 25, 1994," report prepared by the Annenberg Public Policy Center, University of Pennsylvania, funded by the Robert Wood Johnson Foundation, Philadelphia, August 12, 1994; Robin Toner, "Making Sausage: The Art of Reprocessing the Democratic Process," *New York Times*, September 4, 1994, sect. 4, p. 4.

94. Bill Carter, "Buying the Air Time, Foundation Fosters NBC Program on Health," *New York Times*, May 4, 1994, pp. A1, A10.

95. Fox, "Health Policy and the Politics of Research," p. 495.

96. Robert H. Salisbury and Kenneth A. Shepsle, "U.S. Congressman as Enterprise," *Legislative Studies Quarterly*, vol. 6 (November 1981), pp. 559–76; Fox, "Health Policy and the Politics of Research," pp. 495–96.

97. Oliver, "Analysis, Advice, and Congressional Leadership," p. 144; also discussed by Weiss, "Congressional Committees as Users of Analysis," pp. 411–31.

98. Alissa J. Rubin, "The Players, the Process," *Congressional Quarterly Weekly Report*, November 6, 1993, p. 3051.

99. Oliver, "Analysis, Advice, and Congressional Leadership," p. 145.

100. Lomas, "Finding Audiences, Changing Beliefs," pp. 534–37.

101. Quoted in Daniel A. Dreyfus, "The Limitations of Policy Research in Congressional Decision Making," in Carol H. Weiss, ed., *Using Social Research in Public Policy Making* (Lexington, Mass.: Lexington Books, 1977), p. 101.

102. Dreyfus, "Limitations of Policy Research," p. 104.

103. Brown, "Knowledge and Power," pp. 26–28.

104. Paul A. Sabatier, "Knowledge, Policy-Oriented Learning, and Policy Change: An Advocacy Coalition Framework," pp. 649–92.

105. Brown, "Knowledge and Power," p. 20.

106. Lomas, "Finding Audiences," p. 527.

107. James G. March, "Ambiguity and Accounting: The Elusive Link between Information and Decision-Making," in James G. March, ed., *Decisions and Organizations* (New York: Basil Blackwell, 1988), p. 387.

108. Peter L. Berger and Thomas Luckmann, *The Social Construction of Reality: A Treatise in the Sociology of Knowledge* (Garden City, N.Y.: Doubleday, 1967).

109. Sabatier, "Knowledge, Policy-Oriented Learning, and Policy Change," pp. 676–78; Dreyfus, "Limitations of Policy Research," pp. 102–103; Klein, "Research Policy," p. 504.

110. Rose, *Lesson-Drawing in Public Policy*; and Mark A. Peterson, "National Health Care Reform and Social Learning: More Than Just the Facts," paper prepared for the 1993 annual meeting of the American Political Science Association.

111. Fox, "Health Policy and the Politics of Research," p. 498.

112. Fox, "Health Policy and the Politics of Research," pp. 490–94; David M. Frankford, "Scientism and Economism in the Regulation of Health Care," *Journal of Health Politics, Policy and Law*, vol. 19 (Winter 1994), pp. 773–99.

113. Robert G. Evans, "Finding the Levers, Finding the Courage: Lessons from Cost Containment in North America," *Journal of Health Politics, Policy and Law*, vol. 11 (1986), p. 610.

114. Brown, "Knowledge and Power," pp. 31–32; Evans, "Finding the Levers," p. 611; Fox, "Health Policy and the Politics of Research," pp. 481, 496; Lomas, "Finding Audiences," p. 528.

115. Hsiao, "Objective Research and Physician Payment," pp. 72–75.

116. Samuelson, "Accounting for Health Care."

117. Clay Chandler, "It's Reischauer's Hour," *Washington Post*, February 11, 1994, p. E1.

118. John D. Rockefeller IV, "The Devilment Is in the Details," *Washington Post*, February 14, 1994, p. A15.

119. Dana Priest and Spencer Rich, "Health Plan Will Swell Deficit, Hill Office Says," *Washington Post*, February 9, 1994, p. A4.

120. Lars-Erik Nelson, "Phil Gramm's Canada Canard," *Washington Post*, August 28, 1994, p. C7.

121. David S. Cloud, "GOP, to Its Own Great Delight, Enacts House Rules Changes," *Congressional Quarterly Weekly Report*, January 7, 1995, pp. 13–15.

122. Mark A. Peterson, "From Vested Oligarchy to Informed Entrepreneurship."

123. Katharine Q. Seelye, "G.O.P. Decides to Halt Money to 28 Caucuses," *New York Times*, December 7, 1994, pp. A1, A11.

124. Peter Passell, "Economic Scene: Lower Income Taxes Stimulate the Economy. The Sequel," *New York Times*, December 22, 1994, p. D2.

Chapter Five

1. *Study on Federal Regulation: Congressional Oversight of Regulatory Agencies, Volume II*, S. Doc. 95-26, 95 Cong. 1 sess. (Government Printing Office, 1977), p. xi.

2. John F. Bibby, "Congress' Neglected Function," in Melvin R. Laird, ed., *Republican Papers* (Garden City, N.Y.: Anchor, 1968), pp. 477–88.

3. *Report on the Activity of the Committee on Energy and Commerce*, for the 103d Congress, 1st Session, H. Rept. 103-417, 103 Cong. 1 sess. (GPO, 1994), p. 19. This formal count is just one indicator of the amount of oversight activity. Disentangling oversight from legislation can be difficult.

4. Joel D. Aberbach, *Keeping a Watchful Eye: The Politics of Congressional Oversight* (Brookings, 1990), p. 191.

5. Allen Schick, "Politics through Law: Congressional Limitations on Executive Discretion," In Anthony King, ed., *Both Ends of the Avenue: The Presidency, the Executive Branch, and Congress in the 1980s* (American Enterprise Institute, 1983), pp. 154–84.

6. Congressional Research Service, *Congressional Oversight Manual*, February 1984, pp. 1–2.

7. See Arthur W. MacMahon, "Congressional Oversight of Administration: The Power of the Purse—II," *Political Science Quarterly*, vol. 58 (1943), p. 380.

8. Richard Fenno, *The Power of the Purse: Appropriations Politics in Congress* (Boston: Little, Brown, 1966), p. 17.

9. *President Clinton's Fiscal Year 1995 Budget: A Summary and Analysis Prepared by the Staff of the House Budget Committee*, Committee Print, House Committee on the Budget (GPO, 1994), pp. 3, 171–73.

10. See Michael W. Kirst, *Government without Passing Laws: Congress' Nonstatutory Techniques for Appropriations Control* (Chapel Hill: University of North Carolina Press, 1969).

11. *Departments of Labor, Health and Human Services, and Education, and Related Agencies Appropriations Bill, 1993*, H. Rept. 102-708, 102 Cong. 2 sess. (GPO, 1992), p. 39.

12. Editorial, "Mr. Stark's Race Backward," *New York Times*, March 10, 1994, p. A24.

13. Aberbach, *Keeping a Watchful Eye*, p. 132.

14. Marsha Gold and others, "Effects of Selected Cost-Containment Efforts: 1971–1993," *Health Care Financing Review*, vol. 14, no. 3 (Spring 1993), pp. 195–98.

15. John K. Iglehart, "Payment of Physicians Under Medicare," *New England Journal of Medicine*, vol. 318 (1988), pp. 863–68.

16. John K. Iglehart, "The Recommendations of the Physician Payment Review Commission," *New England Journal of Medicine*, vol. 320 (April 27, 1989), pp. 1157–58.

17. Ibid., p. 1157.

18. Julie Kosterlitz, "Managing Medicaid," *National Journal*, May 9, 1992, p. 1113.

19. Ibid.

20. Mann and Ornstein, *Renewing Congress: A First Report* (American Enterprise Institute and Brookings, 1992), p. 10.

21. See, for example, Morris S. Ogul, *Congress Oversees the Bureaucracy: Studies in Legislative Supervision* (University of Pittsburgh Press, 1976).

22. *Congressional Quarterly Almanac, 1993* (Washington: CQ Press, 1993), pp. 132–35.

Chapter Six

1. Julie Rovner, "Finance Weighs Benefit Cuts in Catastrophic-Costs Law," *Congressional Quarterly Weekly Report*, September 16, 1989, p. 2397.

2. *1994 Green Book: Background Material and Data on Programs within the Jurisdiction of the Committee on Ways and Means* (Government Printing Office, 1994), p. 172.

3. House Ways and Means Committee, *1993 Green Book*, p. 137; *1994 Green Book*, pp. 123, 135.

4. Based on statistics in *1994 Green Book*, p. 175.

5. John K. Iglehart, "Health Policy Report: The American Health Care System—Medicare," *New England Journal of Medicine*, vol. 327, no. 20 (November 12, 1992), p. 1467.

6. Paul Starr, *The Social Transformation of American Medicine* (Basic Books, 1982), p. 369.

7. *Medicare: Prescription Drug Issues*, PEMD-87-20 (GAO, July 16, 1987), p. 2.

8. The Pepper Commission: U.S. Bipartisan Commission on Comprehensive Health Care, *A Call for Action*, Final Report (GPO, September 1990), pp. 92, 95.

9. Ibid., p. 100.

10. *Medicare Catastrophic Protection Act of 1987*, H. Rept. 100-105, 100 Cong. 1 sess. (GPO, 1987), pt. 1, p. 8.

11. Jennifer O'Sullivan, "Medicare Catastrophic Coverage Act of 1988 (PL 100-360)," Congressional Research Service, Library of Congress, March 3, 1989, p. 17.

12. Press release, American Association of Retired Persons, March 2, 1987.

13. *Catastrophic Illness Expenses*, Hearings before the Subcommittee on Health, U.S. House Committee on Ways and Means, 100 Cong. 1 sess. (GPO, 1987), p. 7.

14. O'Sullivan, "Medicare Catastrophic Coverage Act," p. 20.

15. *Congressional Quarterly Almanac, 1990* (Washington: CQ Press, 1990), p. 572.

16. O'Sullivan, "Medicare Catastrophic Coverage Act," p. 20.

17. Congressional Quarterly, *Aging in America—The Federal Government's Role* (Washington: CQ Press, 1989), p. 5.

18. Ibid., p. 22.

19. *Congressional Quarterly Almanac, 1986*, p. 4-D.

20. Julie Rovner, "Bowen: Expand Medicare to Cover Catastrophes," *Congressional Quarterly Weekly Report*, November 22, 1986, p. 2956.

21. *Congressional Record*, daily ed., July 22, 1987, p. H6462.

22. Ibid., pp. H6461–62.

23. Julie Rovner, "Reagan Sides with Bowen on Medicare Plan," *Congressional Quarterly Weekly Report*, February 14, 1987, p. 297.

24. Julie Rovner, "Panel Considers Alternatives to Bowen Plan," *Congressional Quarterly Weekly Report*, March 7, 1987, p. 434.

25. Alan Ehrenhalt, ed., *Politics in America: The 100th Congress* (Washington: CQ Press, 1987), p. 341.

26. Robert Pear, "Congress Seeks a Fair Way to Pay for Catastrophic Health Insurance," *New York Times*, June 7, 1987, p. E30.

27. *Catastrophic Illness Expenses*, Hearings, p. 145.

28. Ibid., p. 180.

29. Ehrenhalt, "Politics in America," p. 117.

30. *Catastrophic Illness Expenses*, Hearings, p. 183.

31. Rovner, "Panel Considers Alternatives," p. 434; Jacqueline Calmes, "House Panel Backs Big Expansion of Medicare," *Congressional Quarterly Weekly Report*, April 11, 1987, p. 686.

32. Rovner, "Panel Considers Alternatives," p. 434.

33. Julie Rovner, "House Panel Approves Catastrophic Care Plan," *Congressional Quarterly Weekly Report*, May 9, 1987, pp. 915–16.

34. Rovner, "Panel Considers Alternatives," p. 434.

35. Julie Rovner, "New Medicare Plan May Include Drug Coverage," *Congressional Quarterly Weekly Report*, May 23, 1987, p. 1082.

36. Julie Rovner, "House Panel Adds Drug Benefit to Catastrophic-Insurance Bill," *Congressional Quarterly Weekly Report*, June 13, 1987, pp. 1263–64.

37. Julie Rovner, "Two Panels Add Drug Coverage to Medicare," *Congressional Quarterly Weekly Report*, June 20, 1987, p. 1327.

38. Julie Rovner, "Pepper Leaves Mark on Catastrophic-Care Bill," *Congressional Quarterly Weekly Report*, July 18, 1987, p. 1591.

39. Julie Rovner, "Democratic Leaders Slow Pace of Medicare Bill," *Congressional Quarterly Weekly Report*, July 4, 1987, pp. 1437–38.

40. "Catastrophic-Insurance Bill Headed to House Floor," *Congressional Quarterly Weekly Report*, July 11, 1987, p. 1543.

41. *Congressional Record*, July 22, 1987, p. H6471.

42. Julie Rovner, "Senate Panel Approves Medicare Expansion," *Congressional Quarterly Weekly Report*, May 30, 1987, pp. 1136–37.

43. Phillip Longman, "Catastrophic Follies," *New Republic*, August 21, 1989, p. 17.

44. See Julie Rovner, "Senate Leaders Look for Early Action on Medicare," *Congressional Quarterly Weekly Report*, September 5, 1987, p. 2128.

45. Julie Rovner, "Protagonists Still Jockeying Over Catastrophic-Costs Bill," *Congressional Quarterly Weekly Report*, October 10, 1987, p. 2463.

46. Julie Rovner, "Catastrophic-Costs Measure Back on Track Despite Delays," *Congressional Quarterly Weekly Report*, October 31, 1987, pp. 2677–79.

47. Julie Rovner, "Conferees Set to Begin Work on Catastrophic Costs Bill," *Congressional Quarterly Weekly Report*, February 13, 1988, pp. 313–15.

48. For a fuller discussion of conference issues, see Rovner, "Conferees Set to Begin Work"; Julie Rovner, "Conferees Closing Gap on Health-Cost Bill," *Congressional Quarterly Weekly Report*, April 30, 1988, p. 1169.

49. Julie Rovner, "Catastrophic-Costs Measure Ready for Final Hill Approval," *Congressional Quarterly Weekly Report*, June 4, 1988, pp. 1494–95.

50. Julie Rovner, "Long-Term Care: The True Catastrophe?" *Congressional Quarterly Weekly Report*, May 31, 1986, p. 1227.

51. *Catastrophic Illness Expenses*, Hearings, p. 152.

52. Ibid., p. 167.

53. Julie Rovner, "Catastrophic-Costs Conferees Irked by Lobbying Assaults," *Congressional Quarterly Weekly Report*, March 26, 1988, p. 780.

54. Julie Rovner, "Dispute Over Drug Benefit Slows Catastrophic-Costs Bill," *Congressional Quarterly Weekly Report*, May 14, 1988, p. 1290.

55. Rovner, "Catastrophic-Costs Measure Ready," pp. 1494–95.

56. Julie Rovner, "Conferees Nearing Accord on Health-Costs Bill," *Congressional Quarterly Weekly Report*, May 7, 1988, p. 1217.

57. See Julie Rovner, "Catastrophic-Costs Bill Ready for Final Action," *Congressional Quarterly Weekly Report*, May 28, 1988, pp. 1448–49.

58. Rovner, "Catastrophic-Costs Measure Ready."

59. Julie Rovner, "Authors Defend Catastrophic Insurance Law," *Congressional Quarterly Weekly Report*, January 14, 1989, p. 86.

60. Rovner, "Finance Weighs Benefit Cuts in Catastrophic-Costs Law," p. 2397.

61. Julie Rovner, "Catastrophic-Coverage Law Narrowly Survives Test," *Congressional Quarterly Weekly Report*, June 10, 1989, pp. 1400–1401.

62. See Julie Rovner, "Senate Finance Tries Revision of Catastrophic-Costs Law," *Congressional Quarterly Weekly Report*, September 9, 1989, p. 2316; Rovner, "Finance Weighs Benefit Cuts in Catastrophic-Costs Law," p. 2397.

63. Julie Rovner, "Senate Finance Tilting Toward a Cut in Medicare Surtax," *Congressional Quarterly Weekly Report*, June 3, 1989, p. 1329.

64. Rovner, "Catastrophic-Coverage Law Narrowly Survives Test," p. 1401.

65. Ibid., p. 1400.

66. Ibid., p. 1401.

67. Julie Rovner, "Authors Defend Health-Costs Law," *Congressional Quarterly Weekly Report*, June 3, 1989, p. 1330.

68. Julie Rovner, "Catastrophic-Costs Proposal Pleases Almost No One," *Congressional Quarterly Weekly Report*, July 29, 1989, p. 1956.

69. Ibid., pp. 1958–59.

70. Julie Rovner, "Panel May Pave Way for Death of Catastrophic-Costs Law," *Congressional Quarterly Weekly Report*, July 15, 1989, p. 1781.

71. Julie Rovner, "Catastrophic Coverage Law Dismantled by Congress," *Congressional Quarterly Weekly Report*, November 25, 1989, p. 3239.

72. Julie Rovner, "The Catastrophic-Costs Law: A Massive Miscalculation," *Congressional Quarterly Weekly Report*, October 14, 1989, p. 2715.

73. Ibid., p. 2714.

74. Ibid.

75. Marilyn Moon, *Medicare Now and in the Future* (Washington: Urban Institute Press, 1993), p. 130.

76. Ibid., p. 129.

Chapter Seven

1. Richard Lacayo, "Down for the Count?", *Time*, August 22, 1994, p. 34.

2. Doris Kearns Goodwin, *No Ordinary Time: Franklin and Eleanor Roosevelt and the Home Front in World War II* (Simon and Schuster, 1994), p. 11.

3. Department of Health and Human Services, "National health expenditures for 1993," press release, November 22, 1994.

4. See Julie Rovner, "Governors Ask for Relief . . . From Burdensome Medicaid Mandates," *Congressional Quarterly Weekly Report*, February 16, 1991, pp. 414, 416.

5. Beth Donovan, "The Victory Heard 'Round the Hill," *Congressional Quarterly Weekly Report*, November 9, 1991, p. 3303.

6. Theda Skocpol, "The Rise and Resounding Demise of the Clinton Plan," *Health Affairs*, vol. 14 (Spring 1995), pp. 66–85.

7. Gov. Bill Clinton, "A Healthy Nation," transcript from campaign headquarters, Rahway, N.J., September 24, 1992.

8. President Clinton, "Address Before a Joint Session of Congress on Administrative Goals," February 17, 1993, *Weekly Compilation of Presidential Documents*, vol. 29, no. 7 (February 22, 1993), p. 218.

9. President Clinton, "Remarks on Health Care Reform and an Exchange with Reporters," *Weekly Compilation of Presidential Documents*, vol. 29 (February 1, 1993), p. 96.

10. Dana Priest and Michael Weisskopf, "Health Care Reform: The Collapse of a Quest," *Washington Post*, October 11, 1994, p. A6.

11. Kathleen Day, "Executives Said to Back Clinton on Health Care," *Washington Post*, February 12, 1993, p. B3; Frank Swoboda, "'AFL-CIO Backs Tax for Health Care," *Washington Post*, February 17, 1993, p. F3; Spencer Rich, "Chamber Backs 'Managed Competition," *Washington Post*, March 9, 1993, p. A11.

12. Dana Priest, "Health Reform Fever?", *Washington Post*, Health Section, April 6, 1993, pp. 7–8.

13. Alissa J. Rubin, "Are U.S. Taxpayers Ready for Health Care Reform?," *Congressional Quarterly Weekly Report*, April 17, 1993, p. 955.

14. Alissa J. Rubin, "Hush-Hush Ruled a No-No," *Congressional Quarterly Weekly Report*, March 13, 1993, p. 598.

15. Dana Priest, "GOP Congressman Questions Hillary Clinton's Closed-Door Meetings," *Washington Post*, February 10, 1993, p. A5.

16. Medical News Network, author's interview with Bob Boorstin, air date April 1, 1993.

17. Spencer Rich, "President Blasts Cost of Vaccines," *Washington Post*, February 13, 1993, p. A1.

18. Medical News Network, author's interview with Pete Stark, air date April 8, 1993.

19. Media stakeout with Sen. Phil Gramm after meeting between Hillary Rodham Clinton and Congressional Leaders, April 30, 1993.

20. Medical News Network, author's interview with John Chafee, April 29, 1993.

21. Alissa J. Rubin, "Budget War Casts Shadow on Overhaul Plans," *Congressional Quarterly Weekly Report*, August 14, 1993, p. 2225.

22. National Federation of Independent Business, "Health plans put millions of jobs 'at risk', small business study finds," press release, May 20, 1993.

23. President Clinton, "Address to a Joint Session of the Congress on Health Care Reform, September 22, 1993," *Weekly Compilation of Presidential Documents*, vol. 29, September 22, 1993, pp. 1837–38.

24. *The New Yorker*, October 25, 1993, p. 128.

25. Robert J. Samuelson, "Care: How We Got Into this Mess," *Newsweek*, October 4, 1993, p. 34.

26. These numbers are from briefing materials provided by the White House press office.

27. Rubin, "Budget War Casts Shadow on Overhaul Plans," pp. 2225–26.

28. Special Report, *Congressional Quarterly Weekly Report*, September 4, 1993, p. 2319.

29. Alissa J. Rubin, "Cooper-Grandy Fills a Void," *Congressional Quarterly Weekly Report*, October 9, 1993, p. 2738.

30. Thomas H. Moore, "No Shortage of GOP Input," *Congressional Quarterly Weekly Report*, September 18, 1993, p. 2456.

31. Alissa J. Rubin, "Mrs. Clinton Conquers Hill, Sets Debate in Motion," *Congressional Quarterly Weekly Report*, October 2, 1993, p. 2640.

32. Author's notes from Citizens Jury press conference, October 14, 1993.

33. Drew E. Altman and Robert J. Blendon, *Kaiser Health Reform Project: Kaiser/Harvard/PSRA Survey of Public Knowledge* (Henry J. Kaiser Family Foundation: Menlo Park, Calif.), October 1993.

34. Author's interview with Robert J. Blendon, October 19, 1993.

35. Alissa J. Rubin, "Jurisdictional Power Struggle Slows Overhaul in Senate," *Congressional Quarterly Weekly Report*, November 27, 1993, p. 3274.

36. Alissa J. Rubin, "Members' Health Concerns Now Center on Turf Wars," *Congressional Quarterly Weekly Report*, October 9, 1993, p. 2734.

37. Ibid., p. 2735.

38. Memorandum from Judy Schneider, Congressional Research Service, "Referral of the Clinton Administration's Health Security Act and Other Health Care Reform Measures to Committees of the House and the Senate," February 24, 1994.

39. Ibid.

40. *Congressional Quarterly Almanac, 1988* (Washington: CQ Press, 1988), p. 313; *Congressional Quarterly Almanac, 1989*, p. 171; *Congressional Quarterly Almanac, 1992*, p. 401.

41. Karen Tumulty, "The Lost Faith of Daniel Patrick Moynihan," *Los Angeles Times* Magazine, June 19, 1994.

42. Ibid.

43. Schneider, "Referral."

44. Julie Kosterlitz, "Itching for a Fight," *National Journal*, January 15, 1994, p. 108.

45. Ibid.

46. Health Insurance Association of America, "HIAA lauds Clinton's commitment to health care reform, endorses mandates to assure universal coverage," press release, February 18, 1993.

47. Priest and Weisskopf, "Health Care Reform," p. A1.

48. Howard Wolinsky and Tom Brune, *The Serpent on the Staff: The Unhealthy Politics of the American Medical Association* (G. P. Putnam's Sons, 1994), p. 24.

49. Ibid.

50. Ibid, p. 29.

51. Julie Rovner, "Rx for Care: Competing Plans," *Congressional Quarterly Weekly Report*, February 16, 1991, p. 419.

52. James A. Barnes, "Selling Ideas," *National Journal*, August 13, 1994, p. 1944.

53. Michael Weisskopf and Dana Priest, "AMA Steps Back from Major Part of Clinton Health Reform," *Washington Post*, December 8, 1993, p. A3.

54. Michael Weisskopf, "Health Care Lobbies Lobby Each Other," *Washington Post*, March 1, 1994, p. A8.

55. Memorandum from William Kristol, "Defeating President Clinton's Health Care Proposal," Dec. 2, 1993.

56. James A. Barnes, "Selling Ideas," *National Journal*, August 13, 1994, p. 1944.

57. Dana Priest, "Health Groups Launch Ad Blitzes Criticizing Increased Federal Role," *Washington Post*, January 25, 1994, p. A8.

58. See David S. Hilzenrath, "Health Care Cost Growth Slowing Down," *Washington Post*, December 22, 1993, p. A1.

59. President Clinton, "Address Before a Joint Session of the Congress on the State of the Union, January 25, 1994," *Weekly Compilation of Presidential Documents*, vol. 30, January 31, 1994.

60. For text of the Republican response to the president's State of the Union address, see "Dole: Nation 'Has Health Care Problems, but no Health Care Crisis'," *Washington Post*, January 26, 1994, p. A13.

61. Priest and Weisskopf, "Health Care Reform," p. A6.

62. Spencer Rich and Ann Devroy, "Chamber of Commerce Opposes Clinton Health Plan," *Washington Post*, February 4, 1994, p. A12.

63. Congressional Budget Office, "An Analysis of the Administration's Health Proposal" (Government Printing Office, 1994), p. 36.

64. Ibid., p. xv.

65. Alissa J. Rubin, "GOP Seeks Unity to Bargain with Democrats," *Congressional Quarterly Weekly Report*, March 5, 1994, p. 550.

66. Hilary Stout, "Many Don't Realize It's the Clinton Plan They Like," *Wall Street Journal*, March 10, 1994, p. B1.

67. House Committee on Energy and Commerce, "Joint Statement of Congressman John D. Dingell, Congressman Henry Waxman, and Congresswoman Cardiss Collins," press release, March 2, 1994.

68. Author's notes from House Ways and Means Health Subcommittee markup, March 15, 1994.

69. Ceci Connolly, "Panel Enhances Premium Subsidies, Adds More Benefits to Measure," *Congressional Quarterly Weekly Report*, May 28, 1994, p. 1390.

70. Elizabeth A. Palmer, "Subcommittee Becomes First Panel to Approve Single Payer Plan," *Congressional Quarterly Weekly Report*, June 11, 1994, p. 1530.

71. Alissa J. Rubin and others, "Rostenkowski Sets Markup to Get Panel on Track," *Congressional Quarterly Weekly Report*, May 14, 1994, p. 1223.

72. Author's notes from Senate Finance Committee Hearing, May 4, 1994.

73. David S. Cloud, "Congress Takes on the Explosive Issue of Taxing Health Care Benefits," *Congressional Quarterly Weekly Report*, May 14, 1994, p. 1218.

74. Author's notes from Senate Labor and Human Resources Committee markup, May 18, 1994.

75. David S. Broder and Dana Priest, "Health Bill Funding Snarls House Panel," *Washington Post*, June 16, 1994, p. A1.

76. As quoted in David S. Cloud, "Democrats Band Together to Repel Assault on Employer Mandates," *Congressional Quarterly Weekly Report,* June 18, 1994, p. 1615.

77. Author's notes from June 22, 1994, media stakeout.

78. "Ways and Means' Health Reform Bill Leaves Vast Shortfall," Reuters News Service, June 10, 1994.

79. Elizabeth A. Palmer, "First House Panel Finishes Work, Gains Leverage by its Actions," "Single-Payer Goes to the Floor," both in *Congressional Quarterly Weekly Report,* June 25, 1994, pp. 1710–12, p. 1711.

80. Letter from John Dingell to Speaker Tom Foley, June 28, 1994; Nita Lelyveld, "Will Health Reform Pass John Dingell By?", Associated Press, June 28, 1994.

81. Author's notes from June 14, 1994, media stakeout.

82. See Julie Kosterlitz, "The Sounds of Two Senators Waffling," *National Journal,* August 13, 1994, p. 1945.

83. Author's notes from Senate Finance Committee markup, July 1, 1994.

84. Alissa J. Rubin and Beth Donovan, "Leaders Tell Clinton Measure Must Have Slower Approach," *Congressional Quarterly Weekly Report,* July 23, 1994, p. 2041.

85. Dana Priest, "Mitchell's Health Bill Aims for 95% Coverage," *Washington Post,* August 3, 1994, p. A1.

86. Ann Devroy and Dan Balz, "Clinton Backs 95% for Health Target," *Washington Post,* August 4, 1994, p. A1.

87. Adam Clymer, "The Health Care Debate: The Legislation," *New York Times,* August 5, 1994, p. A1.

88. Author's notes from August 9, 1994, media stakeout.

89. Notes from author's interview with Dave Durenburger, August 11, 1994.

90. *Congressional Record,* August 9, 1994, p. S11028.

91. Ibid, p. S11036.

92. For Gramm's comments, see *Congressional Record,* August 11, 1994, p. S11196; for Kassebaum's comments, see *Congressional Record,* August 9, 1994, p. S11029.

93. Author's notes from interview with Senator Wellstone, August 19, 1994. See Alissa J. Rubin and David S. Cloud, "Doubt Surfaces on Bill Passage as Senate Struggle Continues," *Congressional Quarterly Weekly Report,* August 20, 1994, p. 2458.

94. Robin Toner, "Health Impasse Souring Voters," *New York Times,* September 13, 1994, p. A1.

95. Letter to President Clinton from John D. Dingell, House Committee on Energy and Commerce, September 20, 1994.

96. Adam Clymer, "Clinton is Urged to Abandon Fight Over Health Bill," *New York Times,* September 21, 1994, p. A1.

97. Federal News Service transcript of news conferences with Senate Majority Leader George Mitchell and Senator Bob Dole, September 26, 1994.

98. Michael Wines, "Washington Really is in Touch. We're the Problem," *New York Times,* October 16, 1994, section 4, p. 1.

Chapter Eight

1. See Sven Steinmo and Jon Watts, "It's the Institutions, Stupid: Why the United States Can't Pass Comprehensive Health Reform," *Journal of Health Politics, Policy and Law*, vol. 20 (Summer 1995), pp. 329–72.

2. John W. Kingdon, *Agendas, Alternatives, and Public Policies* (Boston: Little, Brown, 1984), especially chapters 1 and 2.

3. Kingdon concludes that "setting the agenda and getting one's way . . . are two very different things. The president may be able to dominate and even determine the policy agenda, but is unable to dominate the alternatives that are seriously considered, and is unable to determine the final outcome." Ibid., p. 26.

4. See Charles O. Jones, *The Presidency in a Separated System* (Brookings, 1994), especially chapter 6 (pp. 182–207).

5. In dollar amounts and in the distribution of deficit reduction between spending cuts and revenue increases, Congress gave Clinton just about all he requested. The main change was substitution of a tax on gasoline for a tax on the Btu content of energy sources.

6. Clinton won the 1993 budget fight by a 218 to 216 vote in the House and with two 50–50 tiebreakers in the Senate. These votes provided no basis for thinking that the health care reform battle would be easy.

7. President Clinton, "Address Before a Joint Session of the Congress on the State of the Union," *Weekly Compilation of Presidential Documents*, vol. 30 (January 31, 1994), p. 153.

8. In a speech to the National Governors' Association on July 19, 1994, Clinton said he could accept coverage of "somewhere in the ballpark of 95 percent upwards." The very next day, however, Clinton issued a statement declaring "My goal is universal coverage," adding, "if we tinker around with the system and don't try to do something comprehensive, we could actually make it worse." See Ann Devroy and David Broder, "Clinton Affirms his Goal is Universal Coverage'," *Washington Post*, July 21, 1994, p. A1.

9. The Budget Enforcement Act does not bar consideration of entitlement legislation that would cause a rise in the deficit; it does, however, provide for such an increase to be offset by revenue increases, spending cuts, or sequestration.

10. President Clinton, "Address to a Joint Session of the Congress on Health Care Reform," *Weekly Compilation of Presidential Documents*, vol. 29 (September 27, 1993), p. 1845.

11. The data in this sections draw heavily from Karlyn H. Bowman, *Public Attitudes on Health Care Reform: Are the Polls Misleading the Policy Makers?* (American Enterprise Institute, 1994). Reviewing the use of polls in the health care debate, Bowman believes that "pollsters are going beyond areas where opinion can be useful to policy makers" (p. 1).

12. Between 1973 and 1993, the Roper Poll reported a drop from 83 percent to 73 percent in the proportion of Americans who expressed satisfaction with their medical care. Between 1983 and 1993, the Harris Poll found a 9 percentage-point rise (from 75 percent to 84 percent) in those believing that the health care

system had to be completely rebuilt or needed fundamental changes. Ibid., tables 1, 3, pp. 3, 5.

13. In 1993, according to Yankelovich Partners, almost two-thirds of those surveyed said they could meet the expenses of major illness with difficulty or not at all. Ibid., table 4, p. 6.

14. Bowman notes that poll data are highly sensitive to the wording of questions on whether there is a health care crisis. A January 1994 survey found 84 percent agreeing that there was a health care crisis; but another differently worded poll, taken less than one month later, reported only 43 percent believing that health care was in crisis. Ibid., p. 2, and table 2, p. 4.

15. In both 1938 and 1991, 80 percent or more agreed in a Gallup Poll that government should be responsible for providing medical care for those who are unable to pay for it. Ibid., table 6, p. 10. Despite these findings, Bowman notes that Americans are profoundly ambivalent about government and skeptical of its effectiveness. "On the one hand, they think that government should do many things in such a rich and powerful country as our own. On the other, they see government as problem causing, wasteful, inefficient, and expensive. The weight of polling evidence today is clearly on the latter view of government. . . . Seven in ten believe government creates more problems than it solves" (p. 16).

16. Bowman, *Public Attitudes*, table 7, p.11. This poll, conducted by Gallup for *USA Today* and CNN, also found 72 percent supporting guaranteed coverage even if they thought that individual taxes would go up.

17. Maureen Dowd, "The Health Care Debate: The Public," *New York Times*, July 20, 1994, p. A1. Despite this overwhelming endorsement of universal coverage, Robert Blendon and others warned that it was "not enough to generate popular support for a national health care program." Robert Blendon and others, "The Beliefs and Values Shaping Today's Health Reform Debate," *Health Affairs*, vol. 13 (Spring 1994), pp. 274–84 (quote on pp. 282–83).

18. For example, the Harry and Louise ads warned that the Clinton reform plan would limit the choice of medical services available to Americans. In fact, as introduced in Congress, the Clinton proposal would have expanded the options available to the many millions of Americans who are given only one or two choices by their employers.

19. Blendon and others, "The Beliefs and Values," pp. 277–80.

20. *Washington Post*-ABC News Poll, David S. Broder and Richard Morin, "Poll Finds Public Losing Confidence in Clinton, Economy," *Washington Post*, June 28, 1994, p. A4. In this poll, respondents were asked: "From what you know of it, do you approve or disapprove of President Clinton's health care plan?" Polls using different questions reported substantially different results. For example, Gallup asked whether "Congress should pass the health care plan basically as Bill Clinton has proposed it; pass it, but only after making major changes; or reject this plan?" In September 1993, 69 percent said that Congress should reject the plan or make major changes; by March 1994 it was 73 percent.

21. A *Washington Post*-ABC News survey conducted on June 26, 1994, found that 44 percent trusted Congress to do a better job than Clinton in handling

health reform. Thirty-six percent said that Clinton would do a better job. See Broder and Morin, "Poll Finds Public Losing Confidence in Clinton, Economy."

22. Maureen Dowd, "The Health Care Debate," *New York Times*, July 20, 1994, p. A1; NBC-*Wall Street Journal* poll, July 23–26, 1994, see *American Enterprise*, vol. 5 (September/October 1994), p. 109.

23. Hyperpluralism and its impact on American government and public policy are examined in Jonathan Rauch, *Demosclerosis: The Silent Killer of American Government* (Time Books, 1994).

24. David Rogers, "Battle Lines on Health Care Drawn in House," *Wall Street Journal*, August 12, 1994, p. A3.

25. The American Hospital Association was the key group in this alliance. It vigorously opposed the Clinton administration's effort to finance part of the cost of universal coverage through cuts in medicare payments to hospitals and other providers. See David Rogers and Hilary Stout, "Health Plans by Democrats Differ Widely," *Wall Street Journal*, August 1, 1994, p. A3.

26. In August 1994, as the health reform debate neared its futile end, the AMA endorsed the bipartisan bill as "the most realistic hope . . . for significant health system reform of all the bills currently under consideration." AMA News Release, August 10, 1994.

27. Quoted in Jeanne Saddler, "Chamber Poll Finds Opposition to Health Mandates," *Wall Street Journal*, April 27, 1994, p. B2.

28. The ad, which appeared in the *Washington Post* (p. A27) and other papers on July 21, 1994, also endorsed "a required level of employer contributions," assurance that patients would have freedom to "choose from a wide range of physicians and health plans," reliance on "governmental action and market forces" to slow health care inflation, and "achieves universal coverage with a standard set of comprehensive health benefits."

29. Quoted in Robert Pear, "The Health Care Debate: The Doctors," *New York Times*, August 5, 1994, p. A18.

30. Spencer Rich and Ann Devroy, "Chamber of Commerce Opposes Clinton Health Plan," *Washington Post*, February 4, 1994, p. A12.

31. Quoted in Saddler, "Chamber Poll Finds Opposition."

32. Ibid.

33. Michael Weisskopf, "Lobbyists Shift into Reverse," *Washington Post*, May 13, 1994, p. A3.

34. According to Weisskopf, four Republicans on the House subcommittee with jurisdiction over telecommunications legislation wrote the president of Ameritech, one of the regional telephone companies, after he endorsed employer mandates: "From our recent discussions with you on telecommunications legislation, we were under the impression that you believed that government regulations hindered competitiveness and true competition. Thus, your support for a proposal that will result in a tremendous burden on American businesses is surprising." Ibid.

35. Surveys of small business owners show "an overwhelming hatred of government mandates" and a distrust of government promises to lower their health care costs. An NFIB spokesman noted, "They're asking us to rely on a

government $4 trillion in debt to come through on subsidies. That's a gamble our members aren't willing to take." Quoted in Michael Selz, "Health Care Compromises Appeal to Some Small Firms," *Wall Street Journal*, April 21, 1994, p. B2.

36. Hilary Stout, "In Health Care Debate, Small Business Benefits at the Expense of Big," *Wall Street Journal*, July 21, 1994, p. A1.

37. The reconciliation process is described in Allen Schick, *The Federal Budget: Politics, Policy, Process*, (Brookings, 1994), pp. 82–86.

38. See Adam Clymer, "Health Care Plan is One Thing; Passing It is Another," *New York Times*, March 14, 1993, sec. 1, p. 30. Clymer reported that Rostenkowski and others opposed linking health reform and reconciliation, arguing that it would be even more difficult to pass if it had to carry the added burden of deficit reduction.

39. Memorandum from William Kristol to Republican leaders, "Defeating President Clinton's Health Care Proposal," Project for the Republican Future, December 2, 1993, p. 2. See also op-ed article by Kristol, "Pricing Health Care: How to Oppose the Health Plan—and Why," *Wall Street Journal*, January 11, 1994, p. A14.

40. Quoted in *1992 Congressional Quarterly Almanac*, p. 22-B.

41. During the 1993 session, House or Senate Democrats voted unanimously 42 times on partisan votes (in which a majority of Democrats opposed a majority of Republicans), up from 30 the previous year. House or Senate Republicans voted unanimously 122 times on such votes, up from 57 times in the previous session. See *Congressional Quarterly Almanac, 1993* (Washington: CQ Press, 1993), p. 17-C.

42. See tables 8-4 and 8-5.

43. The stimulus appropriations bill proposed by Clinton and passed by the House would have provided $16 billion for various public works, a summer jobs program, expansion of several social programs, and unemployment benefits. When passed by the Senate and enacted into law, only $4 billion in unemployment benefits remained.

44. This maneuver and the Republican reaction are described in the *Congressional Quarterly Almanac, 1993*, pp. 708–09.

45. Ibid, p. 709.

46. David S. Cloud, "Gibbons' Patched-Together Health Bill Now Faces Test on the Floor," *Congressional Quarterly Weekly Report*, July 2, 1994, p. 1793. Representative Benjamin Cardin (D.-Md.), one of the bill's supporters, remarked at the time the Ways and Means Committee reported the bill, "There's going to be changes. We knew that. We all expect that." Ibid.

47. According to John Motley, the Federation's chief lobbyist, "We chose to fight in Energy and Commerce first and Finance second and Ways and Means third." Quoted in Neil A. Lewis, "Lobby for Small-Business Owners Puts Big Dent in Health Care Bill," *New York Times*, July 6, 1994, p. A1.

48. *Congressional Quarterly Weekly Report*, May 21, 1994, p. 1298.

49. *Congressional Quarterly Weekly Report*, June 11, 1994, p. 1522. The article in which Kennedy was quoted noted that if the effort to enact health reform fails,

the Finance Committee "and the Massachusetts Democrat will share the blame for failing to craft a bill that could win GOP support."

50. *Congressional Quarterly Weekly Report*, July 30, 1994, p. 2144.

51. See Allen Schick, "Distributive Legislation," in Allen Schick, ed., *Making Economic Policy in Congress* (Washington: American Enterprise Institute, 1983), pp. 257–73.

52. The story of how tax reform was enacted is recounted in Jeffrey Birnbaum and Alan S. Murray, *Showdown at Gucci Gulch: Lawmakers, Lobbyists, and the Unlikely Triumph of Tax Reform* (Random House, 1987).

53. These scores are percentiles—each member of the House is compared to every other member on selected votes. Moreover, the scores are the sum of separate measures of economic and social conservatism. The data are taken from Richard E. Cohen and William Schneider, "Choosing Sides," *National Journal*, January 22, 1994, pp. 170–89.

54. See Norman J. Ornstein, Thomas E. Mann, and Michael J. Malbin, *Vital Statistics on Congress: 1993–1994* (Washington: CQ Press, 1994), table 8-6, pp. 204–05.

55. Representative Jim McDermott's single-payer bill had more than ninety House sponsors, almost as many as Clinton's proposal; Representative Jim Cooper's bill had almost fifty sponsors.

Index